Springer Optimization and Its Applications

Volume 216

Aims and Scope

Optimization has continued to expand in all directions at an astonishing rate. New algorithmic and theoretical techniques are continually developing and the diffusion into other disciplines is proceeding at a rapid pace, with a spot light on machine learning, artificial intelligence, and quantum computing. Our knowledge of all aspects of the field has grown even more profound. At the same time, one of the most striking trends in optimization is the constantly increasing emphasis on the interdisciplinary nature of the field. Optimization has been a basic tool in areas not limited to applied mathematics, engineering, medicine, economics, computer science, operations research, and other sciences.

The series **Springer Optimization and Its Applications (SOIA)** aims to publish state-of-the-art expository works (monographs, contributed volumes, textbooks, handbooks) that focus on theory, methods, and applications of optimization. Topics covered include, but are not limited to, nonlinear optimization, combinatorial optimization, continuous optimization, stochastic optimization, Bayesian optimization, optimal control, discrete optimization, multi-objective optimization, and more. New to the series portfolio include Works at the intersection of optimization and machine learning, artificial intelligence, and quantum computing.

Volumes from this series are indexed by Web of Science, zbMATH, Mathematical Reviews, and SCOPUS.

Richard B. Berry • Panos M. Pardalos •
Xiaochen Xian
Editors

Handbook of AI and Data Sciences for Sleep Disorders

Springer

Editors
Richard B. Berry
Department of Medicine
UF Health Sleep Disorders Center
Gainesville, FL, USA

Panos M. Pardalos
Department of Industrial and Systems Engineering
University of Florida
Gainesville, FL, USA

Xiaochen Xian
H. Milton Stewart School of Industrial and Systems Engineering
Georgia Institute of Technology
Atlanta, GA, USA

ISSN 1931-6828 ISSN 1931-6836 (electronic)
Springer Optimization and Its Applications
ISBN 978-3-031-68262-9 ISBN 978-3-031-68263-6 (eBook)
https://doi.org/10.1007/978-3-031-68263-6

This Springer imprint is published by the registered company Springer Nature Switzerland AG
The registered company address is: Gewerbestrasse 11, 6330 Cham, Switzerland

Preface

Welcome to the "Handbook of AI and Data Sciences for Sleep Disorders," a comprehensive exploration of the fusion of artificial intelligence (AI) and data science within the realm of sleep disorders. In recent years, the convergence of AI and data science has sparked unprecedented advancements across various fields, and the domain of sleep disorders is no exception. This timely book arrives at a crucial juncture when sleep-related issues are increasingly recognized as significant public health concerns worldwide. With the rise of modern lifestyles characterized by constant connectivity, irregular work schedules, and heightened stress levels, sleep disorders have become alarmingly prevalent. Moreover, the global COVID-19 pandemic has further exacerbated sleep disturbances, with widespread reports of disrupted sleep patterns and heightened insomnia rates due to increased anxiety and lifestyle changes. In this context, the handbook emerges as a beacon of hope, offering a comprehensive resource for researchers, clinicians, and policymakers striving to address the burgeoning challenges in sleep medicine.

By harnessing the transformative potential of AI and data science, this book not only enhances our understanding of sleep disorders but also presents innovative approaches to diagnosis, treatment, and personalized care. From leveraging machine learning algorithms to analyze sleep patterns and predict disorder risk factors to utilizing big data analytics for large-scale epidemiological studies, the methodologies and applications outlined in this handbook promise to reshape the landscape of sleep medicine. Furthermore, the interdisciplinary nature of this endeavor underscores its relevance in fostering collaboration between experts from diverse fields, including computer science, engineering, neuroscience, medicine, and public health. As we navigate the complexities of the digital age and confront the profound impact of sleep disorders on individual well-being and societal productivity, the insights gleaned from this handbook are not only timely but also indispensable for shaping the future of sleep medicine in the twenty-first century.

The enduring clinical challenge of sleep medicine lies in accurately diagnosing and effectively treating a wide range of sleep disorders. These disorders can be complex and often present with overlapping symptoms, making accurate diagnosis challenging. Furthermore, treatment options vary depending on the specific disorder and may involve lifestyle modifications, behavioral therapy, medical interventions, or a combination thereof. Additionally, access to specialized sleep clinics and resources may be limited in certain regions, further complicating the management of sleep disorders. The challenge of precision medicine is to match an individual with the unique treatments that will be of most benefit. For example, while two individuals might have the same frequency of respiratory events, they may differ in the amount of sleep disturbance, cardiovascular changes, and impairment of oxygenation caused by the events. Patients with obstructive apnea may have different underlying characteristics as a cause of the disorder (endotypes), such as a narrow and collapsible upper airway versus patients with instability in ventilatory control or the response of upper airway muscles to airway narrowing. Despite these challenges, advancements in technology, such as AI and data science, offer promising solutions to improve diagnostic accuracy, optimize treatment strategies, and enhance patient outcomes in sleep medicine.

The complexity of sleep disorders demands sophisticated approaches for the analysis and interpretation of the vast array of data generated during sleep studies. Traditional clinical practice for sleep disorders has often relied on subjective assessments, manual scoring of polysomnography data, and limited predictive models based on a few key variables. For example, traditionally sleep is divided into three stages of non-rapid eye movement sleep (stage N1, N2, N3) and REM sleep. Standard sleep reports list the total sleep time and the amount of each sleep stage as a percentage of total sleep time. Sleep is staged in 30-second epochs based on the tradition of paper recording in 30-second pages using the identification of certain features. However, interscorer reliability is not optimal and time-consuming. New AI methods have been developed to stage sleep with good agreement with gold standard human scoring and are fast, and the results are repeatable. Traditional hypnograms display the pattern of the different stages of sleep over the night. While this shows the pattern of sleep across the night, analysis has been limited to identifying the number of sleep stage transitions or latency to the first period of REM sleep. However, using advanced neural network analysis using a parameter based on the overlap of sleep stages, Stephansen and coworkers were able to diagnose narcolepsy by the analysis of a single sleep study. Unfortunately, AI analysis is often a "black box," and clinicians find the results difficult to understand. A real challenge is to correlate identified features with a physiological process that clinicians can understand. Another challenge is the fact that results from a given data set from patients with certain characteristics may not apply to data sets from patients with different characteristics. Clinicians need to understand the limitations of AI and big data analysis. However, with the rapid advancement of AI and data science technologies, the landscape of sleep medicine is undergoing a profound transformation. AI algorithms can now process large volumes of complex sleep data with unprecedented speed and accuracy, enabling clinicians to extract meaningful patterns and insights that were previously inaccessible. For example, one can quickly accurately determine properties of respiration during sleep such as the degree of obstruction for every breath over an entire night and compare the indices between individuals. For instance, machine learning algorithms can analyze multichannel physiological signals from polysomnography recordings to identify subtle patterns indicative of specific sleep disorders, such as obstructive sleep apnea or insomnia. Moreover, AI-driven predictive models can stratify individuals based on their risk of developing certain sleep disorders, allowing for targeted interventions and preventive measures. As a result, the current clinical practice for sleep disorders is evolving toward a more data-driven and personalized approach, where AI serves as a powerful ally in augmenting clinician decision-making and improving patient outcomes.

Furthermore, the development of AI in sleep medicine is prompting a paradigm shift in how clinicians are trained and prepared to leverage these technologies effectively. Training programs are increasingly incorporating curricula on AI and data science principles, equipping future sleep specialists with the skills necessary to harness the full potential of these tools. Additionally, interdisciplinary collaborations between sleep medicine experts, data scientists, computer engineers, and biostatisticians are becoming more commonplace, fostering a culture of innovation and knowledge exchange. By embracing AI and data science, the field of sleep medicine is poised to enter a new era of precision healthcare, where treatments are tailored to individual needs, early detection is enhanced, and the burden of sleep disorders on public health is mitigated.

The chapters in this handbook represent a collaborative effort by leading experts in the fields of AI, data science, and sleep medicine. Each chapter delves into specific aspects of sleep disorder analysis, from the extraction and preprocessing of polysomnography raw data to the application of advanced machine learning algorithms for detecting and characterizing various sleep phenomena. From the identification of REM sleep behavior disorder to the analysis of mandibular jaw movements and the modeling of mechanical work of breathing, the breadth and depth of topics covered in this handbook reflect the multifaceted nature of sleep research.

The journey through these pages begins with an exploration of the fundamental principles underpinning the use of AI and data science in sleep health, setting the stage for a deeper dive into the intricacies of sleep disorder analysis. As you progress through each chapter, you will encounter innovative methodologies, novel insights, and real-world applications that showcase the transformative potential of AI and data science in sleep medicine.

Whether you are a seasoned researcher, a practicing clinician, or a curious enthusiast eager to explore the frontiers of sleep science, this handbook offers something for everyone. We hope that the knowledge contained within these pages will inspire further collaboration, spark new ideas, and ultimately contribute to improved outcomes for individuals suffering from sleep disorders.

We extend our sincere gratitude to the contributors who have shared their expertise and insights, as well as to the readers who embark on this journey with us. Together, let us harness the power of AI and data science to empower sleep health and transform the future of sleep medicine.

Gainesville, FL, USA Richard B. Berry
Gainesville, FL, USA Panos M. Pardalos
Gainesville, FL, USA Xiaochen Xian
May, 2024

Contents

Empowering Sleep Health: Unleashing the Potential of Artificial Intelligence and Data Science in Sleep Disorders

Xin Zan, Feng Liu, Xiaochen Xian, and Panos M. Pardalos

1 Introduction

Sleep is a fundamental component and comprises roughly one-third of our daily lives, profoundly influencing our physical, mental, and emotional well-being. It is the body's natural process of restoration and rejuvenation, playing a vital role for optimal cognitive function, emotional resilience, and overall health [35, 43]. However, in our fast-paced world, where the boundaries between work, leisure, and personal life have blurred, the significance of sleep health has been increasingly overlooked and the prevalence of sleep disorders has surged [84].

Sleep disorders encompass a broad spectrum of conditions, ranging from the seemingly commonplace such as insomnia, to the potentially life-threatening conditions like sleep apnea, which disrupt not only our nocturnal rest but also our daily lives [35, 104]. These disorders, often undiagnosed or undertreated, lead to a range of consequences such as reduced productivity, cognitive impairments, mood

X. Zan
Department of Industrial and Systems Engineering, University of Iowa, Iowa City, IA, USA
e-mail: xin-zan@uiowa.edu

F. Liu
School of Systems and Enterprises, Stevens Institute of Technology, Hoboken, NJ, USA
e-mail: fliu22@stevens.edu

X. Xian (✉)
H. Milton Stewart School of Industrial and Systems Engineering, Georgia Institute of Technology, Atlanta, GA, USA
e-mail: xxian@gatech.edu

P. M. Pardalos
Department of Industrial and Systems Engineering, University of Florida, Gainesville, FL, USA
e-mail: pardalos@ufl.edu

R. B. Berry et al. (eds.), *Handbook of AI and Data Sciences for Sleep Disorders*,
Springer Optimization and Its Applications 216,
https://doi.org/10.1007/978-3-031-68263-6_1

disorders, and even an increased risk of chronic diseases such as hypertension, diabetes, and cardiovascular conditions [25, 96]. Beyond individual suffering, sleep disorders also place a substantial burden on global healthcare systems and economies [19]. In the United States alone, according to the Center for Disease Control and Prevention, sleep disorders are affecting 50–70 million adult population, contributing to approximately 40,000 deaths annually due to cardiovascular problems and incurring healthcare system costs of more than 16 billion dollars [76]. In today's society, sleep disorders have emerged as a pressing health concern that affects millions of people worldwide in pursuing and maintaining optimal sleep health [84, 108].

Sleep disorders manifest in various forms, including complaints of insufficient sleep, excessive amount of perceived sleep, or abnormal movements during sleep [25, 104]. Although sleep disorders have been identified for centuries, the extended research to categorize them has taken place primarily in the last decades and continue to evolve as our understanding of sleep disorders progresses. The American Academy of Sleep Medicine (AASM) has developed a widely acknowledged classification of different sleep disorder types, known as the International Classification of Sleep Disorders (ICSD; [125]). In the latest version ICSD-3, over 80 sleep disorders are categorized into seven types.

- *Insomnia*, a condition of having trouble falling asleep and/or staying asleep. It is defined as a repeated difficulty with sleep initiation, maintenance, consolidation, or quality despite adequate time and opportunity for sleep. As many as 95% of Americans have reported an episode of insomnia at some point during their lives [29, 109].
- *Sleep-related breathing disorders*, a condition of abnormal and difficult respiration during sleep. Approximately one-seventh of the world's adult population is estimated to have obstructive sleep apnea (OSA), the most common type of sleep-related breathing disorders [82, 107].
- *Central disorders of hypersomnolence*, characterized by excessive daytime sleepiness despite normal quality and timing of nocturnal sleep [126, 138].
- *Circadian rhythm sleep-wake disorders*, characterized by a disturbance in the normal circadian rhythm that result in the patient experiencing excessive daytime sleepiness, insomnia, or even both [92].
- *Parasomnias*, characterized by abnormal, unpleasant motor verbal, or behavioral events that occur during sleep or wake to sleep transitions, including walking and talking [135]. Although more common in children, parasomnias can occur at any age [48].
- *Sleep-related movement disorders*, characterized by simple, usually stereotyped movements that disrupt nocturnal sleep and may thus lead to daytime sleepiness and fatigue [8].
- *Other sleep disorders*, which do not belong to any of the abovementioned categories.

Table 1 Types of sleep disorders

Type	Major subtypes
Insomnia	Chronic insomnia, short-term insomnia
Sleep-related breathing disorders	Obstructive sleep apnea (OSA), central sleep apnea (CSA)
Central disorders of hypersomnolence	Narcolepsy type 1 or 2, idiopathic hypersomnia
Circadian rhythm sleep-wake disorders	Advanced or delayed sleep-wake phase disorder, irregular or non–24-hour sleep-wake rhythm disorder, jet lag disorder
Parasomnias	Non-rapid eye movement (NREM)-related parasomnias or rapid eye movement (REM)-related parasomnias (e.g., REM sleep behavior disorder, nightmare disorder, and sleep paralysis)
Sleep-related movement disorders	Restless legs syndrome, periodic limb movement disorder

All these seven types of sleep disorders encompass various subtypes, each characterized by more specific symptoms. Table 1 lists the six main types and their most prevalent subtypes.

Traditionally, the diagnosis and treatment of sleep disorders have heavily relied on subjective assessments, laborious manual monitoring, and limited interventions according to AASM guidelines [17, 25]. However, as we stand on the cusp of the fourth industrial revolution, a new era in sleep health is dawning marked by the convergence of digital technologies and unprecedented access to sleep disorder data. Artificial Intelligence (AI) and Data Science (DS), two pillars of this technological revolution, are poised to unleash their transformative power in the multifaceted realm of sleep disorders [11]. With an ever-increasing prevalence of sleep-related issues affecting individuals worldwide, the integration of AI and DS in sleep disorders has the potential to provide significant advancements in the field, revolutionizing the way we understand, diagnose, and treat these complex conditions [115, 143].

In particular, AI excels in the analysis of large-scale sleep data, automating complex tasks with remarkable efficiency. Sleep studies, such as polysomnography (PSG) and actigraphy, generate vast amounts of data that challenge human experts to process efficiently [18, 106]. AI algorithms, specifically machine learning (ML) models, have the capability to process and interpret these datasets with remarkable speed and accuracy. Strictly speaking, ML is a subset of AI, playing a pivotal role to make AI possible by enabling computers to learn and perform human-like tasks using experience and data without hard-coded rules and instructions. The two terms are now often used interchangeably since ML have long come to dominate AI [53]. Deep Learning (DL), a specialized branch of ML, is adept at handling complex tasks by learning from data independently without human interventions, and thus gaining increasing research attention in recent years. By automatically identifying patterns, anomalies, and subtle variations in sleep patterns, AI significantly enhances clinicians' efficiency in diagnosing various sleep disorders, including sleep apnea, insomnia, narcolepsy, and restless leg syndrome [11, 70, 143].

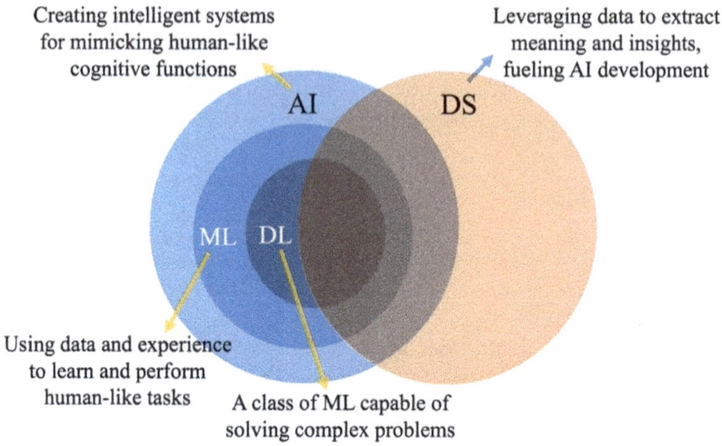

Fig. 1 Venn diagram representing the relationships between DS, AI, ML, and DL

DS, on the other hand, complements AI in sleep disorder research by facilitating the integration of diverse data sources. By combining clinical data, genetic information, lifestyle factors, and even environmental data, researchers can gain a comprehensive understanding of the factors influencing sleep disorders [115]. This interdisciplinary approach not only enhances diagnostic accuracy but also aids in the discovery of novel biomarkers and potential therapeutic targets, thereby paving the way for more effective and personalized treatment strategies [108]. DS and AI, in this context, complement each other in a symbiotic relationship, with DS providing the data-driven foundation and AI harnessing advanced algorithms for ultimately enhancing the value and applicability of data-driven solutions. Consequently, the synergy of AI and DS represents a transformative opportunity to not only unravel the complex tapestry of sleep disorders but also to illuminate the path toward more accurate diagnosis, personalized treatment strategies, and a profound understanding on enhancing sleep health [11, 21, 119]. The relationships between DS, AI, ML, and DL are demonstrated in Fig. 1 through a Venn diagram.

This chapter provides an extensive review of the latest advancements of AI and DS in sleep disorders. Figure 2 visualizes the scope of this chapter, focusing on both applications and methods of AI and DS in sleep disorders. The remainder of this chapter is organized as follows: Section 2 explores AI and DS applications in sleep disorders, categorized by clinical tasks and by different sleep disorders, respectively. Section 3 presents a comprehensive review of the AI and DS methods applied in sleep disorders research throughout the entire data lifecycle, including data types, data preprocessing, and AI and DS techniques. Section 4 discusses the challenges and opportunities of harnessing AI and DS in sleep disorders to enhance sleep health. Section 5 finally concludes this chapter.

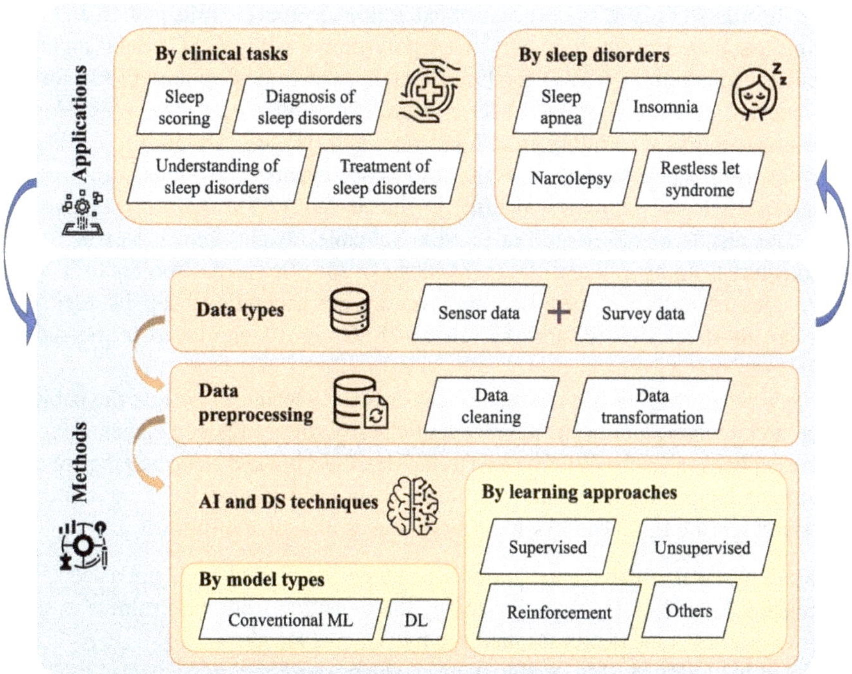

Fig. 2 Applications and methods of AI and DS in sleep disorders

2 AI and DS Applications in Sleep Disorders

This section unravels the profound potential of AI and DS applications in sleep disorders for empowering sleep health from two distinct perspectives: by clinical tasks in Sect. 2.1 and by specific sleep disorders in Sect. 2.2. On the clinical task side, we discuss the critical roles of AI and DS to empower healthcare professionals in automating and improving sleep scoring, precise diagnosis, personalized treatment, and deepening our comprehension of sleep disorders. We then narrow our attention to several key sleep disorders that are most widely investigated in the current research and illustrate the primary clinical tasks where AI and DS methods have been applied and hold potential in studying specific sleep disorders.

2.1 By Clinical Tasks

2.1.1 Sleep Scoring

Sleep scoring is a fundamental task and crucial to understand sleep in sleep research, constituting one of the most important and explored clinical tasks in the realm of sleep disorders [114]. It is a process of extracting sleep cycle information and identifying associated events typically from polysomnography (PSG) data, including electroencephalogram (EEG) for brain activity, electrooculogram (EOG) for eye movements, electromyogram (EMG) for muscle activity, and other physiological measures such as respiratory rate, heart rate, and oxygen saturation [10]. During sleep scoring, sleep stages, arousals, respiratory events, movements, and cardiac events need to be correctly identified, guided by AASM scoring manual [17, 19]. The results of sleep scoring provide valuable insights into a patient's sleep architectures, aiding in the accurate diagnosis of specific sleep disorders [47]. Table 2 provides a summary of sleep scoring tasks, the corresponding sleep disorder types they are most relevant to, and the relevant PSG signals employed in the scoring tasks.

Sleep stage scoring is an essential task in sleep scoring to decode the subject's sleep architecture, aiming to identify and classify different sleep stages using 30-second epochs in sleep [20]. The two terms sleep scoring and sleep staging are often used interchangeably in the current literature as sleep staging has long dominated the sleep scoring task. The five main sleep stages include the following:

1. Stage W (Wakefulness), the period when a person is awake and not asleep.
2. Stage N1 (NREM 1), characterized by the transition from wakefulness to sleep, when muscle tone decreases, and eye movements are slow.
3. Stage N2 (NREM 2), a deeper stage of sleep where eye movements stop, heart rate and body temperature decrease.
4. Stage N3 (NREM 3), a deep and restorative stage characterized by slow, high-amplitude brain waves.
5. Stage R (REM), characterized by REMs, increased brain activity, and vivid dreaming, when muscle tone is greatly reduced during REM sleep, often leading to temporary paralysis.

Associated event scoring involves the scoring of arousals, respiratory events, movements, and cardiac events during sleep [11, 17]. All these events may occur during any sleep stage, including the sophisticated NREM and REM sleep, and the detection of each type of event can particularly enhance the diagnosis of corresponding sleep disorders as summarized in Table 2.

Table 2 Summary of sleep scoring tasks

Sleep scoring tasks	Relevant sleep disorders	Relevant PSG signals
Sleep stage scoring	Insomnia, sleep-related breathing disorders, narcolepsy, parasomnias	EEG, EOG, EMG
Arousal scoring	Insomnia, sleep-related breathing disorders, narcolepsy, parasomnias	EEG, EOG, EMG
Respiratory event scoring	Sleep-related breathing disorders	Respiratory rate, oxygen saturation
Movement scoring	Sleep-related movement disorders	EMG, body movements
Cardiac event scoring	Circadian rhythm sleep-wake disorders	ECG, heart rate

The sleep scoring procedure is very complex, time-consuming, and labor-intensive with many physiological parameters in PSG to be considered simultaneously as well as taking previous and future epoch scoring into account [47]. The heterogeneity of the subjects and of the sleep epochs are also quite difficult to be comprehensively described in a manual [4, 11]. AI and DS are promising tools to overcome these challenges. To be specific, both sleep staging and associated event scoring belong to a classification problem, which is well suited for applying AI algorithms. They can automate sleep scoring, reducing the reliance on manual scoring, and minimizing inter-rater variability [4, 53, 80]. The integration of AI and DS algorithms are also capable of processing vast amounts of sleep data rapidly, allowing for efficient and objective sleep scoring.

ML algorithms have indeed been applied to automating sleep scoring for many years. One of the first evaluations of AI sleep scoring dated back to mid-1990s with the use of a learning vector quantizer and the induction of decision trees for sleep staging in infants [75]. Since 1996, plenty of works have focused on developing various AI models to continuously improve the accuracy of automatic scoring results in agreement to human experts [127]. Several studies have continued to employ AI models to study sleep scoring in different populations, e.g., in infants and in patients with different diseases such as OSA and Parkinson's disease [34, 42]. Meanwhile, some studies have focused on investigating different sleep features for staging [65], and some others have focused on integrating event scoring results to diagnose specific sleep disorders [116]. A systematic review of literature on automated sleep scoring can be found in Alsolai et al. [3].

While ML algorithms can undoubtedly reach a high accuracy for sleep scoring in specific situations, the learning processes based on feature extraction guided by high-level expert knowledge are sophisticated. Recent progress in AI sleep staging has been centralized on DL models which are powerful in extracting complex information directly from a large amount of raw data, particularly focusing on convolutional, recurrent neural networks, or a combination of both [118]. In addition to widely employed PSG data in sleep scoring, DL model further paves the way for automatic sleep scoring using other sensor data such as Videosomnography (VSG; [32]). A thorough review of evaluating DL in sleep scoring can be found in Fiorillo et al. [47] and Loh et al. [81].

2.1.2 Diagnosis of Sleep Disorders

The diagnosis of sleep disorders stands as another one of the most crucial and extensively studied clinical tasks, serving as a cornerstone for better sleep health [53]. Early and accurate diagnosis of specific sleep disorders, such as sleep apnea, insomnia, narcolepsy, and restless leg syndrome, is essential for the subsequent effective management and treatment [22, 25]. It not only identifies and addresses individual sleep issues but also contributes to broader public health initiatives aimed at improving sleep quality and overall well-being.

However, the diagnosis of sleep disorders presents a multifaceted challenge in clinical practice due to labor-intensive and subjective processes. AI and DS have emerged as a transformative solution, automating and streamlining the manual procedures to provide accurate, efficient, and cost-effective diagnosis [21, 95, 143]. AI and DS efficiently handle vast amounts of sleep datasets and enable automatic and efficient diagnosis of sleep disorders on a large scale with significantly reduced manual efforts and time, thereby extending the reach to a larger population [53, 108]. In addition, AI and DS are able to provide objective and precise evaluations that significantly reduce inter- and intra-variability among different healthcare providers subject to manual evaluation [53, 143]. To be specific, the diagnosis of sleep disorders generally belongs to a classification or a regression problem depending on the diagnosis metric, which is well suited for AI algorithms.

In the current literature, diagnosis is the most studied clinical task in sleep disorders by applying AI and DS techniques. Considerable research endeavors have been dedicated to developing different AI and DS methods that integrate different types of sleep data to diagnose different specific disorders, aimed at improving the diagnosis accuracy and efficiency. A more detailed review about different techniques in terms of diagnosing specific sleep disorders is present in Sect. 2.2.

2.1.3 Understanding of Sleep Disorders

There is growing evidence that, traditional clinical practice has not adequately explored the underlying etiology (i.e., endotype), clinical manifestation (i.e., phenotype), and potential healthcare complications associated with different sleep disorders in different individuals [11, 40]. AI and DS have paved the way for advancing the understanding of sleep disorders by improving phenotyping, endotyping, and complication profiling in different sleep disorders. AI and DS play a crucial role in leveraging large-scale data to uncover intricate patterns and associations that were previously challenging to detect through traditional methods [53, 119]. This deeper understanding of sleep disorders forms the foundation of enhanced diagnosis and personalized treatment for the corresponding disorders, ultimately promoting better sleep health.

Phenotyping involves categorizing sleep disorders mainly based on patients' observable clinical characteristics and symptoms. It focuses on identifying common traits and patterns within a group of individuals who share similar symptoms. Phenotyping helps clinicians to recognize distinct subtypes of a sleep disorder [54]. For example, within insomnia, phenotyping may distinguish between individuals who have difficulty falling asleep (initiation insomnia) and those who struggle to maintain sleep (maintenance insomnia; [16]). This differentiation leads to more precise diagnosis and tailored treatments of specific subtypes of sleep disorders, which is crucial for promoting precision medicine as treatment strategies may vary depending on the subtype [49]. By identifying subtle patterns in symptoms, sleep patterns, and responses to treatment, AI algorithms can identify unique clusters of symptoms that suggest a specific subtype of a sleep disorder, thereby creating more refined and accurate phenotypes and helping clinicians tailor interventions more precisely [18, 91]. To be specific, phenotyping typically belongs to an unsupervised clustering problem.

In addition to the aforementioned clinical phenotyping based on clinical characteristics and symptoms, there are many studies focusing on other forms of phenotyping based on a wide range of non-clinical factors to gain insights into sleep disorder patients. For example, some studies have examined the relationship between sleep disorders and such factors as lifestyle habits, competition activities, psychological distress to study potential factors that may lead to a higher risk of sleep disorders [93]. In addition, plenty of works investigate sleep disorders in different population groups, including the elderly, children, pregnant individuals, and different genders [7, 37, 41, 56, 98]. These studies have shown that different demographic and geographic characteristics in different population groups lead to different risk levels of sleep disorder incidence. AI and DS techniques play a pivotal role in analyzing these intricate relationships within datasets, contributing to a deeper understanding of sleep disorders. This enhanced understanding empowers healthcare professionals to effectively screen, diagnose, and provide early interventions. It also enhances our ability to tailor healthcare strategies to specific population groups by addressing their unique needs and risk factors, thereby promoting personalized healthcare and medicine.

Endotyping goes beyond phenotyping and seeks to understand the underlying biological mechanisms or causes (endotypes) that lead to a specific sleep disorder. It aims to uncover the distinct pathways or mechanisms responsible for a sleep disorder at a molecular or physiological level [11]. For example, within OSA, endotyping may distinguish between cases caused by upper airway anatomical abnormalities and those related to neuromuscular control issues [40]. Identifying endotypes can also inform targeted treatments [16, 143]. By analyzing extensive biological and physiological data, such as genetic information, biomarkers, and neuroimaging results, AI can reveal previously unrecognized associations between specific biological factors and sleep disorders, advancing our understanding of their root causes [11].

Complication profiling involves assessing secondary health issues or comorbidities that may arise as a result of untreated or poorly managed sleep disorders. It aims to identify the health risks and consequences associated with a specific sleep disorder, which is vital for comprehensive patient care and ultimately enhances patient's health [35]. Existing studies have shown that untreated sleep disorders may have wide-ranging effects on the cardiovascular, endocrine, immune, and nervous systems, leading to severe health complications such as cardiovascular diseases, suicidal ideation, and mental disorders [31, 35, 63, 100]. AI and DS are capable of analyzing extensive patient data to uncover correlations between untreated sleep disorders and different health complications. These technologies can help predict which individuals with specific sleep disorders are at a higher risk of developing certain comorbidities. Such insights empower clinicians to initiate preventive measures and interventions to reduce the impact of complications on patients' health [53].

2.1.4 Treatment and Management of Sleep Disorders

The treatment and management of sleep disorders represent a challenging task, given the diversity of their conditions and the importance of tailoring interventions to individualized needs. The uniqueness of each individual and their particular set of genetic polymorphisms and gene expression regulatory elements affect how they respond to treatments distinctly [143]. Even with the same sleep disorders, different health profiles of patients may necessitate different treatments. Many existing studies have investigated the treatment of sleep disorders in a wide range of patient populations, e.g., in co-occurring PTSD, in dementia, and in patients with Parkinson's disease [36, 102, 140]. Personalization and precision are key themes in this domain, and AI and DS technologies are instrumental in achieving these objectives [11]. The application of AI and DS in the treatment should inform treatment selection, predict treatment success, evaluate ongoing treatment and compliance, and lead to personalized treatment approach [22, 143].

In the current literature, not many studies have been done in the task of personalizing the treatment and management of sleep disorders. A few recent AI studies have employed reinforcement learning to help optimize and personalize treatment for individuals, allowing patients to connect with treatment methods that would be most effective on an individual basis [22, 30, 53, 88].

2.2 *By Sleep Disorders*

2.2.1 Sleep Apnea: OSA and CSA

Among various sleep disorders, sleep apnea, especially the most common obstructive type OSA, is increasingly prevalent in a large population and has received the most attention in the literature. Existing research shows that ML (including DL) models have been effectively used for diagnosing sleep apnea [15]. Specifically, ML models have demonstrated strong performance in diagnosing sleep apnea by using readily available features from signal data such as ECG, SPO2, and snoring, as well as from survey data corresponding to the patients such as demographic characteristics and symptoms presence. Similarly, ML models have also been successfully applied in classifying sleep apnea into OSA and CSA and predicting the apnea severity. Given its extensive study in the literature, a wide range of AI and DS techniques have been utilized in the field of sleep apnea. The most efficient and popular algorithms for detecting sleep apnea include support vector machine (SVM; [2, 148]), K-nearest neighborhood (KNN; [97]), and neural networks (NNs; [57, 142]). Existing studies also present promising results of ML in guiding treatment of sleep apnea, such as predicting treatment outcomes of different treatment options (e.g., surgical treatment and CPAP therapy), evaluating and improving treatment, and personalizing treatment with enhanced understanding of underlying mechanisms of OSA [15, 22]. ML has also demonstrated potential in better prediction of treatment adherence. For example, compliance classifiers with CPAP therapy have been shown capable of early prediction of compliant patients [11]. As sleep apnea is the most widely studied sleep disorder, numerous extensive reviews on AI techniques for the detection, diagnosis and/or treatment can be found in the current literature, including the works by Álvarez et al. [6], Mendonça et al. [89], Mostafa et al. [96], Ramachandran and Karuppiah [112], Taweesedt et al. [139], Salari et al. [123], and Brennan and Kirby [22].

In addition, endotyping and phenotyping OSA through PSG have been increasingly recognized as significant aspects in the field. There is a growing interest in making OSA endotyping algorithms accessible, cost-effective, and scalable [46]. ML clustering models have also been applied to OSA phenotyping. For example, Ma et al. [83] have employed a combined unsupervised-supervised ML to cluster 2277 OSA patients into six phenotypes by using PSG data, and the new phenotypes show statistically different comorbidity development for OSA-related cardio-neuro-metabolic diseases in contrast to the conventional single-metric apnea–hypopnea index (AHI)-based phenotype. AI techniques have also been proven useful for enhancing patient risk stratification and screening. For example, Huang et al. [64] have utilized clinical data to develop SVM-based models for early identification of patients at risk for OSA when visiting a primary care clinic, which may potentially prioritize such patients for sleep studies.

2.2.2 Insomnia

Insomnia is a prevalent sleep disorder that can lead to a wide range of symptoms, including difficulty falling asleep and experiencing tiredness at different periods of time. Approximately 95% of Americans have reported an episode of insomnia at some point during their lives [29]. Insomnia is another sleep disorder that has received extensive attention in the literature, with numerous studies focusing on the assessment and treatment. Existing studies have demonstrated that the utilization of common signals and typical ML techniques holds promise for predicting insomnia.

ML techniques are widely applied for predicting insomnia by using patients' survey data such as questionnaires. For example, Seth et al. [132] have developed a NN model for predicting insomnia on the basis of depression, anxiety, stress, and the social adjustment of an individual by leveraging their survey data including the Insomnia Severity Index and the Athens Insomnia Scale. Islam et al. [69] have utilized questionnaire data to predict chronic insomnia based on different ML models for comparison, and the results show that the logistic regression model dearly performs best than the other models with the highest prediction accuracy.

Considering the utilization of sensor data, Shahin et al. [133] have analyzed the EEG signal to evaluate characteristics throughout the entire sleep recording and during insomnia-impacted sleep stages. The proposed method has employed a deep NN model and obtained a high classification accuracy of 92%, demonstrating the effectiveness of DL in diagnosing insomnia. Angelova et al. [9] have utilized actigraphy data and applied random forest (RF) and SVM classifiers for identifying the insomnia and the normal sleep, yielding satisfactory classification accuracy. In addition, Kuo and Chen [77] have utilized a single-channel EOG combined with a refined composite multiscale entropy analysis to efficiently detect insomnia with high accuracy in a relatively short time.

There are also other interesting studies associated with insomnia in addition to the classification and prediction. For example, Park et al. [103] have focused on clustering the insomnia patterns by using data obtained from wearable devices. The findings have highlighted the potential of unsupervised learning in enabling healthcare practitioners to develop precise and personalized interventions tailored to data-driven user clusters, offering a promising new approach to insomnia treatment.

2.2.3 Narcolepsy

Narcolepsy is a little-known sleep disorder characterized by abnormal regulation of sleep and wakefulness, causing drowsiness and sleep episodes during the day [78, 125]. This neurological condition is divided into two recognized types with and without cataplexy: narcolepsy type 1, caused by the loss of hypothalamic neurons that produce the neuropeptides orexin-A and -B and type 2, which presents in a very similar way but with an unknown cause [76, 126]. Thus, the existing studies primarily focus on type 1.

Diagnosing narcolepsy type 1 requires a sleep study during which trained scoring technicians visually analyze PSG and manually identify transitions between sleep and wakefulness, and thus sleep staging becomes extremely critical for accurate narcolepsy diagnosis. By identifying sleep-wake transitions and classifying sleep stages, SVM [71] and NNs [138] are the two widely applied and most efficient methods for diagnosing narcolepsy, similar to other sleep disorders. The incorporation of additional patients' survey data has also been shown to increase the NN model performance for detecting narcolepsy [138]. Buettner et al. [24] have also successfully employed the RF model to distinguish between narcolepsy and idiopathic hypersomnia using EEG, achieving high accuracy rates. This study highlights the capability of ML techniques not only in diagnosing specific sleep disorders, but also in distinguishing between various types of disorders that necessitate different treatment approaches.

2.2.4 Restless Legs Syndrome

Restless legs syndrome is characterized by uncomfortable but not painful paresthesia in the lower limbs that tends to occur during rest, significantly disrupting the patient's sleep. Several studies have focused on identifying and diagnosing this syndrome [68, 151]. For example, Iftikhar et al. [68] have successfully employed AI techniques for early detection of restless legs syndrome in patients with type 2 diabetes mellitus who are more susceptible to this condition. This early detection is crucial as it allows patients to take necessary measures in time to prevent potential complications in the future.

As a summary, the prevailing sleep disorders explored in the current literature encompass sleep apnea, insomnia, and narcolepsy. While there are some studies delving into disorders such as restless legs syndrome, parasomnias, and circadian rhythm disorders, many other types and subtypes of sleep disorders still remain underexplored [25, 104]. Factors influencing this discrepancy include data availability, disorder severity, and AI's potential for impactful contributions to diagnosis and treatment [53]. As the field of AI in sleep disorders is continually evolving, we may expect the research to expand to encompass a wide range of sleep disorders over time with the emergence of new technologies and clinical insights.

3 AI and DS Methods in Sleep Disorders

This section presents a comprehensive introduction and review of AI and DS methods in sleep disorders, particularly in applications of sleep scoring, and the diagnosis, understanding, and treatment of sleep disorders by leveraging vast amounts of sleep data. Section 3.1 first examines a diverse range of data types commonly used in sleep disorder research empowered by AI and DS. Section 3.2 then delves into the critical processes of data preprocessing, an essential facet of DS, which plays a pivotal role in enhancing the quality and utility of sleep disorder data to be applied into AI and DS techniques. Section 3.3 finally discusses a wide range of AI and DS techniques employed in sleep disorder analysis from two different perspectives.

3.1 Data Types

AI and DS excel in efficient analysis and integration of large-scale sleep data that encompasses a diverse range of data types and formats. The advancement of AI and DS, together with the evolution of sensor technology, has facilitated the acquisition and utilization of an increasingly diverse range of data types. Sleep data related to disorders is mainly collected by two sources: sensors, which autonomously capture data through various devices and surveys, which necessitate manual reporting by healthcare professionals or patients. Table 3 provides a summary of the major data types employed for studying several key sleep disorders.

3.1.1 Sensor Data

The utilization of sensors for sleep study has been a practice for several decades. PSG, coupled with clinical evaluation, has served as the traditional gold standard

Table 3 Summary of major data types employed for several sleep disorders in the literature

Sleep disorder	Major data types
Sleep apnea	Sensor data: mostly PSG including ECG, SPO2, snoring, respiratory rate and effort; and CPAP
Insomnia	Mostly survey data: sleep questionnaires
	Some sensor data: EEG and EOG in PSG
Narcolepsy	Sensor data: mostly PSG including EEG, EOG, EMG
Restless leg syndrome	Mostly survey data
	Some sensor data: EMG, body movements in EEG
Parasomnias	Sensor data: PSG, VSG, and actigraphy

for examining sleep and diagnosing sleep disorders in clinical laboratory [17]. In recent years, both industry and academia have made substantial investments in developing smaller, less obtrusive, and more portable devices for the continuous sleep monitoring both within and outside laboratory [61, 108]. This progress is driven by the aspiration to facilitate data collection among larger participant groups for extended periods and in more natural settings, thereby reducing monitoring costs and participant burden [108]. Sensor data is generally considered as objective.

3.1.1.1 PSG

PSG provides the most detailed information on sleep architecture and clinical diagnosis of sleep disorders, remaining a gold standard to diagnose various sleep disorders [138]. It involves the recording of multiple digital physiological signals, including brain activity electroencephalography (EEG), eye movement electrooculography (EOG), muscle activity electromyography (EMG), heart activity electrocardiography (ECG), heart rate, oxygen saturation (SPO2), respiratory effort and airflow, and snoring [108].

PSG is the primary sleep data type explored in AI and DS methods for sleep disorder study. Existing AI and DS methods either employ one single PSG signal or a combination of multiple PSG signals depending on different types of disorders. Typically, different PSG signals are utilized based on the specific sleep disorder under investigation. For OSA, the most studied sleep disorder in the literature, ECG is the most commonly applied single-channel signal [141]. Various parameters useful in the OSA diagnosis can be derived from the ECG signal, e.g., Heart Rate Variability (HRV) measuring the variation in the time interval between consecutive heartbeats (known as the RR intervals) and ECG derived respiration (EDR) measuring respiratory activity from ECG [113]. SPO2, snoring, respiratory effort, and airflow are also useful signals that can aid in assessing OSA [96, 117]. For insomnia, the most widespread disorder, actigraphy and EOG signals are commonly employed in many studies [9, 76, 77]. For many other sleep disorders such as narcolepsy, sleep staging has been demonstrated as an essential task to diagnose and treat disorders [76, 138]. Most studies have focused on utilizing single-channel EEG or even on single-channel EOG for sleep staging, while several studies have combined EEG with EMG and EOG signals [33, 47]. Despite the general consensus that the use of multiple signals improves performance for sleep staging, the incorporation of multiple channels can be computationally expensive and may compromise the efficiency of the algorithm without leading to a far better performance [11, 47, 108].

Evolving Sensing Technology Although traditional PSG necessitates that participants sleep in a laboratory environment, the advent of portable PSG devices has enabled home-based testing, making PSG testing increasingly prevalent. This home PSG approach facilitates the monitoring of patients with sleep disorders that may not be easily assessed within a clinical setting [23]. For example, ambulatory PSG serves as an alternative method for home testing, employing a reduced number of sensors [111].

Limitations PSG recordings, conducted either in a laboratory or at home, are typically subject to meticulous analysis by certified technicians who visually inspect the data on standardized screens. This process requires significant manual efforts for scoring. In addition, PSG may pose challenges when applied to young children and is less informative for assessing daytime sleep, regular nighttime awakenings, behavioral insomnia, and schedule-related sleep disorders [121].

3.1.1.2 VSG

VSG is another conventional method for sleep evaluation, encompassing a range of video-based methods for recording an individual during sleep. VSG offers a non-invasive means of documenting specific sleep behaviors, which can be particularly valuable in diagnosing parasomnia. It is often used in conjunction with PSG for comprehensive sleep disorder study [131]. Compared to PSG, VSG presents several advantages in terms of ease of use, particularly for infants and preschool children [121]. Recent advancements in telemedicine have also facilitated the utilization of VSG in home-based settings [108].

Limitations VSG necessitates the installation of equipment at home, followed by the labor-intensive processes of visual inspection and manual scoring. These requirements can be time-consuming and potentially raise privacy concerns. Furthermore, VSG is influenced by the sleeping positions and locations of individuals, potentially affecting the accuracy of sleep assessments and particularly posing challenges in sleep scoring for older children [121].

3.1.1.3 Actigraphy

Actigraphy is a non-invasive method for monitoring human activity and rest cycles, which is recognized as a valid assessment method by the AASM [17, 137]. It is cost-effective and allows for continuous tracking of individuals over extended periods in a home-based setting, making it ideal for large-scale population studies [121, 130]. Actigraphy has advantages over VSG in terms of user-friendliness, especially for children, as it requires no specialized installation and its sleep-wake scoring is relatively straightforward [27, 136].

Limitations Actigraphy only measures physical activity and lacks the capacity to provide detailed information about sleep stages, respiratory patterns, or specific behaviors during sleep. Consequently, it may not be suitable for diagnosing certain disorders like sleep apnea and narcolepsy, which demand more comprehensive physiological data [108, 121]. In addition, actigraphy data is prone to contamination by large amounts of artifacts stemming from external movements, device removal, and instances of motionless wakefulness [136]. This necessitates significant efforts to meticulously identify and eliminate these artifacts to maintain data validity [121].

3.1.1.4 Continuous Positive Air Pressure (CPAP)

CPAP is a widely employed treatment method for sleep apnea, involving information about breathing patterns, airflow, and pressure levels during sleep. It can also serve as a valuable source of data for sleep disorder study. CPAP data can be utilized to classify and track sleep for monitoring the progress and effectiveness of CPAP treatment in sleep apnea patients [1].

Limitations CPAP data falls short in providing a comprehensive view of all aspects of sleep, such as sleep staging or detailed behavioral information. In addition, its primary use is focused on monitoring sleep apnea treatment, making it less suitable for studying other sleep disorders that require other types of data.

3.1.1.5 Other Emerging Sensors

In recent years, there has been a notable increase in home testing and monitoring for sleep disorders, enabled by the development of affordable and scalable sensors. This trend marks a shift from traditional laboratory-based assessment to encompass non-obtrusive methods in free-living environments [108, 119]. These technological advancements have expanded the types of sensor data available for studying sleep disorders, thus opening new possibilities for research in this field.

Low-cost wearable sensors have emerged as promising tools for studying sleep architectures and disorders. These sensors are often complemented by other minimally invasive devices, such as heart rate monitors, miniaturized ECG systems, pulse-oximeters, blood pressure monitors, galvanic skin conductance sensors, light sensors, gyroscopes, barometric altimeters, and GPS trackers [108]. The rise of wearable devices, such as smartwatches, fitness trackers, and smartphone sensing, has made them widely accessible to large populations for the collection of large-scale sleep data. Researchers have tapped into the potential of lifelog data collected from daily digital activities recorded by smartphones, and such data has proven valuable for large-scale sleep disorder screening [50, 74]. In addition, AI-powered wearable devices have revolutionized the consumer market by enabling individuals to monitor their sleep patterns and receive personalized insights into their sleep quality. These devices leverage advanced data analysis and machine learning techniques to provide actionable recommendations for improving sleep hygiene and overall well-being [108]. As AI algorithms continue to evolve, they hold the promise of developing adaptive interventions that dynamically adjust sleep therapy based on real-time data. This dynamic approach customizes treatment plans to each patient's unique needs, ultimately enhancing patient outcomes and empowering healthcare professionals to deliver more effective and patient-centered care. An extensive review of various types of data collected from emerging sensors for sleep disorder study can be found in Perez-Pozuelo et al. [108].

Besides wearable sensors, a more recent development in sensor technology also includes the use of three-dimensional (3D) facial photography, obtained through 3D scan displays, to analyze and predict sleep apnea based on craniofacial features associated with the condition [39, 60, 94]. This advancement reflects the ongoing evolution of sensor data collection and its potential in sleep disorder prediction and screening.

3.1.2 Survey Data

Survey data, which complements sensor data, represents another essential type of information used to study sleep disorders and establish diagnosis.

3.1.2.1 Sleep Diaries and Questionnaires

Sleep diaries and questionnaires are both common and cost-effective sources of data containing comprehensive information for analyzing and diagnosing sleep disorders [67]. Sleep diaries provide self-reported data on sleep schedules, night wakings, and related disturbances. Sleep questionnaires are structured assessment tools that contain questions to collect subjective information about an individual's sleep patterns, sleep quality, sleep-related behaviors, and any sleep-related problems they may be experiencing [16, 67, 121]. Many questionnaires have undergone validation through extensive statistical studies, and they are commonly employed as screening tools to complement sleep disorder diagnosis. These subjective reports are frequently used alongside sensor data like PSG, VSG, or actigraphy for a more robust evaluation of sleep disorders [69, 74]. In addition, sleep diaries are also used to quality-check actigraphy data by helping identify and remove artifacts [121].

Limitations Sleep diaries and questionnaires rely on subjective information provided by patients or caregivers for infants and children, making them susceptible to bias and inaccuracies. While reported sleep schedules tend to be reliable, measures of sleep quality such as night wakings, are less valid [14, 121]. Responses can vary based on an individual's mood, memory, or interpretation of questions, leading to inconsistencies. In addition, sleep diaries and questionnaires often provide qualitative or semi-quantitative data, making it challenging to perform rigorous statistical analysis. Furthermore, while they can help identify sleep-related issues, they alone may not provide a complete picture of sleep disorders and offer precise diagnostic information required for clinical assessments [101].

3.1.2.2 Life History

Patients' life history encompasses their demographic characteristics, clinical history, and physical examinations, such as mental and physical health, trauma, and life events [15, 16]. Demographic characteristics, objective in nature, have been shown to play a crucial role in analyzing risks and personalizing sleep disorder treatments, with factors like age and gender influencing the assessment of sleep disorders in various population groups [76]. Considerable studies have investigated sleep disorders in different population groups, including the elderly, children, pregnant individuals, and those with depression [7, 36, 37, 41, 56, 98]. The awareness of demographic characteristics and health profiles within these groups has proven highly valuable for assessing and managing sleep disorders.

Limitations While demographic information can provide insights into population-level trends, it may not offer specific and accurate diagnostic details for sleep disorders. Demographic characteristics and health histories can also vary widely among individuals, making it challenging to generalize findings or establish causality [16]. In addition, life history data may not capture all relevant aspects of an individual's medical or psychological history, potentially missing critical factors that contribute to sleep disorders. Individuals may not remember or disclose certain health-related events or conditions. Furthermore, life history data alone typically lacks critical sleep-related physiological parameters, such as brain activity or respiratory patterns, for accurate diagnosis of sleep disorders [15].

In summary, many studies often combine multiple sources of sleep data to enhance the understanding, diagnosis, treatment, and screening of sleep disorders. While multiple sources may estimate the same sleep variables, their accuracy may not always align. For example, Camerota et al. [27] have conducted an analysis using sleep data from VSG, actigraphy, and sleep diaries in infant sleep studies. The results indicate that actigraphy and sleep diaries, compared to VSG, have significantly overestimated sleep period duration and underestimate the number of night waking episodes. Actigraphy and sleep diaries demonstrated higher agreement with each other than with VSG. Further epoch-by-epoch analyses indicated that actigraphy had low sensitivity to detect wakefulness. In this context, the utilization of AI and DS techniques holds tremendous potential in handling such heterogeneous data. These technologies can effectively resolve inconsistencies across diverse data sources and extract valuable insights for advancing the understanding of sleep disorders and patient care.

3.2 *Data Preprocessing*

Data preprocessing is a crucial step in sleep data analysis to empower the potential of AI and DS techniques in sleep disorders, especially in the context of the growing trend in integrating sleep data from a multitude of sensors. It refines the quality of sleep data by addressing potential errors, inconsistencies, or noise in raw data that may adversely affect the subsequent analysis and compromise the integrity of AI and DS outcomes. Effective data preprocessing is essential to ensure the reliability and effectiveness of AI and DS models and to provide more accurate insights into sleep patterns and disturbances [33, 96]. AI and DS techniques not only facilitate the seamless integration of multi-source sleep data to improve the understanding, diagnosis, treatment, and screening of sleep disorders, but also streamline the preprocessing phase with reduced need of extensive manual intervention, marking a shift toward more efficient data preprocessing in sleep studies.

This section discusses several pivotal processes in data preprocessing, with a particular focus on two major steps: data cleaning and data transformation. Specifically, data cleaning is the process of repairing or removing incorrect, corrupted, poorly formatted, redundant, mislabeled, or incomplete data within a dataset. After data cleaning, data transformation then serves as the process of converting the shape and structure of raw data into a functional format that can be explored in the following AI and DS techniques. These processes collectively pave the way for comprehensive and reliable sleep data analysis, ultimately advancing the study of sleep disorders to empower sleep health.

3.2.1 Data Cleaning

Noise Reduction Sensor data often contains noise due to measurement errors, and signal processing methods like smoothing or filtering can reduce noise in sensor data. Filtering can not only remove unwanted noise but also enhance the signal to better extract desired features. Several key filters include low pass, high pass, bandpass, and notch filters, each designed to pass specific frequencies that are desired [33, 108]. For raw PSG, the AASM recommends using routine low and high pass filter settings [17].

Outlier Detection Sensor data, especially physiological measurements, is prone to outliers that significantly differ in multiple aspects from the other data in a population. The sources of outliers in the dataset include human errors, system maintenance, and sampling errors such as including a pediatric sample in adult research [3]. Detecting and removing these outliers is vital for learning a robust and generalizable ML model [66]. Clustering algorithms like DBSCAN or isolation forests are typically tools to identify outliers [128, 134].

Artifact Rejection Artifact rejection can be complex as every system, experiment, and subject may vary in number, magnitude, and type of artifacts. Researchers use different criteria for artifact rejection. Some simply reject trials with artifacts, while others may use techniques like independent component analysis (ICA) that breaks up a mixture of signals into their distinct sources to correct movement artifacts [105]. Certain artifacts, like spikes, might be easy to detect because of their distinct signal properties, while others are more challenging. Traditional artifact detection methods are deficient because they assume very typical and well-described artifacts and require experts to manually explore and annotate data for artifact segments [120]. Several advanced unsupervised EEG artifact detection and correction have been evolving in recent years [122].

Missing Data Handling Missing data is a widespread phenomenon in both sensor and survey data, either because it exists and was not collected or never existed. Simply ignoring missing data fails many ML models, and the model results can easily be biased if missing records are not appropriately handled. There are two major methods to deal with missing values: simply dropping observations that have missing values or filling missing values based on other similar observations, using techniques such as linear or higher-order interpolation. If any of the PSG epochs contains a null value or a missing segment, the common practice is to remove it from the dataset [55, 86].

3.2.2 Data Transformation

Categorical Data Encoding Survey data often includes categorical variables like gender or education level, and sleep data also comes with categorical labels. Most ML models can only handle numeric variables, and therefore categorical data has to be transformed into numeric form before applying any ML model. Common techniques for encoding categorical data into numerical format include one-hot encoding, label encoding, or embedding layers in NNs [38, 59].

Normalization (Standardization) Data normalization or standardization severs as a critical and commonly employed preprocessing step to improve data integrity and consistency and thus ensures the stability, accuracy, and generalization of ML models by transforming raw data into one uniform scale. A wide array of sensor and survey data with different units and scales benefits from normalization. The two most common normalization methods are min–max normalization and z-score standardization, which can suppress noise levels and variability in sleep data [26]. Normalization can also be done automatically by incorporating batch normalization layers in DL models [4].

Dimensionality Reduction High-dimensional data, often encountered in sleep sensor data, improves the models' accuracy but pose challenges such as model overfitting and high storage demands. Depending on the dataset, while reducing dimensionality does cause some data loss that might lead to slightly worse model performance, it can speed up model training and improves visualization. Principal component analysis (PCA) is by far the most popular dimensionality reduction algorithm by projecting the data onto the closest hyperplane [47, 66]. Autoencoders are also powerful tools to automatically reduce the dimensionality while preserving essential information [44]. Downsampling is also a common tool for dimensionality reduction particularly in high-resolution PSG signal data by reducing the signal resolution [44].

Feature Extraction Feature extraction sometimes overlaps with dimensionality reduction. The key difference is that feature extraction requires knowledge to ensure the extracted features preserve relevant information desired for later sleep disorder analysis. It is particularly important for extracting relevant information from sensor data, where raw signals can be vast and complex and can significantly improve model accuracy and efficiency. Following the AASM manual guidelines, various important features can be extracted from PSG signals through statistical analysis [33, 47]. AI techniques, such as convolutional neural networks (CNNs) and recurrent neural networks (RNNs), allows for automatic feature extraction from sensor data. For example, in PSG, CNNs can identify specific sleep stage patterns and RNNs can capture temporal dependencies in sleep data [112].

3.3 *AI and DS Techniques*

In this section, we will review the diverse spectrum of AI and DS techniques employed in sleep disorder analysis, uncovering their potential in transforming sleep health in multiple aspects from sleep scoring to the diagnosis, treatment, and deeper understanding of sleep disorders. This comprehensive review will be organized from two perspectives, by learning approaches and by model types in Sects. 3.3.1 and 3.3.2, respectively.

3.3.1 By Learning Approaches

Broadly speaking, AI techniques, particularly ML models, utilize sleep data and knowledge to intelligently learn and perform human-like clinical tasks in the realm of sleep disorders. Based on the learning approaches, most AI (or interchangeably, ML) techniques, often empowered by DS, can be divided into supervised, unsupervised, and reinforcement learning, as shown in Fig. 3. The basic structures of the three learning paradigms are demonstrated in Fig. 4. It should be noted that recent advancements have seen a growing trend toward the development of novel AI algorithms that may not clearly fit in these traditional categories [11, 112].

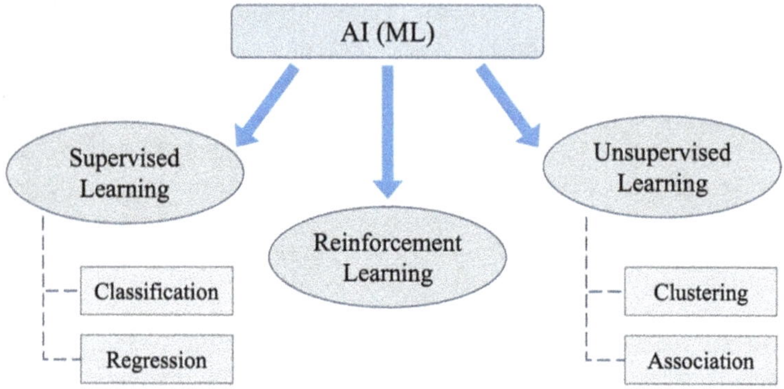

Fig. 3 Categories of AI (ML) by learning tasks

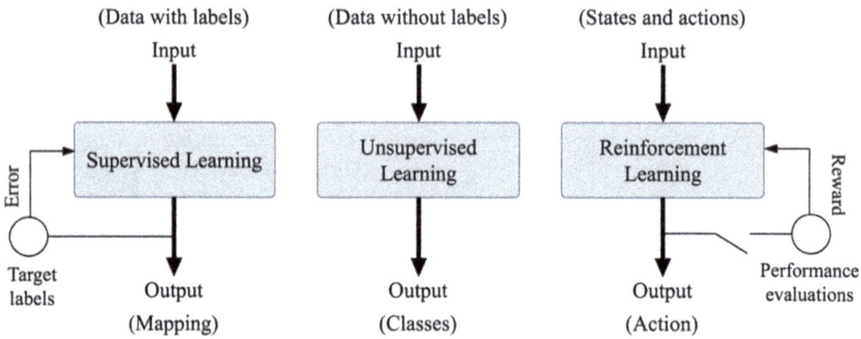

Fig. 4 Basic structures of supervised, unsupervised, and reinforcement learning paradigms

Table 4 Summary of ML learning approaches and tasks for different clinical tasks in the literature

Clinical tasks	Employed learning approaches	Performed ML tasks
Sleep stage scoring	Supervised, unsupervised, semi-supervised, self-supervised, or reinforcement learning	Classification
Diagnosis of sleep disorders	Supervised learning	Classification or regression
Understanding of sleep disorders	Unsupervised or self-supervised learning	Clustering or association
Treatment and management of sleep disorders	Reinforcement learning	–

Different learning approaches are applied targeting different clinical tasks. Table 4 provides a summary of employed ML learning approaches and tasks for different clinical tasks.

3.3.1.1 Supervised Learning

Supervised learning algorithms take data with labels as training input and aim to learn the appropriate relationship mapping the input data to the target output labels, e.g., predicting human-scored sleep stages from PSG signals.

A substantial portion of existing research in the realm of sleep disorders belongs to supervised learning, most in classification problem for sleep scoring and the diagnosis of sleep disorders [108, 112, 141]. Specifically, the majority of studies is to perform binary or multiple classification for identifying and classifying sleep disorders [96, 144] as well as for classifying sleep stages that can enhance the diagnosis and treatment of specific sleep disorders for individuals [33, 47]. The developed techniques continue to improve model accuracy and efficiency for the diagnosis of different sleep disorders, significantly reducing the need for manual interventions and associated costs. There are also some studies focusing on regression problems, where the objective is to derive certain diagnostic metrics of sleep disorders from an individual's sleep data, e.g., predicting the overall AHI measure to evaluate the sleep apnea severity of one patient [96]. Extensive reviews on applying supervised AI techniques to sleep stage scoring and diagnosing sleep disorders can be found in Fiorillo et al. [47], Chriskos et al. [33], Mostafa et al. [96], etc.

In the literature, most of the developed AI models typically fall under the umbrella of supervised learning. These methods are designed to learn the best model that effectively maps the relationship between input data and output labels for accurately classifying new data relevant to specific tasks, such as the classification of sleep stages and sleep disorders. The specific models will be discussed later in Sect. 3.3.2.

3.3.1.2 Unsupervised Learning

Unsupervised learning takes data without labels as training input, and the major task is to identify patterns or clusters within the data. Most unsupervised learning studies are focused on clustering or association analysis [11].

Clustering in unsupervised learning plays a pivotal role in subtyping sleep disorders and discovering novel disorder phenotypes, extending beyond simplistic conventional diagnostic criteria [83, 103]. For example, Park et al. [103] have developed a NN-based unsupervised clustering method tailored to individuals with insomnia to identify distinctive characteristics of each resulting cluster by using a multitude of information sources from smart bands and neural-nets. This study demonstrates that unsupervised learning of insomnia data gathered from wearable fitness devices could identify meaningful clusters. It also underscores the potential of unsupervised learning in allowing healthcare practitioners to design precise and personalized interventions at the level of data-driven population clusters, which could be a novel approach for the treatment of insomnia and other mental health disorders [103]. In another notable example, Ma et al. [83] have developed a comprehensive multimeric phenotyping framework that combines both supervised and unsupervised learning techniques to cluster 2277 patients with OSA into six distinct phenotypes based on their PSG data. The proposed method has not only identified previously unrecognized phenotypes but also revealed statistically significant variations in the development of comorbidities related to OSA-induced diseases. This phenotyping framework can automatically classify new patients and predict their comorbidity risks based solely on their PSG data, demonstrating potential applications in phenotyping other complex diseases and identifying critical high-risk patient features [83].

In unsupervised learning, association analysis plays a crucial role in sleep disorder endotyping and complication profiling, thus facilitating the screening of high-risk patients with certain diseases. For example, Christensen et al. [34] have employed unsupervised learning to uncover sleep stage features indicative of neurodegeneration directly from EEG or EOG data. The study suggests that patients with idiopathic REM (iRBD) sleep disorder are at an increased risk of developing Parkinson's disease.

In addition, recent endeavors have also integrated unsupervised learning into automatic sleep staging to address the challenges of limited labeled training data and physiological differences due to subject variability [44, 145, 147, 150]. Many emerging unsupervised methods focus on employing domain adaptation techniques to create a pre-trained network with an existing large-scale dataset (source domain) that is applicable to smaller datasets (target domain). The results conclusively demonstrate that the suggested domain adaptation substantially enhances sleep staging performance across various model transfer tasks without the requirement of labeled sleep data in the target domain [145, 150].

3.3.1.3 Reinforcement Learning

Reinforcement learning typically has a feedback ingredient and learns the model based on interacting with the environment and receiving penalties and rewards depending on model prediction performance. Specifically, reinforcement learning is effectively employed to train AI agents to perform sequential actions toward a specific goal, which is well suited for the clinical task of the treatment and management of sleep disorders.

Recent research has embraced reinforcement learning for sleep stage classification [45] and treatment guidance [12, 30], which relies on measurable outcomes to guide the training process rather than predefined expected outcomes for each input. For example, Ferjani et al. [45] have utilized Multi-agent Systems to create a model for classifying sleep stages by using various physiological signals from heterogeneous sources. The proposed model facilitates cooperative learning and achieves high classification accuracy even with unlabeled data. Moreover, existing studies have also explored the potential of reinforcement learning in treatment optimization tailored to multiple sleep disorders due to the trial-and-error mechanism of reinforcement learning [11].

3.3.1.4 Others: Semi- and Self-Supervised Learning

In response to the limitation of labeled sleep data in clinical practice, emerging research has delved into hybrid approaches that may not clearly fit in one of these traditional learning categories to establish relationships between input data and outputs. Novel learning paradigms include semi-supervised learning [62, 73, 79, 146], combining supervised and unsupervised learning with partially labeled data, and self-supervised learning [13, 72, 149], a technique that leverages data structure to generate labels for model training.

The semi-supervised and self-supervised learning methods have been primarily applied to sleep stage classification, significantly enhancing classification accuracy and reducing labeling costs during the training phase. For example, Banville et al. [13] have investigated self-supervised learning to address two clinical challenges: EEG-based sleep staging and pathology detection. The results demonstrate that linear classifiers trained on features learnt by self-supervised learning consistently outperform purely supervised deep NNs especially when labeled data is scarce. The proposed method not only performs high classification accuracy in sleep staging but also uncovers latent physiological and clinical structures, providing insights into aspects like age-related effects.

3.3.2 By Model Types

A wide array of AI and DS models employed in sleep disorder research can be broadly categorized into two groups: conventional ML models that necessitate feature engineering and DL models that operate without this need. Table 5 provides a comparison of conventional ML models and DL models, outlining their differences in the input data, the preprocessing effort, and the need for domain expertise.

Specifically, conventional ML models rely on a set of carefully selected features as their input and demand a deep understanding of domain expertise, often requiring significant efforts to engineer sophisticated features in the step of data preprocessing. Thus, the applicability of conventional ML models is usually restricted to few

Table 5 Comparison of conventional ML models and DL models in sleep disorder research

Model	Input data	Preprocessing	Domain expertise
Conventional ML	Small-scale selected features	Sophisticated, mainly on feature engineering	Significant and high-level
DL	Large-scale sensor and survey data	Less intensive, mainly on data normalization	Moderate to low-level

sleep disorders, including insomnia, sleep apnea, and narcolepsy [144]. By contrast, the recently evolving DL models can excel in large-scale sleep data and complex patterns with automatic feature learning [47, 96, 108]. The powerful ability of DL models makes them suitable for a broader range of sleep disorders and clinical applications [11].

3.3.2.1 Conventional ML Models

Conventional ML models involve prior feature extraction and selection, where extracted features mainly come from patients' demographic characteristics, questionnaires, and physiological signals. With these selected features as input, ML models learn from input data to identify patterns or make predictions regarding the target task, mainly belonging to supervised learning. In the literature, plenty of works have applied numerous conventional ML models to analyze significant features associated with sleep disorders, identify and diagnose sleep disorders, and classify sleep stages. Frequently used ML models include logistic regression [5, 107], SVM [148], KNN [97], RF [9], and decision tree [69] for characterizing and classifying sleep disorders. Among these models, logistic regression and SVM are the most popular and powerful ones in the literature to identify and classify various sleep disorders with the highest classification accuracy [93, 108].

Logistic regression is a simple and efficient model for classification tasks related to sleep disorders. It can not only classify sleep disorders but also identify the most relevant features associated with the output class, effectively estimating parameters for logistic models.

Logistic regression models have been widely employed in uncovering associations and identifying potential factors related to sleep disorders such as sleep apnea and restless leg syndrome [90, 129]. These models are particularly effective in singling out critical features significantly associated with specific sleep disorders. For example, Chellappa and Araújo [31] have applied logistic regression models to explore the multivariate relationships between co-variables and suicidal ideation in patients with major depressive disorder. This study has revealed a significant association between insomnia and suicidal ideation with accounting for potentially confounding factors like medication intake [31].

Logistic regression models have also proven valuable in the direct identification of sleep disorders. For example, Garde et al. [51] have utilized time- and frequency-domain features extracted from SPO2 and ECG signals to apply logistic regression for identifying sleep apnea or hypopnea events. Additionally, Islam et al. [69] have shown the superiority of logistic regression over other ML models in predicting chronic insomnia by using questionnaire data, highlighting its effectiveness of sleep disorder diagnosis in practical clinical applications.

SVM, a supervised learning-based machine learning classifier, employs hyperplanes as decision boundaries to classify data. The dimensionality of the hyperplanes depends on the number of feature vectors, and the optimal hyperplane is the one that maintains the largest margin from the support vectors.

SVM stands out as one of the most widely used and powerful classifiers for predicting several types of sleep disorders, including sleep apnea, insomnia, and narcolepsy. For example, Al-Angari et al. (2012) have effectively applied the SVM classifier to identify sleep apnea events by using HRV, SPO2, and respiratory effort signals. Ahuja et al. (2019) have evaluated 15 different ML algorithms for predicting insomnia, and SVM has emerged as the top performer with the highest prediction accuracy. The study has also underscored the strong relationship between insomnia and such factors as vision problems, mobility issues, and other sleep disorders. Similarly, Jensen et al. [71] have also successfully utilized SVM to accurately identify sleep-wake transitions in patients with narcolepsy.

KNN, a simple ML algorithm suitable for classification, utilizes existing cases to classify new cases based on similarity. It assigns new data points, a category based on their proximity to the K-nearest neighbors, where selecting the right K value is crucial to avoid overfitting and optimize model performance.

In Mendez et al. (2010), KNN and NNs have been applied as two supervised classifiers to classify apnea events by using features extracted from a single-channel ECG signal. The results have indicated comparable classification accuracy between the two classifiers, highlighting the efficacy of KNN in OSA detection from ECG signals. Mostafa et al. [97] have employed the KNN classifier combined with two different feature selection methods based on SPO2 signals, yielding commendable performance in apnea detection. In addition, the study has further incorporated ECG signals into the analysis and demonstrated enhanced apnea detection performance, highlighting the effectiveness of KNN with more features from various signal types.

RF employs an ensemble of decision trees to collectively enhance classification accuracy by breaking down complex problems into hierarchical and manageable stages. The structure and parameters of these decision trees are learnt from a training dataset, and the learnt knowledge is then applied to classify new data. This process makes RF particularly effective for intricate problems that are challenging to manually formulate.

In Boostani et al. [20], a comparative analysis of various ML classifiers for automatic sleep staging has been conducted. By using publicly available PSG data, different combinations of extracted features have been evaluated alongside five classifiers, among which the RF classifier, paired with the wavelet coefficient entropy, has emerged as the most effective and promising combination for accurate sleep stage prediction. This study underscores the significance of RF in automatic sleep staging particularly with useful features.

3.3.2.2 DL Models

DL is part of a broader family of ML that does not require sophisticated feature engineering with high-level domain knowledge like conventional ML and can directly utilize raw signals as input [11]. The major advantage of DL models is the superior capability in extracting complex information from a large amount of data by learning features directly from the raw input data with little to no prior

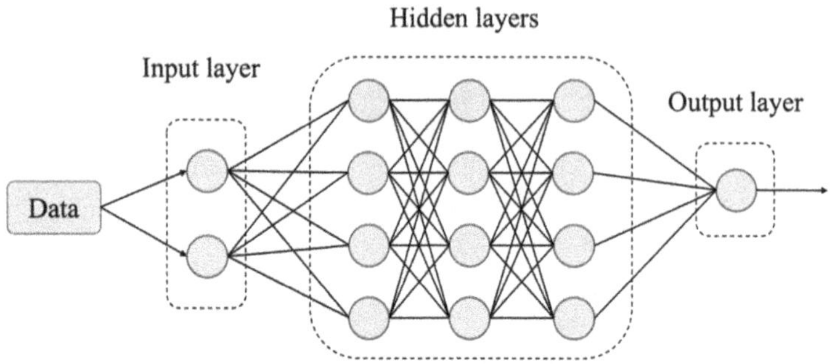

Fig. 5 A schematic diagram of a basic NN architecture

knowledge. While DL models may lack result, interpretability, and demand longer computational time, the large volume and high heterogeneity of sleep data provide great potential for DL models. In recent years, DL has emerged as one of the most popular and powerful tool for automating sleep staging and investigating various sleep disorders directly from raw signal data. Generally, DL models outperform conventional ML models in terms of (i) classification accuracy of sleep staging and sleep disorders; (ii) reduced need for handcrafted feature engineering; (iii) capability of handling diverse and novel signals collected from a multitude of emerging sensors; and (iv) capability of diagnosing and treating a broad range of disorders including insomnia, sleep apnea, parasomnia, rest leg syndrome, and narcolepsy [76, 96].

DL can be seen as an AI function that mimics the human brain's processing of data, and such biologically inspired computational networks are referred to as NNs [11, 124]. Founded on artificial NNs, DL models differ primarily in the architecture that is determined by the arrangement and connections of neurons [47, 124]. Neurons within the same level collectively form a layer, and the network comprises numerous neurons. Each neuron performs a linear combination of inputs followed by a non-linear transformation, as illustrated in Fig. 5.

Standard deep NNs (DNNs) typically consist of multiple fully connected layers arranged sequentially. Within the realm of DL, several noteworthy DNN architectures have emerged, including convolutional NNs (CNN; [99]), recurrent NNs (RNN; [19]), and long short-term memory (LSTM; [52]). Below we will briefly introduce the architecture of each and how it works. Numerous studies have extensively reviewed on applying DL in the diagnosis and treatment of sleep disorders, especially for sleep apnea, e.g., Álvarez et al. [6], Stephansen et al. [138], Mostafa et al. [96], Ramachandran and Karuppiah [112], Salari et al. [123], and Brennan and Kirby [22].

CNN is a typical supervised classification model for processing inputs like raw signals and spectrogram images. The network is commonly composed by a combination of four different types of layers: input; convolution followed by activation functions such as rectified linear units (ReLU); pooling or sub sampling;

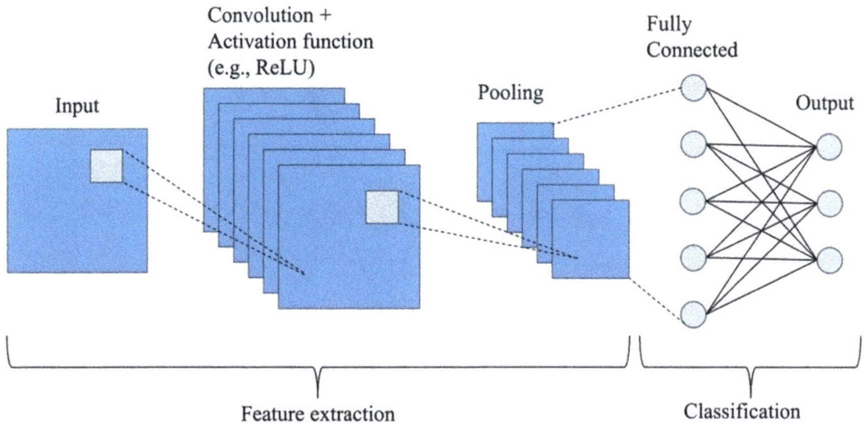

Fig. 6 A schematic diagram of a basic CNN architecture

and classification (commonly a fully connected layer with the softmax function in the end). Batch normalization and dropout layers may also be incorporated into CNN architecture. Each filter layer can be regarded as a feature identifier, and pooling layers reduce the dimensionality while preserving important information. Stacking more layers can generate more complex features. The last layer computes the output probability of identifying the target task, e.g., a specific sleep disorder or each sleep stage. A schematic diagram of a basic CNN is provided in Fig. 6. During the training phase, the weights and biases of the neuron filters are fine-tuned to achieve the target probability class for the input data. Once trained, the CNN model is ready for classifying new input data with such applications as sleep staging and sleep disorder diagnosis [47, 96].

While CNN is primarily designed for image classification, some studies have adapted the concept to one-dimensional CNN (CNN1D) for signal classification with one or multiple signals, which is well suited for sleep data [96]. For example, Urtnasan et al. [141] have employed CNN1D with varying numbers of layers to classify sleep apnea using a single-channel ECG signal, among which a six-layer model has achieved the highest classification accuracy. Haidar et al. [57] have applied a CNN1D model with three-channel inputs for apnea event detection by using three one-dimensional signals. Furthermore, a few studies have employed two-dimensional CNN (CNN2D) models for apnea event detection by using the spectrogram or wavelet transform of signals like nasal airflow and SPO2 as inputs [28, 87].

RNN differs from CNN by considering not only the current input but also the previously received inputs. The principle of RNN is saving the output of a layer and feeding it back to the input to predict the future output of the layer. A schematic diagram of a basic RNN architecture is provided in Fig. 7. Compared to CNNs, RNNs further introduce recurrent connections and are capable of handling sequential data, making them particularly useful in sleep stage classification, where

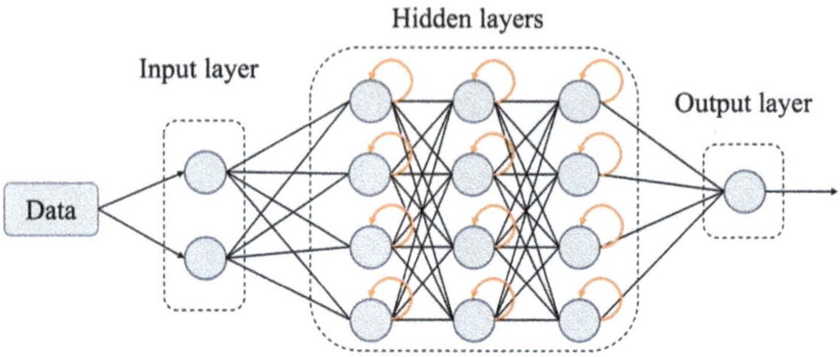

Fig. 7 A schematic diagram of a basic RNN architecture

the temporal dynamics of sleep stages need to be considered as the staging of each 30-second epoch is strongly related to the preceding and following epochs [47].

For example, Aggarwal et al. [1] have combined deep convolution and recurrent neural networks (RCNNs) to extract high-level features from raw flow signals for sleep staging. The proposed model has incorporated a structured output layer based on a conditional random field to effectively model the temporal transition structure of sleep stages. It not only enhances sleep staging classification performance but also enables accurate tracking of sleep metrics, which can be valuable for monitoring the response of CPAP therapy in sleep apnea patients [1]. Similarly, Biswal et al. [19] have also employed an RCNN for supervised learning tasks that involve clinical labels of sleep stages, sleep apnea events, and limb movements. The proposed RCNN model has consistently achieved high accuracy across all three tasks, demonstrating its effectiveness in various clinical classification tasks [19].

LSTM is a specialized type of RNN designed for effective processing and memory retention in time series data. Compared to a basic RNN, a typical LSTM architecture involves a set of gates: an input gate processing the input data, a memory cell storing the temporal data, an output gate controlling the flow of output activations, and most importantly, a forget gate allowing the unit to discard the unwanted time series data that need not be considered as part of the series. Overall, the LSTM network maps the input and output using various activation units inside the cell [76]. This unique architecture empowers LSTM models with the ability to predict sequences over defined time intervals, making them exceptionally well suited for handling sequential inputs like sleep epochs in automatic sleep staging [47, 76]. In the literature, various LSTM configurations have been employed often with multiple stacked layers to achieve accurate sleep stage classification and predict various sleep disorders [52, 96, 142].

In addition to these established NN architectures, recent advances in DL have led to the development of more advanced and specified architectures building upon traditional NNs. Such examples include RobustSleepNet [55] and XSleepNet [110], designed specifically for automated sleep stage classification and sleep disorder diagnosis.

4 Challenges and Opportunities

4.1 Challenges

4.1.1 Challenges Posed by the Inherent Complexity of Sleep Disorders

Multifaceted Nature of Sleep Disorders Sleep disorders manifest in diverse ways and often co-occur with other medical conditions, making it challenging to isolate the symptoms and effects of the sleep disorder itself. This complexity complicates the development of diagnostic tools and interventions that can address the full spectrum of sleep-related issues.

Subject Heterogeneity and Personalization Different genetic backgrounds and environmental factors contribute to the diversity in how sleep disorders manifest in individuals. The subject heterogeneity includes each individual's unique sleep patterns, manifest symptoms, and their responses to treatments, which necessitates developing AI tools that can tailor precise diagnosis and personalized treatment to the specific needs of patients.

4.1.2 Challenges in Sleep Data Handling and Analysis

Data Heterogeneity and Quality Sleep data originates from various sources, including polysomnography, wearable devices, and clinical records. This diversity introduces challenges related to data heterogeneity, variability, and inconsistency. Furthermore, data quality, including noise, artifacts, and missing values, poses challenges in conducting efficient and reliable analyses.

Temporal and Source Variability Sleep data exhibits temporal variations both within and across individuals. Understanding and characterizing these variations are crucial for accurate analysis. Additionally, different sources of sleep data, such as clinical records and wearable devices, may have distinct temporal patterns, which necessitates careful consideration.

Data Representation and Integration Effectively representing and integrating data and metadata from different sensors and sources are essential steps in harnessing the full potential of sleep data. Developing common representation spaces and fusion techniques is a challenge to unlock shared latent information among various data distributions.

4.1.3 Challenges in Integrating AI into Clinical Practice

Data Ethics, Privacy, and Security Integrating AI into clinical practice involves handling sensitive patient data and should be approached cautiously. It is paramount to protect those sensitive health data and to ensure data privacy and security. AI applications must adhere to regulations such as the Health Insurance Portability and Accountability Act (HIPAA), and General Data Protection Regulation (GDPR). Stringent security measures must be implemented to protect patient information.

Model Bias and Accuracy It is crucial to ensure that AI models are accurate and free from biases to ensure they perform reliably across diverse datasets and different patient demographics. This is essential to provide fair, equitable, and effective treatments to all individuals.

Logistical Challenges The introduction of AI technologies into sleep laboratories poses logistical challenges. Increased IT support is required, and healthcare providers and systems need training mechanisms to effectively integrate AI software into existing care pathways. Ensuring that AI-driven solutions align with clinical workflows is vital.

Regulation and Standardization There is an urgent need for the regulation and standardization of developed AI algorithms before their integration into sleep clinics. This challenge encompasses establishing robust regulatory frameworks, ethical guidelines, and safety measures to ensure the responsible and effective use of AI in clinical practice.

Validation Standards Adapting validation requirements based on the end-use of the technology is crucial, especially for new sensing technologies in clinical settings. It is essential to ensure reliability and validity testing of these emerging sensing technologies.

4.2 Opportunities

4.2.1 Opportunities for Enhancing AI and DS Techniques

Combinatorial Approach with Clinical Knowledge A combinatorial approach that integrates ML with clinical information holds the potential for enhanced success, particularly in addressing mild OSA [37]. This approach leverages the wealth of clinical expertise and domain knowledge to augment AI and DS solutions, leading to more accurate and context-aware sleep disorder assessments.

Model Personalization Personalization represents a promising avenue for improving the performance of AI-based sleep modeling systems, especially when dealing with data from noisy modalities like wearable devices. This approach, successfully employed in other fields such as mood recognition and seizure detection, has untapped potential in sleep science. Recent research has demonstrated the feasibility of personalization through transfer learning, where DNNs are initially trained on a large population and then fine-tuned at the subject level [108].

Model Generalization Another way of enhancing AI-based systems' performance includes improving the model generalization by reducing the effects of contextual information. Methods that focus on learning representative features less sensitive to contextual factors can enhance the robustness of sleep classification tasks across various complexities [108]. These approaches aim to increase the generalization capabilities of AI models, making them applicable to diverse sleep-related scenarios and diverse population groups.

Model Interpretability It is crucial for AI systems to not only be effective but also understandable, especially in a clinical context where decision rationale is important [21]. Efforts to enhance the interpretability of AI models can lead to greater trust and integration in clinical practice, as healthcare providers are better able to understand and rationalize the AI's decision-making process.

4.2.2 Opportunities for Advancing Clinical Understanding and Practice

Research Advancements AI and DS techniques can expedite sleep disorder research by automating data analysis and uncovering previously unrecognized patterns. This can lead to breakthroughs in understanding the underlying mechanisms of sleep disorders.

Drug Discovery and Treatment Development AI and DS can sift through extensive genetic and molecular data to identify new therapeutic targets for sleep disorders. These techniques can significantly speed up the drug development process, paving the way for innovative treatment options.

Precision Medicine AI and DS have the potential to transform sleep disorder diagnosis and treatment by analyzing individual sleep patterns, therapy responses, and patient-specific data. This personalized approach, facilitated by DS's ability to integrate diverse data sources, holds promise for optimizing treatment outcomes and improving patient well-being.

Patient Engagement AI-driven applications and devices can actively engage patients in managing their sleep health. With user-friendly interfaces, educational resources, and interactive feedback systems, these tools can motivate patients to follow their treatment plans and adopt healthier sleep habits.

Healthcare Delivery AI can streamline healthcare delivery by automating routine tasks, such as data analysis and report generation. This allows healthcare providers to allocate more time to patient care and clinical decision-making, making the healthcare delivery more patient-focused and responsive.

Continuous Sleep Tracking AI-powered wearable devices and home monitoring tools enable continuous tracking of sleep patterns outside the laboratory setting. These devices use ML to provide personalized insights and recommendations for improving sleep quality, promoting better sleep habits and overall health. It also allows for long-term monitoring and the collection of valuable real-world data, facilitating more comprehensive assessments [85].

Telemedicine and Remote Monitoring AI-powered telemedicine platforms enable remote consultations and monitoring of patients with sleep disorders. This technology allows for continuous assessment and adjustment of treatment plans without the need for frequent in-person visits. This also extends access to care, particularly in underserved areas, and provides convenience for both patients and healthcare providers.

4.2.3 Opportunities for Improving Public Health

Health Equity Sleep disorders are not evenly distributed across the population, and addressing sleep health is a crucial step toward achieving health equity [58]. AI and DS can play a vital role in this endeavor by providing accessible, personalized, and cost-effective solutions that cater to individuals from diverse backgrounds and circumstances. For example, by analyzing large datasets, AI can identify patterns and risk factors specific to different demographic groups, facilitating targeted interventions that advance health equity.

Economic Efficiency AI can optimize resource allocation in sleep clinics, streamline workflows, and enhance patient care, leading to significant cost savings. Automated data analysis and predictive modeling can help identify which patients are most likely to benefit from specific interventions, reducing unnecessary spending and improving the allocation of healthcare resources.

Public Health Outcomes The widespread adoption of AI and DS in sleep medicine has the potential to mitigate the public health burden of sleep disorders. AI-driven tools can assist in early detection and more effective management of sleep conditions, potentially decreasing the risk of associated chronic diseases and improving overall health outcomes.

4.2.4 Opportunities for Collaboration for AI Development and Implementation

Collaboration Across Scientific Disciplines Uniting diverse scientific expertise catalyzes the development and implementation of AI in sleep medicine. By harmonizing clinical insights, genetic research, and environmental data, multi-disciplinary teams, including medical professionals, computer scientists, biologists, and data analysts, craft AI tools with a nuanced understanding of sleep disorders. This cross-disciplinary alliance is key to creating innovative, effective AI solutions that address the complex challenges of sleep health.

Collaboration Across Stakeholders The journey from conceptual AI frameworks to clinically impactful applications in sleep medicine requires collaborative efforts involving industry, academia, public policy makers, and clinical stakeholders [108]. This collaborative approach ensures that emerging technologies are rigorously validated, ethically applied, and seamlessly integrated into healthcare practices, ultimately leading to truly personalized and effective digital health solutions.

5 Conclusion

Driven by the fusion of digital technologies and unprecedented access to sleep data in the transformative landscape, AI and DS have emerged as formidable allies in studying and addressing sleep disorders, marking a new era of empowering sleep health on an unprecedented scale. This chapter provides an extensive review of recent advancements in both AI and DS applications and methods within multifaceted realm of sleep disorders, organized from different perspectives.

On the application side, the overarching clinical tasks include enhancing the accuracy and efficiency of both sleep scoring and sleep disorder diagnosis, personalizing treatment strategies to individuals, and fostering a deeper understanding of the disorders. Specifically, most existing AI and DS study initiatives have placed a significant emphasis on automating and enhancing sleep staging and the diagnosis of several specific sleep disorders. It is noteworthy that sleep staging has demonstrated as a valuable task for facilitating not only the accurate diagnosis of sleep disorders such as sleep apnea and narcolepsy and but also the personalized treatment strategies tailored to individuals. Some AI and DS studies also aspire to elevate our comprehension of sleep disorders by advancing phenotyping and endotyping various sleep disorders. A deeper understanding of the specific disorders, in turn, constitutes a stepping stone for enhanced diagnosis and personalized treatment. By contrast, not many AI and DS studies have delved into the clinical task of personalizing treatment and management of sleep disorders in the current literature. Furthermore, only several major disorders have received significant attention to enhance the diagnosis, treatment, and understanding in the application of AI and DS, including sleep apnea, insomnia, narcolepsy, and restless leg syndrome, whereas many other types of sleep disorders still remain underexplored.

From the methodological point of view, AI and DS exhibit remarkable capabilities in handling vast and diverse arrays of sensor and survey data in the current era. The rapid evolution of sensor technologies has given rise to increasingly varied and novel data types, underscoring the need for proper data preprocessing to ensure the effectiveness and reliability of AI techniques. Certain AI and DS tools can be further employed to streamline the data preprocessing phase, e.g., the incorporation of batch normalization layers within DL models has proven beneficial. Supervised learning stands out as the most frequently studied AI technique, primarily aimed at improving the classification of sleep stages and the diagnosis of sleep disorders. Unsupervised learning techniques often focus on clustering and association analysis to enhance our understanding of the sleep disorders through phenotyping and endotyping. Reinforcement learning, on the other hand, holds promise for the personalized treatment and management of sleep disorders tailored to individuals. To combat the significant challenge of limited labeled data in the current era, several emerging unsupervised, semi-supervised, and self-supervised learning techniques have been developed for automating sleep staging. Notably, recent advancements have witnessed a shift away from conventional ML and DL models toward more advanced NN-based models. These models are increasingly being developed to further automate and enhance the diagnosis and management of a wide range of sleep disorders while reducing associated manual costs and facilitating large-scale analysis.

It is evident that both challenges and opportunities coexist in the field of AI and DS techniques applied in sleep disorders. The challenges primarily revolve around the integration of developed AI algorithms into clinical practice and handling the ever-increasing complexity of sleep data. Overcoming these challenges is crucial for the seamless integration of AI into clinical practice, ultimately benefitting both patients and healthcare providers. Indeed, despite the powerful capabilities and recent advancements of AI and DS techniques in studying sleep disorders, it is evident that there is still untapped potential. The ever-emerging, ever-expanding data and ever-evolving technology continue to offer fertile ground for future research on advancing AI and DS in the realm of sleep disorders to ultimately empower sleep health.

References

1. Aggarwal, K., Khadanga, S., Joty, S., Kazaglis, L., & Srivastava, J. (2018, December). A structured learning approach with neural conditional random fields for sleep staging. In *2018 IEEE International Conference on Big Data (Big Data)* (pp. 1318–1327). IEEE.
2. Al-Angari, H. M., & Sahakian, A. V. (2012). Automated recognition of obstructive sleep apnea syndrome using support vector machine classifier. *IEEE Transactions on Information Technology in Biomedicine*, *16*(3), 463–468.
3. Alsolai, H., Qureshi, S., Iqbal, S. M. Z., Vanichayobon, S., Henesey, L. E., Lindley, C., & Karrila, S. (2022). A Systematic Review of Literature on Automated Sleep Scoring. *IEEE Access*.
4. Alvarez-Estevez, D., & Fernández-Varela, I. (2020). Addressing database variability in learning from medical data: An ensemble-based approach using convolutional neural networks and a case of study applied to automatic sleep scoring. *Computers in Biology and Medicine*, *119*, 103697.
5. Álvarez, D., Cerezo-Hernández, A., Crespo, A., Gutiérrez-Tobal, G. C., Vaquerizo-Villar, F., Barroso-García, V., … & Del Campo, F. (2020). A machine learning-based test for adult sleep apnoea screening at home using oximetry and airflow. *Scientific reports*, *10*(1), 5332.
6. Álvarez, D., Cerezo-Hernández, A., López-Muñiz, G., Castro, T. Á.-D., Ruiz-Albi, T., Hornero, R., & Campo, F. del. (2017). Usefulness of Artificial Neural Networks in the Diagnosis and Treatment of Sleep Apnea-Hypopnea Syndrome. In *Sleep Apnea—Recent Updates*. IntechOpen. doi:https://doi.org/10.5772/66570.
7. Ancoli-Israel, S., & Ayalon, L. (2006). Diagnosis and treatment of sleep disorders in older adults. *The American journal of geriatric psychiatry*, *14*(2), 95–103.
8. Anees, S., Wu, W. P., & Thorpy, M. J. (2013). Sleep-Related Movement Disorders. In *Encyclopedia of Sleep* (pp. 37–42). Elsevier Inc.
9. Angelova, M., Karmakar, C., Zhu, Y., Drummond, S. P., & Ellis, J. (2020). Automated method for detecting acute insomnia using multi-night actigraphy data. *IEEE Access*, *8*, 74413–74422.

10. Arslan, R. S., Ulutaş, H., Köksal, A. S., Bakır, M., & Çiftçi, B. (2022). Automated sleep scoring system using multi-channel data and machine learning. *Computers in Biology and Medicine*, *146*, 105653.
11. Bandyopadhyay, A., & Goldstein, C. (2023). Clinical applications of artificial intelligence in sleep medicine: a sleep clinician's perspective. *Sleep and Breathing*, *27*(1), 39–55.
12. Banerjee, P. S., Mandal, S. N., De, D., & Maiti, B. (2020). RL-sleep: Temperature adaptive sleep scheduling using reinforcement learning for sustainable connectivity in wireless sensor networks. *Sustainable computing: Informatics and systems*, *26*, 100380.
13. Banville, H., Chehab, O., Hyvärinen, A., Engemann, D. A., & Gramfort, A. (2021). Uncovering the structure of clinical EEG signals with self-supervised learning. *Journal of Neural Engineering*, *18*(4), 046020.
14. Bauer, K. M., & Blunden, S. (2008). How accurate is subjective reporting of childhood sleep patterns? A review of the literature and implications for practice. *Current Pediatric Reviews*, *4*(2), 132–142.
15. Bazoukis, G., Bollepalli, S. C., Chung, C. T., Li, X., Tse, G., Bartley, B. L., ... & Armoundas, A. A. (2023). Application of artificial intelligence in the diagnosis of sleep apnea. *Journal of Clinical Sleep Medicine*, jcsm-10532.
16. Benjamins, J. S., Migliorati, F., Dekker, K., Wassing, R., Moens, S., Blanken, T. F., ... & Van Someren, E. J. (2017). Insomnia heterogeneity: characteristics to consider for data-driven multivariate subtyping. *Sleep Medicine Reviews*, *36*, 71–81.
17. Berry, R. B., Budhiraja, R., Gottlieb, D. J., Gozal, D., Iber, C., Kapur, V. K., ... & Tangredi, M. M. (2012). Rules for scoring respiratory events in sleep: update of the 2007 AASM manual for the scoring of sleep and associated events: deliberations of the sleep apnea definitions task force of the American Academy of Sleep Medicine. *Journal of clinical sleep medicine*, *8*(5), 597–619.
18. Bianchi, M. T., Russo, K., Gabbidon, H., Smith, T., Goparaju, B., & Westover, M. B. (2017). Big data in sleep medicine: prospects and pitfalls in phenotyping. *Nature and science of sleep*, 11–29.
19. Biswal, S., Sun, H., Goparaju, B., Westover, M. B., Sun, J., & Bianchi, M. T. (2018). Expert-level sleep scoring with deep neural networks. *Journal of the American Medical Informatics Association*, *25*(12), 1643–1650.
20. Boostani, R., Karimzadeh, F., & Nami, M. (2017). A comparative review on sleep stage classification methods in patients and healthy individuals. *Computer methods and programs in biomedicine*, *140*, 77–91.
21. Brennan, H. L., & Kirby, S. D. (2022). Barriers of artificial intelligence implementation in the diagnosis of obstructive sleep apnea. *Journal of Otolaryngology-Head & Neck Surgery*, *51*(1), 1–9.
22. Brennan, H. L., & Kirby, S. D. (2023). The role of artificial intelligence in the treatment of obstructive sleep apnea. *Journal of Otolaryngology-Head & Neck Surgery*, *52*(1), 1–6
23. Bruyneel, M., & Ninane, V. (2014). Unattended home-based polysomnography for sleep disordered breathing: current concepts and perspectives. *Sleep medicine reviews*, *18*(4), 341–347.
24. Buettner, R., Fuhrmann, J., & Kolb, L. (2019, October). Towards high-performance differentiation between Narcolepsy and Idiopathic Hypersomnia in 10 minute EEG recordings using a Novel Machine Learning Approach. In *2019 IEEE International Conference on E-health Networking, Application & Services (HealthCom)* (pp. 1–7). IEEE.
25. Bukhari, M. A. A., Alghtani, M. A. M., Sultan, Z., Aljohani, A. A. A., & Alhazmi, I. H. M. (2021). Diagnosis and treatment of sleep disorders: A brief review. *Int. J. Med. Dev. Ctries*, *5*, 364–369.
26. Cabello-Solorzano, K., Ortigosa de Araujo, I., Peña, M., Correia, L., & J. Tallón-Ballesteros, A. (2023, August). The Impact of Data Normalization on the Accuracy of Machine Learning Algorithms: A Comparative Analysis. In *International Conference on Soft Computing Models in Industrial and Environmental Applications* (pp. 344–353). Cham: Springer Nature Switzerland.

27. Camerota, M., Tully, K. P., Grimes, M., Gueron-Sela, N., & Propper, C. B. (2018). Assessment of infant sleep: how well do multiple methods compare?. *Sleep*, *41*(10), zsy146.
28. Cen, L., Yu, Z. L., Kluge, T., & Ser, W. (2018, July). Automatic system for obstructive sleep apnea events detection using convolutional neural network. In *2018 40th annual international conference of the IEEE engineering in medicine and biology society (EMBC)* (pp. 3975–3978). IEEE.
29. Chawla, J. (2022, August 31). Insomnia. Medscape. Retrieved from https://emedicine.medscape.com/article/1187829.
30. Che, N., Zhang, T., Li, Y., Yu, F., & Wang, H. (2023). RLSF: Multimodal Sleep Improvement Algorithm based Reinforcement Learning. *IEEE Access*.
31. Chellappa, S. L., & Araújo, J. F. (2007). Sleep disorders and suicidal ideation in patients with depressive disorder. *Psychiatry research*, *153*(2), 131–136.
32. Choe, J., Schwichtenberg, A. J., & Delp, E. J. (2019, March). Classification of sleep videos using deep learning. In 2019 IEEE Conference on Multimedia Information Processing and Retrieval (MIPR) (pp. 115–120). IEEE.
33. Chriskos, P., Frantzidis, C. A., Nday, C. M., Gkivogkli, P. T., Bamidis, P. D., & Kourtidou-Papadeli, C. (2021). A review on current trends in automatic sleep staging through bio-signal recordings and future challenges. Sleep medicine reviews, 55, 101377.
34. Christensen, J. A., Zoetmulder, M., Koch, H., Frandsen, R., Arvastson, L., Christensen, S. R., ... & Sorensen, H. B. (2014). Data-driven modeling of sleep EEG and EOG reveals characteristics indicative of pre-Parkinson's and Parkinson's disease. *Journal of neuroscience methods*, *235*, 262–276.
35. Colten, H. R., & Altevogt, B. M. (2006). Extent and health consequences of chronic sleep loss and sleep disorders. *Sleep Disorders and Sleep Deprivation: An Unmet Public Health Problem. Washington, DC: Institute of Medicine of the National Academies*, 55–135.
36. Colvonen, P. J., Straus, L. D., Stepnowsky, C., McCarthy, M. J., Goldstein, L. A., & Norman, S. B. (2018). Recent Advancements in Treating Sleep Disorders in Co-Occurring PTSD. *Current Psychiatry Reports*, *20*(7), 48.
37. Combs, D., & Parthasarathy, S. (2017). Machines Learning to Detect Obstructive Sleep Apnea in Children. Are We There Yet? *American Journal of Respiratory and Critical Care Medicine*, *196*(12), 1506–1507.
38. Dahouda, M. K., & Joe, I. (2021). A deep-learned embedding technique for categorical features encoding. *IEEE Access*, *9*, 114381–114391.
39. Eastwood, P., Gilani, S. Z., McArdle, N., Hillman, D., Walsh, J., Maddison, K., ... & Mian, A. (2020). Predicting sleep apnea from three-dimensional face photography. *Journal of Clinical Sleep Medicine*, *16*(4), 493–502.
40. Edwards, B. A., Redline, S., Sands, S. A., & Owens, R. L. (2019). More than the sum of the respiratory events: personalized medicine approaches for obstructive sleep apnea. *American journal of respiratory and critical care medicine*, *200*(6), 691–703.
41. El Shakankiry, H. M. (2011). Sleep physiology and sleep disorders in childhood. *Nature and Science of Sleep*, *3*, 101–114.
42. El-Solh, A. A., Mador, M. J., Ten-Brock, E., Shucard, D. W., Abul-Khoudoud, M., & Grant, B. J. (1999). Validity of neural network in sleep apnea. *Sleep*, *22*(1), 105–111.
43. Eugene, A. R., & Masiak, J. (2015). The neuroprotective aspects of sleep. *MEDtube science*, *3*(1), 35.
44. Fan, J., Zhu, H., Jiang, X., Meng, L., Chen, C., Fu, C., ... & Chen, W. (2022). Unsupervised domain adaptation by statistics alignment for deep sleep staging networks. *IEEE Transactions on Neural Systems and Rehabilitation Engineering*, *30*, 205–216.
45. Ferjani, R., Rejeb, L., & Said, L. B. (2020, February). Cooperative Reinforcement Multi-Agent Learning System for Sleep Stages Classification. In *2020 International Multi-Conference on: "Organization of Knowledge and Advanced Technologies" (OCTA)* (pp. 1–8). IEEE.
46. Finnsson E, Ólafsdóttir GH, Loftsdóttir DL, Jónsson S, Helgadóttir H, Ágústsson JS, et al. A scalable method of determining physiological endotypes of sleep apnea from a polysomnographic sleep study. Sleep. 2021;44(1).

47. Fiorillo, L., Puiatti, A., Papandrea, M., Ratti, P. L., Favaro, P., Roth, C., ... & Faraci, F. D. (2019). Automated sleep scoring: A review of the latest approaches. *Sleep medicine reviews*, 48, 101204.
48. Fleetham, J. A., & Fleming, J. A. (2014). Parasomnias. *Cmaj*, *186*(8), E273-E280.
49. Gaines, J., Vgontzas, A. N., Fernandez-Mendoza, J., & Bixler, E. O. (2018). Obstructive sleep apnea and the metabolic syndrome: the road to clinically-meaningful phenotyping, improved prognosis, and personalized treatment. *Sleep medicine reviews*, *42*, 211–219.
50. Gan, W., Dao, M. S., & Zettsu, K. (2022). Monitoring and Improving Personalized Sleep Quality from Long-Term Lifelogs. *arXiv preprint arXiv:2211.12778*.
51. Garde, A., Dekhordi, P., Ansermino, J. M., & Dumont, G. A. (2016, August). Identifying individual sleep apnea/hypoapnea epochs using smartphone-based pulse oximetry. In *2016 38th Annual International Conference of the IEEE Engineering in Medicine and Biology Society (EMBC)* (pp. 3195–3198). IEEE.
52. Gokulan, S., Narmadha, S., Pavithra, M., Rajmohan, R., & Ananthkumar, T. (2020, July). Determination of various deep learning parameter for sleep disorder. In *2020 international conference on system, computation, automation and networking (ICSCAN)* (pp. 1–6). IEEE.
53. Goldstein, C. A., Berry, R. B., Kent, D. T., Kristo, D. A., Seixas, A. A., Redline, S., ... & Shelgikar, A. V. (2020). Artificial intelligence in sleep medicine: an American Academy of Sleep Medicine position statement. *Journal of Clinical Sleep Medicine, 16*(4), 605–607.
54. Gool, J. K., Zhang, Z., Oei, M. S., Mathias, S., Dauvilliers, Y., Mayer, G., ... & Lammers, G. J. (2022). Data-driven phenotyping of central disorders of hypersomnolence with unsupervised clustering. *Neurology*, *98*(23), e2387-e2400.
55. Guillot, A., & Thorey, V. (2021). RobustSleepNet: Transfer learning for automated sleep staging at scale. *IEEE Transactions on Neural Systems and Rehabilitation Engineering*, *29*, 1441–1451.
56. Gulia, K. K., & Kumar, V. M. (2018). Sleep disorders in the elderly: A growing challenge. *Psychogeriatrics*, *18*(3), 155–165.
57. Haidar, R., McCloskey, S., Koprinska, I., & Jeffries, B. (2018, July). Convolutional neural networks on multiple respiratory channels to detect hypopnea and obstructive apnea events. In *2018 International Joint Conference on Neural Networks (IJCNN)* (pp. 1–7). IEEE.
58. Hale, L., Troxel, W., & Buysse, D. J. (2020). Sleep health: an opportunity for public health to address health equity. *Annual review of public health*, *41*, 81–99.
59. Hancock, J. T., & Khoshgoftaar, T. M. (2020). Survey on categorical data for neural networks. *Journal of Big Data*, *7*(1), 1–41.
60. Hanif, U., Leary, E. B., Schneider, L. D., Paulsen, R. R., Morse, A. M., Blackman, A., ... & Mignot, E. J. (2021). Estimation of apnea-hypopnea index using deep learning on 3-D craniofacial scans. *IEEE Journal of Biomedical and Health Informatics*, *25*(11), 4185–4194.
61. Hao, Y., & Foster, R. (2008). Wireless body sensor networks for health-monitoring applications. *Physiological measurement*, *29*(11), R27.
62. Haoran, B., & Guanze, L. (2021, January). Semi-Supervised End-to-End Automatic Sleep Stage Classification Based on Pseudo-Label. In *2021 IEEE International Conference on Power Electronics, Computer Applications (ICPECA)* (pp. 83–87). IEEE.
63. Hertenstein, E., Feige, B., Gmeiner, T., Kienzler, C., Spiegelhalder, K., Johann, A., Jansson-Fröjmark, M., Palagini, L., Rücker, G., Riemann, D., & Baglioni, C. (2019). Insomnia as a predictor of mental disorders: A systematic review and meta-analysis. *Sleep Medicine Reviews*, *43*, 96–105.
64. Huang, W. C., Lee, P. L., Liu, Y. T., Chiang, A. A., & Lai, F. (2020). Support vector machine prediction of obstructive sleep apnea in a large-scale Chinese clinical sample. *Sleep*, *43*(7), zsz295.
65. Huupponen, E., Saastamoinen, A., Niemi, J., Virkkala, J., Hasan, J., Värri, A., & Himanen, S. L. (2005). Automated frequency analysis of synchronous and diffuse sleep spindles. *Neuropsychobiology*, *51*(4), 256–264.
66. Ian Goodfellow, Y. Bengio, and A. Courville, Deep Learning. MIT Press, 2016. [Online]. Available: http://www.deeplearningbook.org

67. Ibáñez, V., Silva, J., & Cauli, O. (2018). A survey on sleep questionnaires and diaries. *Sleep medicine*, *42*, 90–96.
68. Iftikhar, S., Shahid, S., Hassan, M. U., & Ghias, M. (2020). Assessment and prediction of restless leg syndrome (RLS) in patients with diabetes mellitus type II through artificial intelligence (AI). *Pakistan Journal of Pharmaceutical Sciences*, *33*.
69. Islam, M. M., Masum, A. K. M., Abujar, S., & Hossain, S. A. (2020, July). Prediction of chronic insomnia using machine learning techniques. In *2020 11th International Conference on Computing, Communication and Networking Technologies (ICCCNT)* (pp. 1–7). IEEE.
70. Jacobowitz, O., & MacKay, S. (2020). The faces of sleep apnea in the age of machine learning. *Journal of Clinical Sleep Medicine*, *16*(4), 469–470.
71. Jensen, J. B., Sorensen, H. B., Kempfner, J., Sørensen, G. L., Knudsen, S., & Jennum, P. (2014). Sleep–Wake transition in narcolepsy and healthy controls using a support vector machine. *Journal of Clinical Neurophysiology*, *31*(5), 397–401.
72. Jiang, X., Zhao, J., Du, B., & Yuan, Z. (2021, July). Self-supervised contrastive learning for eeg-based sleep staging. In *2021 International Joint Conference on Neural Networks (IJCNN)* (pp. 1–8). IEEE.
73. Kazemi, A., McKeown, M. J., & Mirian, M. S. (2022). Sleep staging using semi-unsupervised clustering of EEG: Application to REM sleep behavior disorder. *Biomedical Signal Processing and Control*, *75*, 103539.
74. Kim, J., & Park, M. (2023). A Study on ML-Based Sleep Score Model Using Lifelog Data. *Applied Sciences*, *13*(2), 1043.
75. Kubat, M., Pfurtscheller, G., & Flotzinger, D. (1994). AI-based approach to automatic sleep classification. *Biological Cybernetics*, *70*(5), 443–448.
76. Kumar, M. R., Kumar, R., & Vaithiyanathan, D. (Eds.). (2021). *Advancing the Investigation and Treatment of Sleep Disorders Using AI*. IGI Global.
77. Kuo, C. E., & Chen, G. T. (2020). A short-time insomnia detection system based on sleep EOG with RCMSE analysis. *IEEE Access*, *8*, 69763–69773.
78. Lehert, P., & Falissard, B. (2018). Multiple treatment comparison in narcolepsy: a network meta-analysis. *Sleep*, *41*(12), zsy185.
79. Li, Y., Luo, S., Zhang, H., Zhang, Y., Zhang, Y., & Lo, B. (2022). MtCLSS: Multi-Task Contrastive Learning for Semi-Supervised Pediatric Sleep Staging. *IEEE Journal of Biomedical and Health Informatics*.
80. Liu, G. R., Lin, T. Y., Wu, H. T., Sheu, Y. C., Liu, C. L., Liu, W. T., ... & Lo, Y. L. (2021). Large-scale assessment of consistency in sleep stage scoring rules among multiple sleep centers using an interpretable machine learning algorithm. *Journal of Clinical Sleep Medicine*, *17*(2), 159–166.
81. Loh, H. W., Ooi, C. P., Vicnesh, J., Oh, S. L., Faust, O., Gertych, A., & Acharya, U. R. (2020). Automated detection of sleep stages using deep learning techniques: A systematic review of the last decade (2010–2020). *Applied Sciences*, *10*(24), 8963.
82. Lyons, M. M., Bhatt, N. Y., Pack, A. I., & Magalang, U. J. (2020). Global burden of sleep-disordered breathing and its implications. Respirology, 25(7), 690–702.
83. Ma, E. Y., Kim, J. W., Lee, Y., Cho, S. W., Kim, H., & Kim, J. K. (2021). Combined unsupervised-supervised machine learning for phenotyping complex diseases with its application to obstructive sleep apnea. *Scientific Reports*, *11*(1), 4457.
84. Magnavita, N., & Garbarino, S. (2017). Sleep, health and wellness at work: a scoping review. *International journal of environmental research and public health*, *14*(11), 1347.
85. Martinot, J. B., Le-Dong, N. N., Cuthbert, V., Denison, S., Gozal, D., Lavigne, G., & Pépin, J. L. (2021). Artificial intelligence analysis of mandibular movements enables accurate detection of phasic sleep bruxism in OSA patients: a pilot study. *Nature and science of sleep*, *13*, 1449.
86. Mashrur, F. R., Islam, M. S., Saha, D. K., Islam, S. R., & Moni, M. A. (2021). SCNN: Scalogram-based convolutional neural network to detect obstructive sleep apnea using single-lead electrocardiogram signals. *Computers in Biology and Medicine*, *134*, 104532.

87. McCloskey, S., Haidar, R., Koprinska, I., & Jeffries, B. (2018). Detecting hypopnea and obstructive apnea events using convolutional neural networks on wavelet spectrograms of nasal airflow. In *Advances in Knowledge Discovery and Data Mining: 22nd Pacific-Asia Conference, PAKDD 2018, Melbourne, VIC, Australia, June 3–6, 2018, Proceedings, Part I 22* (pp. 361–372). Springer International Publishing.
88. McLay, L. K., & Lang, R. (2022). The Role of Reinforcement in the Treatment of Sleep Problems. In *Clinical Handbook of Behavioral Sleep Treatment in Children on the Autism Spectrum* (pp. 161–175). Cham: Springer International Publishing.
89. Mendonça, F., Mostafa, S. S., Ravelo-García, A. G., Morgado-Dias, F., & Penzel, T. (2019). A Review of Obstructive Sleep Apnea Detection Approaches. *IEEE Journal of Biomedical and Health Informatics*, *23*(2), 825–837.
90. Merlino, G., Fratticci, L., Valente, M., Giudice, A. D., Noacco, C., Dolso, P., ... & Gigli, G. L. (2007). Association of restless legs syndrome in type 2 diabetes: a case-control study. Sleep, 30(7), 866–871.
91. Messineo, L., Magri, R., Corda, L., Pini, L., Taranto-Montemurro, L., & Tantucci, C. (2017). Phenotyping-based treatment improves obstructive sleep apnea symptoms and severity: a pilot study. *Sleep and Breathing*, *21*, 861–868.
92. Meyer, N., Harvey, A. G., Lockley, S. W., & Dijk, D. J. (2022). Circadian rhythms and disorders of the timing of sleep. *The Lancet*.
93. Monma, T., Ando, A., Asanuma, T., Yoshitake, Y., Yoshida, G., Miyazawa, T., ... & Takeda, F. (2018). Sleep disorder risk factors among student athletes. *Sleep medicine*, *44*, 76–81.
94. Monna, F., Messaoud, R. B., Navarro, N., Baillieul, S., Sanchez, L., Loiodice, C., ... & Pépin, J. L. (2022). Machine learning and geometric morphometrics to predict obstructive sleep apnea from 3D craniofacial scans. *Sleep Medicine*, *95*, 76–83.
95. Moridian, P., Shoeibi, A., Khodatars, M., Jafari, M., Pachori, R. B., Khadem, A., ... & Ling, S. H. (2022). Automatic diagnosis of sleep apnea from biomedical signals using artificial intelligence techniques: Methods, challenges, and future works. *Wiley Interdisciplinary Reviews: Data Mining and Knowledge Discovery*, *12*(6), e1478.
96. Mostafa, S. S., Mendonça, F., G. Ravelo-García, A., & Morgado-Dias, F. (2019). A Systematic Review of Detecting Sleep Apnea Using Deep Learning. *Sensors*, *19*(22), Article 22.
97. Mostafa, S. S., Morgado-Dias, F., & Ravelo-García, A. G. (2020). Comparison of SFS and mRMR for oximetry feature selection in obstructive sleep apnea detection. *Neural Computing and Applications*, *32*(20), 15711–15731.
98. Moturi, S., & Avis, K. (2010). Assessment and treatment of common pediatric sleep disorders. *Psychiatry (Edgmont)*, *7*(6), 24–37.
99. Mousavi, Z., Rezaii, T. Y., Sheykhivand, S., Farzamnia, A., & Razavi, S. N. (2019). Deep convolutional neural network for classification of sleep stages from single-channel EEG signals. *Journal of neuroscience methods*, *324*, 108312.
100. Nutt, D., Wilson, S., & Paterson, L. (2008). Sleep disorders as core symptoms of depression. *Dialogues in Clinical Neuroscience*, *10*(3), 329–336.
101. O'Sullivan, R., Bissell, S., Hamilton, A., Bagshaw, A., & Richards, C. (2023). Concordance of objective and subjective measures of sleep in children with neurodevelopmental conditions: A systematic review and meta-analysis. *Sleep Medicine Reviews*, 101814.
102. Ooms, S., & Ju, Y.-E. (2016). Treatment of Sleep Disorders in Dementia. *Current Treatment Options in Neurology*, *18*(9), 40.
103. Park, S., Lee, S. W., Han, S., & Cha, M. (2019). Clustering Insomnia Patterns by Data From Wearable Devices: Algorithm Development and Validation Study. *JMIR MHealth and UHealth*, *7*(12), e14473.
104. Pavlova, M. K., & Latreille, V. (2019). Sleep disorders. *The American Journal of Medicine*, 132(3), 292–299.
105. Peng, F., Zhang, Z., Gou, X., Liu, H., & Wang, W. (2014). Motion artifact removal from photoplethysmographic signals by combining temporally constrained independent component analysis and adaptive filter. *Biomedical engineering online*, *13*(1), 1–14.

106. Pépin, J. L., Bailly, S., & Tamisier, R. (2020). Big Data in sleep apnoea: Opportunities and challenges. *Respirology*, *25*(5), 486–494.
107. Peppard, P. E., Young, T., Barnet, J. H., Palta, M., Hagen, E. W., & Hla, K. M. (2013). Increased prevalence of sleep-disordered breathing in adults. *American journal of epidemiology*, *177*(9), 1006–1014.
108. Perez-Pozuelo, I., Zhai, B., Palotti, J., Mall, R., Aupetit, M., Garcia-Gomez, J. M., Taheri, S., Guan, Y., & Fernandez-Luque, L. (2020). The future of sleep health: A data-driven revolution in sleep science and medicine. *Npj Digital Medicine*, *3*(1), Article 1.
109. Perlis, M. L., Posner, D., Riemann, D., Bastien, C. H., Teel, J., & Thase, M. (2022). Insomnia. *The Lancet*, *400*(10357), 1047–1060.
110. Phan, H., Chén, O. Y., Tran, M. C., Koch, P., Mertins, A., & De Vos, M. (2021). XSleepNet: Multi-view sequential model for automatic sleep staging. *IEEE Transactions on Pattern Analysis and Machine Intelligence*, *44*(9), 5903–5915.
111. Phelps, A. J., Kanaan, R. A., Worsnop, C., Redston, S., Ralph, N., & Forbes, D. (2018). An ambulatory polysomnography study of the post-traumatic nightmares of post-traumatic stress disorder. *Sleep*, *41*(1), zsx188.
112. Ramachandran, A., & Karuppiah, A. (2021). A Survey on Recent Advances in Machine Learning Based Sleep Apnea Detection Systems. *Healthcare (Basel, Switzerland)*, *9*(7), 914.
113. Ramachandran, A., Pant, A. K., & Karuppiah, A. (2022). Performance Analysis of Machine Learning Algorithms for Sleep Apnea Detection Using ECG. In Y.-D. Zhang, T. Senjyu, C. So-In, & A. Joshi (Eds.), *Smart Trends in Computing and Communications* (pp. 485–493). Springer.
114. Rayan, A., Szabo, A. B., & Genzel, L. (2023). The pros and cons of using automated sleep scoring in sleep research: Comparative analysis of automated sleep scoring in human and rodents: advantages and limitations. *Sleep*, zsad275.
115. Redline, S., & Purcell, S. M. (2021). Sleep and Big Data: harnessing data, technology, and analytics for monitoring sleep and improving diagnostics, prediction, and interventions—an era for Sleep-Omics?. *Sleep*, *44*(6), zsab107.
116. Redmond, S. J., & Heneghan, C. (2006). Cardiorespiratory-based sleep staging in subjects with obstructive sleep apnea. *IEEE Transactions on Biomedical Engineering*, *53*(3), 485–496.
117. Roebuck, A., Monasterio, V., Gederi, E., Osipov, M., Behar, J., Malhotra, A., Penzel, T., & Clifford, G. (2014). A review of signals used in sleep analysis. *Physiological Measurement*, *35*(1), R1–57. doi:https://doi.org/10.1088/0967-3334/35/1/R1
118. Ronzhina, M., Janoušek, O., Kolářová, J., Nováková, M., Honzík, P., & Provazník, I. (2012). Sleep scoring using artificial neural networks. *Sleep medicine reviews*, *16*(3), 251–263.
119. RTSleepWorld. (2020, July 3). Machine Learning in Sleep Medicine: The AI Revolution. *RTSleepWorld*. Retrieved from https://rtsleepworld.com/2020/07/03/machine-learning-in-sleep-medicine-the-ai-revolution/
120. Saba-Sadiya, S., Chantland, E., Alhanai, T., Liu, T., & Ghassemi, M. M. (2021). Unsupervised eeg artifact detection and correction. *Frontiers in Digital Health*, *2*, 608920.
121. Sadeh, A. (2015). III. Sleep assessment methods. *Monographs of the Society for Research in Child Development*, *80*(1), 33–48.
122. Sadiya, S., Alhanai, T., & Ghassemi, M. M. (2021, May). Artifact detection and correction in eeg data: a review. In *2021 10th International IEEE/EMBS Conference on Neural Engineering (NER)* (pp. 495–498). IEEE.
123. Salari, N., Hosseinian-Far, A., Mohammadi, M., Ghasemi, H., Khazaie, H., Daneshkhah, A., & Ahmadi, A. (2022). Detection of sleep apnea using Machine learning algorithms based on ECG Signals: A comprehensive systematic review. *Expert Systems with Applications*, *187*, 115950.
124. Sarker, I. H. (2021). Deep learning: a comprehensive overview on techniques, taxonomy, applications and research directions. *SN Computer Science*, *2*(6), 420.
125. Sateia, M. J. (2014). International classification of sleep disorders. *Chest*, *146*(5), 1387–1394.
126. Scammell, T. E. (2015). Narcolepsy. *New England Journal of Medicine*, *373*(27), 2654–2662.

127. Schaltenbrand, N., Lengelle, R., Toussaint, M., Luthringer, R., Carelli, G., Jacqmin, A., ... & Macher, J. P. (1996). Sleep stage scoring using the neural network model: comparison between visual and automatic analysis in normal subjects and patients. *Sleep*, *19*(1), 26–35.
128. Schindler, T. F., Schlicht, S., & Thoben, K. D. (2023). Towards Benchmarking for Evaluating Machine Learning Methods in Detecting Outliers in Process Datasets. *Computers*, *12*(12), 253.
129. Schlesinger, I., Erikh, I., Avizohar, O., Sprecher, E., & Yarnitsky, D. (2009). Cardiovascular risk factors in restless legs syndrome. *Movement disorders: official journal of the Movement Disorder Society*, *24*(11), 1587–1592.
130. Schoch, S. F., Kurth, S., & Werner, H. (2021). Actigraphy in sleep research with infants and young children: Current practices and future benefits of standardized reporting. *Journal of sleep research*, *30*(3), e13134.
131. Schwichtenberg, A. J., Choe, J., Kellerman, A., Abel, E. A., & Delp, E. J. (2018). Pediatric videosomnography: can signal/video processing distinguish sleep and wake states?. *Frontiers in pediatrics*, *6*, 158.
132. Seth, A., Babu, B. S., & Iyenger, S. S. (2019, December). Machine learning model for predicting insomnia levels in Indian college students. In *2019 4th International Conference on Computational Systems and Information Technology for Sustainable Solution (CSITSS)* (pp. 1–6). IEEE.
133. Shahin, M., Ahmed, B., Hamida, S. T. B., Mulaffer, F. L., Glos, M., & Penzel, T. (2017). Deep learning and insomnia: assisting clinicians with their diagnosis. *IEEE journal of biomedical and health informatics*, *21*(6), 1546–1553.
134. Sikder, M. N. K., & Batarseh, F. A. (2023). Outlier detection using AI: a survey. *AI Assurance*, 231–291.
135. Singh, S., Kaur, H., Singh, S., & Khawaja, I. (2018). Parasomnias: a comprehensive review. *Cureus*, *10*(12).
136. Sitnick, S. L., Goodlin-Jones, B. L., & Anders, T. F. (2008). The use of actigraphy to study sleep disorders in preschoolers: some concerns about detection of nighttime awakenings. *Sleep*, *31*(3), 395.
137. Smith, M. T., McCrae, C. S., Cheung, J., Martin, J. L., Harrod, C. G., Heald, J. L., & Carden, K. A. (2018). Use of actigraphy for the evaluation of sleep disorders and circadian rhythm sleep-wake disorders: an American Academy of Sleep Medicine clinical practice guideline. *Journal of Clinical Sleep Medicine*, *14*(7), 1231–1237.
138. Stephansen, J. B., Olesen, A. N., Olsen, M., Ambati, A., Leary, E. B., Moore, H. E., ... & Mignot, E. (2018). Neural network analysis of sleep stages enables efficient diagnosis of narcolepsy. *Nature communications*, *9*(1), 1–15.
139. Taweesedt, P., Kim, J., Park, J., Park, J., Sharma, M., & Surani, S. (2021). 414 Deep Neural Networks: A Survey Tool for Obstructive Sleep Apnea Prediction. *Sleep*, *44*(Supplement_2), A164.
140. Trotti, L. M., & Bliwise, D. L. (2014). Treatment of the Sleep Disorders Associated with Parkinson's Disease. *Neurotherapeutics*, *11*(1), 68–77. doi:https://doi.org/10.1007/s13311-013-0236-z
141. Urtnasan, E., Joo, E. Y., & Lee, K. H. (2021). Ai-enabled algorithm for automatic classification of sleep disorders based on single-lead electrocardiogram. *Diagnostics*, *11*(11), 2054.
142. Van Steenkiste, T., Groenendaal, W., Deschrijver, D., & Dhaene, T. (2018). Automated sleep apnea detection in raw respiratory signals using long short-term memory neural networks. *IEEE journal of biomedical and health informatics*, *23*(6), 2354–2364.
143. Watson, N. F., & Fernandez, C. R. (2021). Artificial intelligence and sleep: advancing sleep medicine. *Sleep Medicine Reviews*, *59*, 101512.
144. Xu, S., Faust, O., Silvia, S., Chakraborty, S., Barua, P. D., Loh, H. W., ... & Acharya, U. R. (2022). A review of automated sleep disorder detection. *Computers in Biology and Medicine*, 106100.

145. Yoo, C., Lee, H. W., & Kang, J. W. (2021). Transferring structured knowledge in unsupervised domain adaptation of a sleep staging network. *IEEE Journal of Biomedical and Health Informatics*, *26*(3), 1273–1284.
146. Zhang, C., Yu, W., Li, Y., Sun, H., Zhang, Y., & De Vos, M. (2022). CMS2-Net: Semi-Supervised Sleep Staging for Diverse Obstructive Sleep Apnea Severity. *IEEE Journal of Biomedical and Health Informatics*, *26*(7), 3447–3457.
147. Zhang, J., & Wu, Y. (2018). Complex-valued unsupervised convolutional neural networks for sleep stage classification. *Computer methods and programs in biomedicine*, *164*, 181–191.
148. Zhang, J., Zhang, Q., Wang, Y., & Qiu, C. (2013, April). A real-time auto-adjustable smart pillow system for sleep apnea detection and treatment. In *Proceedings of the 12th international conference on Information processing in sensor networks* (pp. 179–190).
149. Zhao, A., Dong, J., & Zhou, H. (2020). Self-supervised learning from multi-sensor data for sleep recognition. *IEEE Access*, *8*, 93907–93921.
150. Zhao, R., Xia, Y., & Zhang, Y. (2021). Unsupervised sleep staging system based on domain adaptation. *Biomedical Signal Processing and Control*, *69*, 102937.
151. Zhou, P., Huang, L., Zhao, Q., Xiao, W., & Li, S. (2019). A domestic diagnosis system for early restless legs syndrome based on deep learning. *Chinese Journal of Medical Instrumentation*, *43*(2), 79–82.

Polysomnography Raw Data Extraction, Exploration, and Preprocessing

Malak A. Almarshad, Saiful Islam, Sultan Bahammam, Saad Al-Ahmadi, and Ahmed S. BaHammam

1 Introduction

Polysomnography (PSG) remains the fundamental diagnostic testing in sleep medicine and results in vast amounts of raw data, which is well suited for analysis with data science (DS) means. Furthermore, scoring and understanding PSG requires a high level of expertise and training, which might be fulfilled with advanced artificial intelligence (AI) methods. AI is able to explore, recognize patterns, and derive optimized conclusions from big data within a remarkably short time.

M. A. Almarshad
Computer Science Department, College of Computer and Information Sciences, Al-Imam Mohammad Ibn Saud Islamic University, Riyadh, Saudi Arabia

Computer Science Department, College of Computer and Information Sciences, King Saud University, Riyadh, Saudi Arabia
e-mail: malakalmarshad@gmail.com

S. Islam
Department of Computer Engineering, TED University, Ankara, Türkiye
e-mail: saiful.islam@tedu.edu.tr

S. Bahammam · S. Al-Ahmadi
The University Sleep Disorders Center, Department of Medicine, College of Medicine, King Saud University, Riyadh, Saudi Arabia

A. S. BaHammam (✉)
The University Sleep Disorders Center, Department of Medicine, College of Medicine, King Saud University, Riyadh, Saudi Arabia

Strategic Technologies Program of the National Plan for Sciences and Technology and Innovation in the Kingdom of Saudi Arabia, Riyadh, Saudi Arabia
e-mail: ashammam2@gmail.com

R. B. Berry et al. (eds.), *Handbook of AI and Data Sciences for Sleep Disorders*,
Springer Optimization and Its Applications 216,
https://doi.org/10.1007/978-3-031-68263-6_2

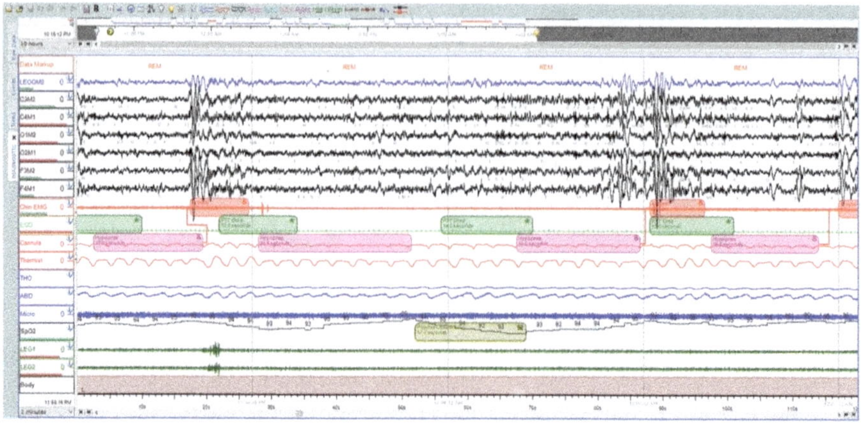

Fig. 1 Polysomnographic recording, scored manually by a professional technician at the University Sleep Disorders Center, at King Saud University Medical City, showing some different obstructive respiratory events, within 2 minutes time window

PSG is the gold-standard diagnostic test for sleep disorders, including sleep-related breathing disorders, such as obstructive sleep apnea (OSA), central disorders of hypersomnolence, unusual behaviors during sleep, and unexplained long-lasting insomnia. PSG contains multiple signals, including eye movements, brain and muscle activity, respiratory effort and airflow, blood oxygen saturation, carbon dioxide, body positioning and movements, snoring, and heart rate [1]. Recorded PSG is scored by a sleep physician or a qualified sleep technologist. Until today, the standard scoring process is done manually, which takes about 4 hours for each patient (Fig. 1).

Laboratory PSG is expensive, with long waiting lists, and needs time and high levels of expertise to score sleep studies; promoting alternative sleep disorders evaluation methods, such as home sleep apnea test (HSAT), which is a limited-channel portable sleep study that is less accurate than laboratory PSG. Medicare [2] approved using HSAT devices with at least three signals. The American Academy of Sleep Medicine (AASM) also approved type III portable sleep study to diagnose patients with a high likelihood of moderate to severe OSA [3].

As scoring sleep studies are time-consuming, a few PSG scoring solutions have evolved over the last 10 years. In practice, Somnolyzer [4] from Philips is the only ready-to-use product. However, there is no available information on how it works or its underlying algorithm.

Furthermore, validating the performance of an automated PSG scoring system is still a work in progress. Nevertheless, manual scoring is still needed [5], and the American Academy of Sleep Medicine still recommends manual scoring for sleep studies [3]. Multiple types of research have been done to resolve PSG, statistical analysis, signal processing, machine learning (ML), and deep learning (DL) methods [6]. It is crucial to preprocess PSG data correctly, as they contain various forms of input signals, which can affect its quality. Preprocessing data is an essential step in any ML workflow, as raw data can be inconsistent, incomplete,

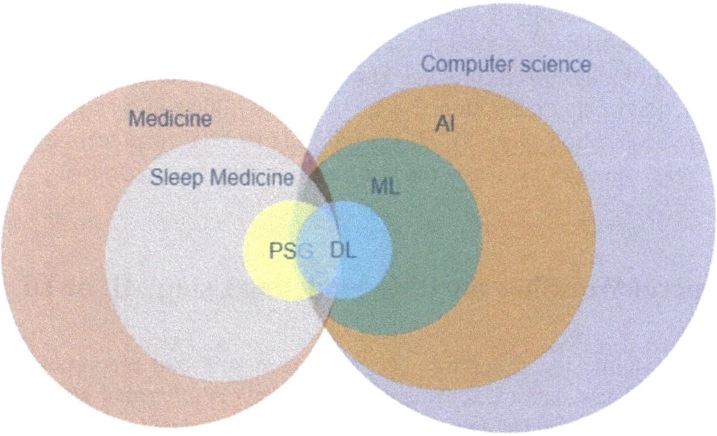

Fig. 2 Polysomnography (PSG) modeling position among other related disciplines

and contain noise. Effectively preprocessing PSG data can enhance the overall ML model accuracy, which increases its reliability in analyzing different sleep disorders.

ML is a specific subfield of AI that aims at automatically learning from data; it was only started in the field of PSG in 2011 [7] (Fig. 2). Examples of popular ML models used in PSG datasets are regression, decision tree, and support vector machine (SVM) [6]. DL is an ML modeling taken to the next level. DL is one of many ML branches that mimic the human brain's learning process. It is a generalized mapping function between a set of inputs and outputs that can be utilized for future observations. Typically, when the term deep learning is used, it refers to deep artificial neural networks (ANN). DL effectively teaches computers to do what humans naturally do; learning by example. In addition, DL performs well on large datasets, compared to ML, such as PSG datasets.

Four different DL models, including PSG, were used widely for time series data, namely, multilayer perceptron (MLP), convolutional neural networks (CNN), recurrent neural network (RNN), and long short-term memory (LSTM) [8–10]. Features in DL are learned during the training process and not handcrafted; this is a big advantage over traditional machine learning algorithms [11].

PSG data is treated as time series data that is recorded over consistent intervals of time. New ML and DL models are usually applied and tested first over natural language processing (NLP) data and then digital image processing (DIP). Finally, the tide is slowly turning to time series classification (TSC).

This chapter explores the most common preprocessing steps for PSG signals. Taking into account that we can execute the ones that suit the problem definition and the nature of the raw data we are dealing with. It is not mandatory to follow these steps in order, but one may take these steps as a general guide that one can start from, though it is likely that one needs to modify them slightly to suit the used PSG dataset and aid in finding what is looked for.

The rest of this chapter is organized as follows: First, we will give an overview of the general workflow of PSG modeling (Sect. 2), and then the first steps of the workflow will be discussed in detail, starting from problem formulation (Sect. 3). After that, PSG dataset curation (Sect. 4) will be followed by data exploration, including visualization (Sect. 5). This is followed by PSG preprocessing, including data cleaning and transformation (Sect. 6), and finally, the conclusion.

2 General Workflow for PSG Modeling Using ML or DL

First, let us define the difference between processing and preprocessing in the context of PSG raw data [12]. Processing PSG data is the actual analysis of PSG signals through ML or DL techniques. PSG preprocessing includes all the steps required to prepare the PSG data for actual analysis. Preprocessing tends to be tedious and time-consuming, there is no standard pipeline for it, and one might need to do it iteratively. This chapter covers the preprocessing part, the first four steps of the general workflow of PSG modeling.

In general, the workflow for PSG modeling using ML or DL is as the following [13] (Fig. 3):

1. *Define the problem:* What is needed to be achieved? What data is available, and what should be estimated? Is the available data labeled or not?
2. *Collect raw data:* Do data need to be collected from the ground up or is it enough to use already available datasets?
3. *Data exploration:* This step is one of the first steps of data analysis utilized to identify patterns and visualize data.

Fig. 3 The workflow of PSG modeling using ML or DL

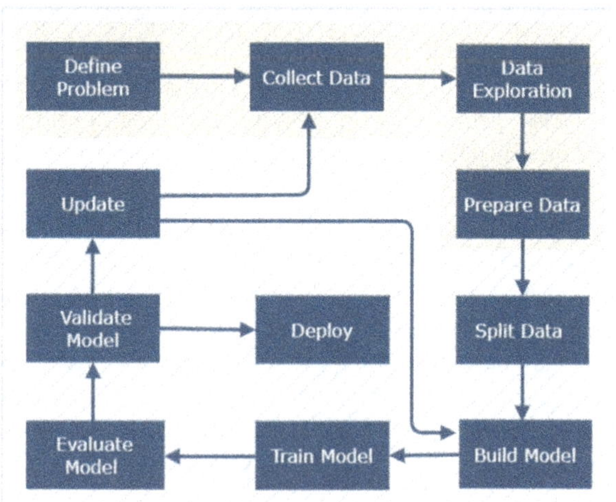

4. *Prepare raw PSG data:* Various processing methods to yield a polished dataset that can be fed to an ML model.
5. *Build a model:* The actual analysis process to solve the problem and deliver a solution.
6. *Split data into three sets (train, validation, and test):* This step aims to train the dataset used for model learning, validation set for unbiased model evaluation, and test set for final model evaluation.
7. *Train the model:* The actual learning process utilized on the training partition of the dataset.
8. *Evaluate the model:* Using the test partition of the dataset to select the single best model for the problem at hand.
9. *Validate and tune the model:* Performed on the validation partition of the dataset.
10. *Deploy the model:* Deploying the ML model in production.
11. *Maintain:* Keeping the model and the data updated.

3 Problem Formulation

ML and DL models can provide robust solutions to a wide range of time series data problems, including biosignals such as PSG, especially areas involving classification, prediction, filtering, regression, pattern recognition, and anomaly detection. Before diving deep into the model building or other phases within an ML or DL project lifecycle, it is sensible to identify the problem clearly and propose a solution plan systematically. The first significant step in any ML or DL project is defining the problem (Fig. 1).

A problem definition is a clear statement describing the initial status of an issue to be solved. In addition, it discusses problem characteristics, overall methodological approach, solution objectives, and the main expected contribution to the field.

In general, ML problems fall under two categories supervised and unsupervised learning, depending on the data available and the nature of the problem to be solved [14]. In a supervised learning problem, there is a ground truth the model needs to learn. This ground truth is a labeled dataset, which might be a label from a set of predefined discrete classes (classification) or a value in a continuous domain (regression) [15]. On the other hand, unsupervised learning tries to discover patterns from an unlabeled dataset, for example, clustering.

The majority of models in the literature on PSG are considered supervised learning. The following are a few examples of different sleep disorders problems that have been addressed using AI, ML, and DL:

3.1 Supervised Learning

Classification:

- Classification of OSA episodes [16, 17]
- Sleep staging [10]

Regression:

- Predicting apnea-hypopnea index (AHI) and oxygen desaturation index (ODI) [18]
- Age estimation [19]

3.2 Unsupervised Learning

Clustering:

- Patient's phenotype clustering [20]

4 PSG Dataset Curation

Data curation is the process of collecting and organizing a dataset to meet the needs of a specific task. Collecting raw data, as it is, is only the beginning. However, making these data useful for a particular model is a critical part of the curation. Data quality highly determines the model's quality [21].

The best way to learn about something is to build it from the ground up. Building a PSG dataset is not easy, although it allows for gaining valuable knowledge, experience, and better insight through the data. PSG channels must be scored by qualified professional technicians who are trained and regularly evaluated by inter-scorer reliability [22]. In addition, as many records as time and resources allow should be collected. Ideally, the dataset has to contain a maximum number of PSG channels.

4.1 Collect the Right Kind of Data

To build ML or DL model that achieves a specific goal, we need the right kind of data that the model can learn from. For example, if the goal is to classify PSG into sleep stages, we need EEG channels from raw PSG recordings labeled with the five sleep stages Wake, N1, N2, N3, and REM [23]. Another example is if the target output is predicting oxygen desaturation index (ODI), then SpO_2 channels for multiple patients are needed; each of them has a different ODI value [24, 25]. However, personal data such as the name of the patients are useless for this task. However, sometimes, it will not be known in ML with 100% confidence what type of raw data will be relevant. It is expected to refine data as the process goes on.

Additionally, PSG data need to be accurate. Therefore, expecting a great model trained on inaccurate PSG data is unfair. Nonetheless, there should be no worry about PSG accuracy if recorded in regular clinical practice, as sleep technologists are mainly responsible for maintaining the integrity of PSG recording [26].

But how much PSG data are needed for ML or DL tasks? There is no single correct answer to this question; it really depends on the type of model to be built. DL models crave for data more than ML models. And it is always a great idea to have as many relevant and reliable samples as possible to receive accurate results.

Moreover, what happens if enough data cannot be obtained? If there are not enough labeled data, great results can be achieved by applying a pre-trained model that is already trained in another similar dataset [27]. Also, the amount of data can be increased by adding slightly modified or shuffled versions of the existing dataset, which is called data augmentation [28].

An imbalanced dataset is where samples on classes are not represented equally or do not reflect the natural distribution of the population. Imbalanced data may result in a biased model with undesirable consequences [13]. For example, the data are imbalanced concerning the number of patients for each sleep disorder. Due to this, for identifying the type of sleep disorder, the model becomes biased toward one type of sleep disorder [29]. This concern is common in a medical dataset, generating models that are biased toward correctly diagnosing a patient as a patient but also mistakenly diagnosing a normal individual as a patient [30].

There are multiple solutions to overcome the imbalanced dataset problem besides collecting more data. The simplest method to balance the dataset is by oversampling the minority class or undersampling the majority class [31]. This can be achieved by choosing shorter epochs [32]. Another way is data augmentation [33]. In addition, choosing different performance metrics, rather than relying on model accuracy, precision, recall, or $F1$ score, may provide fair insight into model performance.

4.2 *Ethical Considerations*

Before building a new dataset using participants from a health institute, it is mandatory to obtain Institutional Review Board (IRB) approval in order to protect participants' interests. In addition, it is mandatory to ensure that patients' private data are completely anonymized or de-identified. Patient consent is not generally necessary after proper anonymization [34]. All patients' private information shall be removed from the study, including patient name, file number, ID, and contact numbers. Also, doctors' and technicians' names need to be removed. Collecting annotated PSG signals is typically enough for this type of study.

4.3 Public Datasets

While some researchers prefer to build their datasets from scratch, many prefer benchmark datasets. Three datasets have been used widely in the literature, namely, St. Vincent's University Hospital/University College Dublin sleep apnea database [35], MIT-BIH polysomnographic database [36], and SRUC-Sleep [37]. In addition, a few other publicly available datasets have physiological signals that can be used for analysis; these include the "PhysioNet," a large collection of physiologic signals that are captured and made available online for free [38]. Additionally, the "National Sleep Research Resource" (NSRR) is a new "National Heart, Lung, and Blood Institute" ad hoc website designed with a single point of access to provide the community of sleep researchers with access to enormous amounts of data (NSRR; R24HL114473) [39]. On the NSRR's free and public web platform, de-identified data for more than 35,000 patients (at the time of writing) associated with sleep medicine are available from 22 US-based datasets. These data include PSGs and links to risk factors and outcome data for research participants [40]. Additionally, the "MrOS dataset" on NSRR (a supporting investigation of the primary study, Osteoporotic Fractures in Men)—whose main focus is PSG data—and the "Multi-Ethnic Study of Atherosclerosis (MESA Sleep)"—which included a sleep questionnaire, actigraphy, and a full overnight unattended PSG—as well as data combining from separate research groups like the "Wisconsin Sleep Cohort"—are both important [38, 41].

Dataset is a crucial part of any successful deep learning model. Many challenges are facing open data in medical research. Evidence-based medical research relies heavily on the availability of sufficient raw data in terms of quantity and quality. In addition, there are patient confidentiality concerns, organizational structures, and legal challenges. The three most used PSG datasets are more than a decade old. Since then, a lot of sleep study standards' practices have changed.

Public datasets can be used as a good starting point for building more tailored solutions, giving a chance to be compared to others' work. A PSG dataset with valid features and labeling is a critical solution for the success of the ML model.

4.4 Digital Specifications for PSG Recordings

PSG is a sequence of multiple simultaneous signals collected in successive order over a period of time. A full PSG is the standard manner to diagnose several sleep disorders accurately. The AASM guidelines for PSG performance include the following [42]:

1. EEG and chin electromyogram (EMG) for sleep staging
2. ECG for heart rate
3. Electromyogram (EMG) for chin and leg movements
4. Thermal airflow sensors and a nasal pressure transducer to monitor breathing
5. PPG for oxygen saturation [43]

Table 1 PSG channels' sampling rates

Signal	Desirable (Hz)	Minimal (Hz)
EEG, EOG, EMG, ECG, snoring sound	500	200
Airflow, nasal pressure, end-tidal PCO_2, PAP device flow, esophageal pressure, rib cage, and abdominal movements	100	25
Oximetry, transcutaneous PCO_2N_8	25	10
Body position	1	1

Note: Adapted from Berry et al. [42] Copyright © 2018 American Academy of Sleep Medicine

4.4.1 Sampling Rates

It is recommended to collect PSG data starting from the AASM guidelines [42]. Recommended minimum analog-to-digital resolution is 12 bits per sample. Sampling rates are given in (Table 1) adapted from [42].

4.4.2 Minimum and Maximum Frequency Filters

When looking at the frequencies of a digital biosignal, EEG, ECG, or PSG, a common thing to do is to filter specific frequencies, either by removing some frequencies band or possibly keeping some filters. Raw PSG signal is commonly contaminated with noise that might affect the model performance. Though it may be assumed to think of noise as discrete elements, noise is a part of every waveform. Some types of noise components are relatively isolated to a distinctive frequency range. The employment of filters can mitigate this issue. There are several types of filters. It is recommended to start exporting raw PSG with the routine low- and high-pass filter settings by the AASM [42]. Low- and high-pass filters are the two main types [8].

Low-pass (high-cut) filter It is a filter that passes low frequencies and attenuates the high ones. The main goal of a low-pass filter is to smooth or denoise the signal. For example, a low-pass filter can partially reduce motion artifacts from the PPG signal [44].

High-pass filter (low-cut) filter Does the opposite of the above, only allowing through frequencies above the cut-off value. The main application of high-frequency filters is to detect the edge amplitude.

Other less commonly used filters are:

Bandpass filter Frequencies within a specific range are passed, and other frequencies are rejected. The opposite is a band-stop filter, which rejects all frequencies in a specific range.

Table 2 Routinely recorded filter settings by AASM

Channel type	Low-frequency filter	High-frequency filter
EEG	0.3 Hz	35 Hz
EOG	0.3 Hz	35 Hz
EMG	10 Hz	100 Hz
ECG	0.3 Hz	70 Hz
Oronasal thermal flow, thoracoabdominal belt signals	0.1 Hz	15 Hz
Nasal pressure	Direct current (DC) or $\leq$0.03 Hz	100 Hz
PAP device flow	DC	DC
Snoring	10 Hz	100 Hz

Note: Adapted from Berry et al. [42] Copyright © 2018 American Academy of Sleep Medicine

Notch filter this is a special band-stop filter that rejects a single frequency rather than a whole bandwidth of different frequencies. It is also possible to combine multiple notch filters, to remove a particular set of single frequencies, which helps remove electricity noise [8]. Details of the digital and filter settings that are recommended for routine PSG recording are listed in Table 2 [42].

5 Data Exploration

Data exploration enhances a deeper understanding of raw PSG datasets. By getting to know PSG data better, data analysis becomes more efficient. Data exploration is performed before, during, and after data analysis; it describes dataset characterizations, such as size, quantity, and accuracy, for a better abstract human understanding through visualization and statistical techniques.

5.1 PSG Visualization

Time series visualization is a rich field of study on its own. A fundamental part of a data scientist's toolkit is data visualization. Although it is pretty easy to create visualizations, producing publication-quality ones is more complicated. In PSG data visualization, using different graphs and plots makes discovering data patterns easier. It even helps to get some insights and a deeper understanding of raw PSG data before the modeling begins.

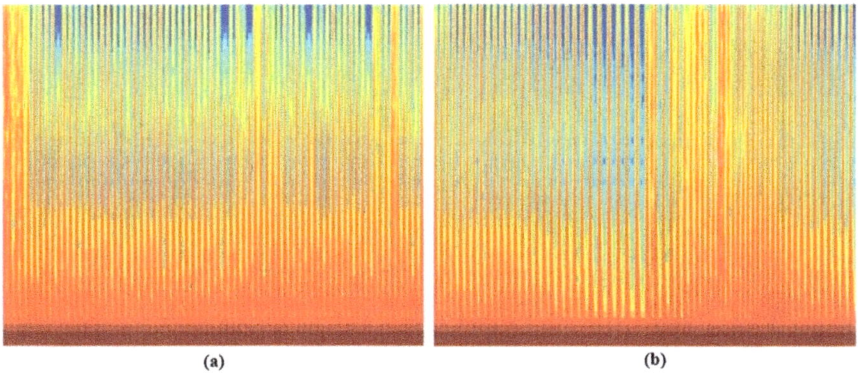

Fig. 4 One-minute ECG segments transformed into Spectrogram to detect OSA: (**a**) Spectrogram of normal ECG segment, (**b**) Spectrogram of an apnea ECG segment. (Note. Adapted from Niroshana et al. [48], Fig. 4. (CC BY 4.0))

5.1.1 Waveform Representation (Time-Domain)

It is the signal's shape over time, showing a temporal representation of the signal's amplitude. It is the most intuitive visualization of signal variations. It can be zoomed in or out to get information about a specific epoch or over a specific time.

5.1.2 Spectrum Representation (Frequency-Domain)

The signal spectrum represents a signal's magnitude and phase characteristics as a function of frequency. One of the primary motivations for using a frequency-domain representation of a signal is to simplify the mathematical analysis. We need the power spectral density (PSD) for frequency-domain analysis [45]. PSD function is useful for knowing the frequencies and amplitudes of PSG signals in a dataset [46]. In addition, the PSD demonstrates the strength of energy as a function of frequency.

5.1.3 Transforming PSG Signal into Image (Both Time and Frequency)

Spectrogram and scalogram are three-dimensional space (3D) views of a signal compromise between time-based and frequency-based representations of a signal.

Spectrogram is a representation of the short-time Fourier transform (STFT) sliding along the signal. Transforming PSG signals to spectrograms is used to distinguish between normal and patients with OSA (Fig. 4) [47, 48].

Scalogram is a scaled representation of a continuous wavelet transformation (CWT) performed on the signal. For example, a model trained on ECG scalograms to extract deep features for OSA detection (Fig. 5) [48, 49].

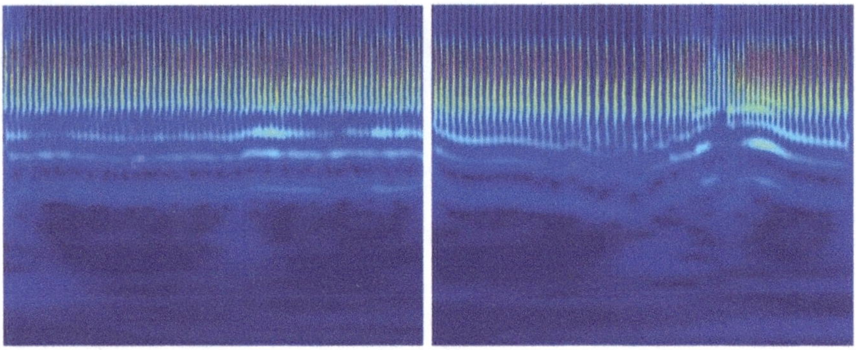

(a) (b)

Fig. 5 One minute ECG segments transformed into Scalogram to detect OSA: (**a**) Scalogram image of normal ECG segment, (**b**) Scalogram image of an apnea ECG segment. (Note. Adapted from Niroshana et al. [48], Fig. 4. (CC BY 4.0))

Whether we describe a phenomenon in the time domain, frequency domain, or both, we describe the same signal's physical nature. Nevertheless, proper choice of description improves our understanding, and modeling outcomes. Transforming a signal into these two representations can be used in applying state-of-the-art image modeling, such as CNN.

6 PSG Preprocessing

It is impossible to cover all feasible sorts of preprocessing, though we will address the most important ones, which are generally used in dealing with time series data, specifically PSG. The primary goal of preprocessing is to remove variations that came from shaping the PSG samples.

What Is PSG Preprocessing?
Generally, preprocessing transforms raw data into a digestible shape that a machine learning model can consume and process efficiently. In the case of PSG data, preprocessing usually refers to removing noise from the data to get closer to the true signals' origins. It transforms raw data into a highly concentrated form to serve a specific task. In practice, preprocessing consumes up to 80% of the project time.

Why Is Preprocessing Needed?
There are several reasons why preprocessing is necessary for PSG data. First, the signals picked up from different body parts are not necessarily an exact representation of the pure signal origin. Second, PSG data tends to contain a lot of noise and artifacts, such as blinking or movement, that distort the signal. Finally,

we need to separate the relevant PSG signals from random noise that might occur during sleep recording.

How Much Preprocessing Is Needed for PSG?
At first, it seems the more preprocessing of data, the better results obtained. On the contrary, overdoing preprocessing might even harm the model results. Researchers have some freedom in choosing how to transform PSG raw data, and no standard adopted PSG preprocessing pipeline exists. However, most successful deep learning-based PSG diagnosing models require a minimum amount of preprocessing [50], while machine learning-based PSG diagnosing models tend to demand heavier preprocessing.

Finally, no matter how good the preprocessing is or how much time is spent doing it, it will not be able to account for bad data, and it will comply with the garbage in and garbage out principle [11].

6.1 *Data Cleaning*

PSG cleaning is the process of repairing or removing incorrect, corrupted, poorly formatted, redundant, mislabeled, or incomplete data within a dataset. It includes picking the right samples from the population, choosing good channels, detecting outliers, and dealing with different types of artifacts and missing values.

6.1.1 Population Selection

Before obtaining PSG raw data, researchers shall specify their protocols and provide a complete description of the study population, namely, covering the targeted population, sample size, and inclusion and exclusion criteria for participation in a study. Inclusion criteria are the features patients must have to be included in the study. Exclusion criteria are features that disqualify patients from inclusion in the study. Inclusion and exclusion criteria may include metadata such as age, gender, race, type, and severity of sleep disorder. An example of inclusion criteria for a study of sleep apnea detection might be the diagnostic part of an overnight sleep study for adults above 16 years who have been diagnosed with OSA with no comorbidities. An example of exclusion criteria for the same research is patients who have done a CPAP titration study.

6.1.2 Channel Selection

The typical PSG has a minimum of 11 channels attached to different body parts. Furthermore, all of them are recorded for approximately 8 hours of sleep. This generates a tremendous amount of data. With a large number of acquired PSG channels, it has become apparent that efficient channel selection is required.

The fundamental reasons for effective channel selection at the beginning of PSG preprocessing are to decrease overall computational complexity, minimize the chance of overfitting that may arise from the use of unnecessary PSG channels, and reduce configuration time.

It is always better to start from the original clinically used channels to evaluate such a specific goal. For example, most sleep staging using machine learning and deep learning literature rely solely on EEG channels and discards the rest of the PSG recording.

Channel selection includes removing bad channels that do not provide accurate information. It is essential to remove malfunctioning channels early before doing further analysis [51, 52]. The channel might be defective for some reasons, such as improper placement, poor skin contact, or saturated electrode. Visualizing raw PSG data can help detect bad channels even before completing data collection. A bad channel usually appears as a flat line or significantly more fluctuated than others. Removing a lot of bad channels from raw data is not the ultimate solution, especially if we do not have many channels. It might be necessary to redo the experiment or repair the bad parts of the channel by filling in the missing values using other similar ones [53, 54].

6.1.3 Outlier Detection

Outliers are those PSG recordings that differ strongly in multiple aspects from the other PSG recordings in a population. Before determining the outliers, it is important to understand the source of outliers. There are various reasons why there can be outliers in the dataset, like human errors, for example, a dummy PSG study that was created for system maintenance and sampling errors, like including a pediatric sample in adult research. Detecting and removing these outliers is vital for learning a robust and generalizable machine learning model [50].

6.1.4 Artifact Rejection

Finding an appropriate approach for artifact rejection is not as simple as it might seem. Every system, every experiment, and every subject will vary in number, magnitude, and type of artifacts. Furthermore, some researchers might be okay with just rejecting trials with any artifacts, while some only if certain events like eye blinks come before a stimulus. In contrast, others might want to correct movement artifacts by using an independent component analysis (ICA) approach [44]. ICA is the process that breaks up a mixture of signals into their distinct sources [55].

Furthermore, some artifacts, like spikes, might be easy to detect because of their signal properties, while others might be much harder to detect. For these reasons, visual inspection of the raw data is important. Full automatic artifact rejection is warranted in rare cases of very typical and well-described artifacts. Early manual inspection of raw data gives a certain sense of data quality.

6.1.5 Dealing with Missing Values

In reality, missing values in a dataset is a widespread phenomenon. Many datasets arrive with missing data, either because it exists and was not collected or never existed. We cannot simply ignore missing data; few ML models will fail if the dataset contains missing values. However, the resulting machine learning model could be biased if missing records are not appropriately handled. Missing records can appear as (NA, null, 0, or NaN) in a database. There are two methods to deal with missing values: The first is simply dropping observations that have missing values. The second option is filing missing values based on other similar observations. If any of the PSG epochs contains a null value or a missing segment, the common practice is to remove it from the PSG dataset [49, 51].

6.2 Data Transformation

Data transformation is the process of converting the shape and structure of raw data into a functional format that can be explored in the ML model. This involves the normalization and aggregation of data according to the needs of the data set.

In the following section, multiple data transformation techniques are discussed.

6.2.1 Dimensionality Reduction

Having more data definitely improves the models' accuracy, but there comes a stage where more data can cause model overfitting. Excessive data can be costly in terms of storage and model efficiency. Dimensionality can be reduced by feature selection or reduction algorithms. Reducing dimensionality speeds up training, but it does cause some data loss, which might lead to slightly worse model performance, and that depends on the dataset. However, dimensionality reduction helps facilitate data visualization. Principal component analysis (PCA) is by far the most popular dimensionality reduction algorithm [50]. In simple words, it projects the data onto the closest hyperplane. PCA shows the ability to detect anomalies in a highly correlated dataset after applying machine learning models [56].

6.2.2 Categorical Variable Transformations

Most ML models can only handle numeric variables. Hence, categorical data has to be transformed into numeric form before applying any ML model. There are multiple methods for categorical data transforming, such as one hot encoding and label encoding. Figure 6 shows a dataset snippet where categorical data are transformed using binary encoding.

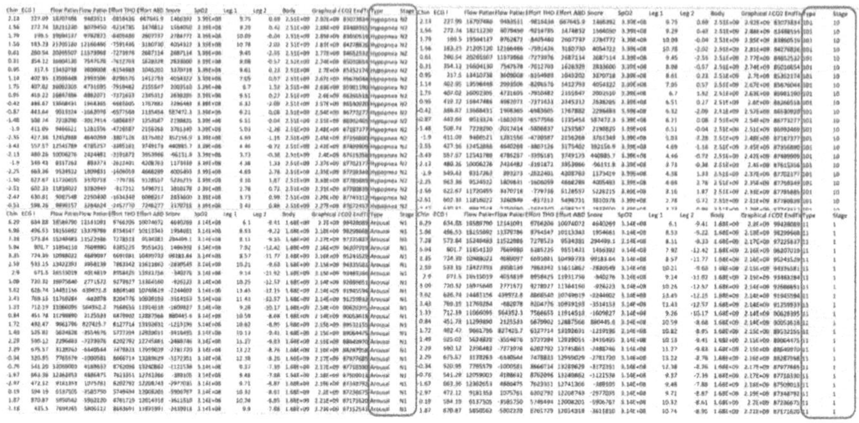

Fig. 6 A random snippet from a PSG dataset, where binary encoding was applied for PSG labels. Arousal and hypopnea are encoded as 110 and 10, respectively. Sleep stages, wake, N1, N2, N3, and REM are encoded to 00, 10, 01, 11, and 001, respectively

6.2.3 Normalization

PSG data normalization is transforming raw data into one uniform scale. Within a PSG recording, there is often a large difference between the maximum and minimum values for different channels, for example, the SpO_2 value can be up to 100, while ECG is between 0.5×10^{-6} and 1×10^{-6}. Normalization magnitudes these values into one unified scale, for example, between 0 and 1. This step is essential for many ML models like the k-nearest neighborhood and SVM and also for deep learning in general. It boosts model training performance and stability.

The two most common normalization methods are [12]:

Min-max normalization Rescales the data set such that all sample values are between 0 and 1, as seen in (1).

$$x' = \frac{x - \min(x)}{\max(x) - \min(x)} \tag{1}$$

Figure 7 abstracts the effect of min-max normalization on PSG data.

Z-Normalization (Standardization) For each PSG channel, the mean and standard deviation are calculated. Then the mean is subtracted from each channel. Subsequently, the result is divided by channels' standard deviation, as in (2).

$$x' = \frac{\mathrm{x} - \mathrm{x}'}{\sigma} \tag{2}$$

Standardization makes the algorithm less sensitive to outliers (noise) in contrast to min-max scaling.

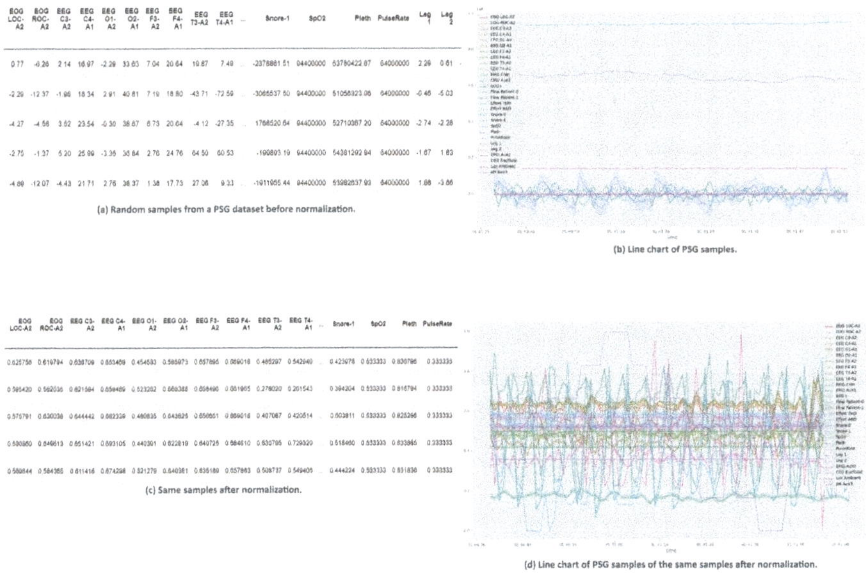

Fig. 7 The effect of Min-max normalization on PSG samples and visualization: (**a**) is a random snippet from a PSG dataset before Min-max normalization, (**b**) the line chart of the same snippet, (**c**) the same set of samples after min-max normalization, and (**d**) shows that all channels are on the same scale

6.2.4 Downsampling

Downsampling or downscaling is the process of reducing PSG signal resolution by selecting a subset from the collected dataset. First, raw PSG data collection should be started according to the AASM sampling rate. Later, experimenting with downsampling can be done, given that PSG raw data are originally high-resolution data. Downsampling can escalate the model speed and makes data visualization easier. Figure 8 displays the same PSG segment before and after downsampling.

6.2.5 Partitioning and Segmentation

Time series segmentation is a process of partitioning continuous time series by dividing them into a sequence of discrete segments. The PSG segmentation problem can be described as, given a continuous PSG raw data *T*, producing the best model results using specific *K* segments from *N* samples. The most common time series segmentation algorithms categories are sliding windows (rolling window), top-down, and bottom-up [57]. Sliding windows is the only type used so far in the PSG literature. The sliding window can be overlapping or non-overlapping, and the window length can be fixed or variable [58].

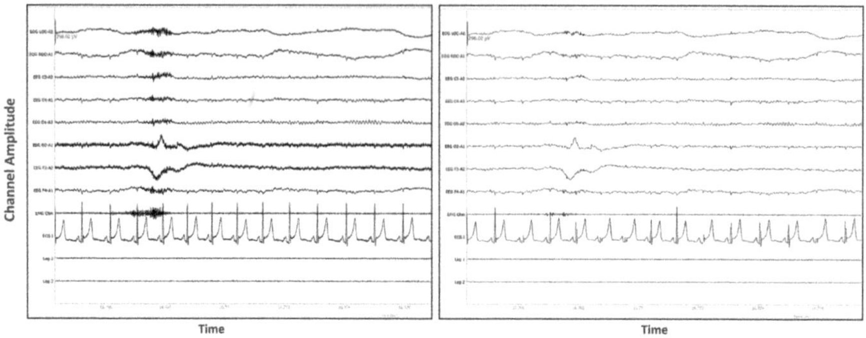

Fig. 8 Same PSG segment with different sampling rates. The original segment on the left, the segment with a reduced sampling rate to the right

7 Conclusion

Proper data preprocessing is essential for the efficient performance of learning algorithms. Machine learning algorithms have proven their ability to extract valuable knowledge from raw PSG data. Unfortunately, their success usually depends on the quality of the PSG data they operate on. Prior preprocessing is necessary to resolve several problems, including noisy channels, redundancy, and missing segments. All ML models rely heavily on the product of this stage, which is the final training set. To achieve the best model performance that serves a specific task, multiple steps are required, including having a clear problem statement, gaining access to a dataset with a sufficient number of samples, and exploring and visualizing the data from multiple perspectives. Finally, it should be noted that even the best preprocessing practices cannot account for insufficient data.

References

1. R. Gupta, Pandi-Perumal, and A. S. BaHammam, *Clinical Atlas of Polysomnography*, 1st Editio. Apple Academic Press, 2018.
2. Carmel Armon, "What are the Medicare guidelines for the use of home-based, limited-channel polysomnography?," 2020. https://www.medscape.com/answers/1188764-193034/what-are-the-medicare-guidelines-for-the-use-of-home-based-limitedchannel-polysomnography-psg
3. I. M. Rosen *et al.*, "Clinical use of a home sleep apnea test: An updated American academy of sleep medicine position statement," *J. Clin. Sleep Med.*, vol. 14, no. 12, pp. 2075–2077, 2018, https://doi.org/10.5664/jcsm.7540.
4. Philips., "Sleepware G3 with integrated Somnolyzer Scoring." https://www.usa.philips.com/healthcare/product/HC1082462/sleepware-g3-sleep-diagnostic-software
5. A. Malhotra, M. Younes, S. T. Kuna, and M. Ruth Benca, MD5; Clete A. Kushida, MD6; James Walsh, PhD7; Alexandra Hanlon3; Bethany Staley3; Allan I. Pack, MD, PhD3; Grace W. Pien, "Performance of an Automated Polysomnography Scoring System Versus Computer-Assisted Manual Scoring," *Sleep*, vol. 388. pp. 539–547, 2013.

6. D. Ferreira-Santos, P. Amorim, T. Silva Martins, M. Monteiro-Soares, and P. Pereira Rodrigues, "Helping early obstructive sleep apnea diagnosis with machine learning: A systematic review (Preprint)," *J. Med. Internet Res.*, vol. 24, pp. 1–23, 2022, https://doi.org/10.2196/39452.
7. M. E. Tagluk and N. Sezgin, "A new approach for estimation of obstructive sleep apnea syndrome," *Expert Syst. Appl.*, vol. 38, no. 5, pp. 5346–5351, 2011, https://doi.org/10.1016/j.eswa.2010.10.022.
8. S. S. Mostafa, F. Mendonça, A. G. Ravelo-García, and F. Morgado-Dias, "A systematic review of detecting sleep apnea using deep learning," *Sensors (Switzerland)*, vol. 19, no. 22, pp. 1–27, 2019, https://doi.org/10.3390/s19224934.
9. C. Sun, S. Hong, J. Wang, X. Dong, F. Han, and H. Li, "A systematic review of deep learning methods for modeling electrocardiograms during sleep," *Physiol. Meas.*, vol. 43, no. 8, 2022, https://doi.org/10.1088/1361-6579/ac826e.
10. T. R. Sri, A. Ravi Raja, J. Madala, S. L. Duddukuru, R. Reddipalli, and P. K. Polasi, "A Systematic Review on Deep Learning Models for Sleep Stage Classification," *2022 6th Int. Conf. Trends Electron. Informatics, ICOEI 2022 – Proc.*, no. ICOEI, pp. 1505–1511, 2022, https://doi.org/10.1109/ICOEI53556.2022.9776965.
11. C. C. Aggarwal, *Neural Networks and Deep Learning*. 2018. https://doi.org/10.1007/978-3-319-94463-0.
12. S. B. Kotsiantis and D. Kanellopoulos, "Data preprocessing for supervised leaning," *Int. J. . . .*, vol. 1, no. 2, pp. 1–7, 2006, https://doi.org/10.1080/02331931003692557.
13. F. Chollet, *Deep Learning with Python*. 3 Lewis Street Greenwich, CT United States: Manning Publications Co., 2017.
14. D. Tovar, E. Cornejo, P. Xanthopoulos, M. R. Guarracino, and P. M. Pardalos, "Data Mining in Psychiatric Research," in *Methods in Molecular Biology*, vol. 531, no. 1, 2009, p. 588. [Online]. Available: http://books.google.com/books?id=Ku2wPAAACAAJ
15. P. M. Pardalos and H. E. Romeijn, *Handbook of optimization in medicine*. 2009. [Online]. Available: http://bvbr.bib-bvb.de:8991/F?func=service&doc_library=BVB01&doc_number=017106536&line_number=0001&func_code=DB_RECORDS&service_type=MEDIA%5Cn; http://deposit.d-nb.de/cgi-bin/dokserv?id=3168944&prov=M&dok_var=1&dok_ext=htm
16. I. De Falco, G. De Pietro, A. Della, G. Sannino, U. Scafuri, and E. Tarantino, "Evolution-based configuration optimization of a Deep Neural Network for the classification of Obstructive Sleep Apnea episodes," *Futur. Gener. Comput. Syst.*, vol. 98, pp. 377–391, 2019, https://doi.org/10.1016/j.future.2019.01.049.
17. A. Ramachandran and A. Karuppiah, "A Survey on Recent Advances in Machine Learning Based Sleep Apnea Detection Systems," *Healthcare*, pp. 1–19, 2021.
18. G. C. Gutiérrez-tobal, D. Álvarez, F. Vaquerizo-villar, and R. Hornero, "Ensemble-learning regression to estimate sleep apnea severity using at-home oximetry in adults," *Appl. Soft Comput.*, vol. 111, p. 107827, 2021, https://doi.org/10.1016/j.asoc.2021.107827.
19. A. Brink-Kjaer *et al.*, "Age estimation from sleep studies using deep learning predicts life expectancy," *npj Digit. Med.*, vol. 5, no. 1, 2022, https://doi.org/10.1038/s41746-022-00630-9.
20. E. Y. Ma, J. W. Kim, Y. Lee, S. W. Cho, H. Kim, and J. K. Kim, "Combined unsupervised-supervised machine learning for phenotyping complex diseases with its application to obstructive sleep apnea," *Sci. Rep.*, vol. 11, no. 1, pp. 1–15, 2021, https://doi.org/10.1038/s41598-021-84003-4.
21. J. M. Cavanillas, E. Curry, and W. Wahlster, *New Horizons for a Data-Driven Economy: A Roadmap for Usage and Exploitation of Big Data in Europe*, no. January. 2016. https://doi.org/10.1007/978-3-319-21569-3.
22. R. S. Rosenberg and S. Van Hout, "the American Academy of sleep Medicine Inter-scorer Reliability Program: sleep stage scoring," *J. Clin. Sleep Med.*, vol. 10, no. 4, pp. 447–454, 2014, https://doi.org/10.5664/jcsm.3630.

23. R. Huttunen *et al.*, "Assessment of obstructive sleep apnea-related sleep fragmentation utilizing deep learning-based sleep staging from photoplethysmography," *Sleep*, Jun. 2021, https://doi.org/10.1093/sleep/zsab142.
24. F. Vaquerizo-villar *et al.*, "A Convolutional Neural Network Architecture to Enhance Oximetry Ability to Diagnose Pediatric Obstructive Sleep Apnea," *IEEE J. Biomed. Heal. Informatics*, vol. 25, no. 8, pp. 2906–2916, 2021.
25. S. S. Mostafa, F. Mendonça, F. Morgado-dias, and A. Ravelo-garcía, "SpO2 based Sleep Apnea Detection using Deep Learning," in *INES 2017, 21st International Conference on Intelligent Engineering Systems*, 2017, pp. 91–96.
26. American Academy of Sleep Technologists, "AAST Technical Guideline," no. July, 2012.
27. M. Radha *et al.*, "A deep transfer learning approach for wearable sleep stage classification with photoplethysmography," *npj Digit. Med.*, vol. 4, no. 1, pp. 1–11, 2021, https://doi.org/10.1038/s41746-021-00510-8.
28. J. W. Ran Wei, Xinghua Zhang, "The research of sleep staging based on single-lead electrocardiogram and deep neural network," *Biomed. Eng. Lett.*, 2018.
29. A. N. Olesen, P. Jennum, P. Peppard, E. Mignot, and H. B. D. Sorensen, "Deep residual networks for automatic sleep stage classification of raw polysomnographic waveforms," *Proc. Annu. Int. Conf. IEEE Eng. Med. Biol. Soc. EMBS*, vol. 2018–July, no. November, pp. 3713–3716, 2018, 10.1109/EMBC.2018.8513080.
30. S. Ryu *et al.*, "Diagnosis of obstructive sleep apnea with prediction of flow characteristics according to airway morphology automatically extracted from medical images: Computational fluid dynamics and artificial intelligence approach," *Comput. Methods Programs Biomed.*, vol. 208, p. 106243, 2021, https://doi.org/10.1016/j.cmpb.2021.106243.
31. H. ElMoaqet, M. Eid, M. Glos, M. Ryalat, and T. Penzel, "Deep Recurrent Neural Networks for Automatic Detection of Sleep Apnea from Single Channel Respiration Signals," *Sensors*, pp. 1–20, 2020, https://doi.org/10.3390/s20185037.
32. H. Korkalainen *et al.*, "Detailed Assessment of Sleep Architecture With Deep Learning and Shorter Epoch-to-Epoch Duration Reveals Sleep Fragmentation of Patients With Obstructive Sleep Apnea," *IEEE J. Biomed. Heal. Informatics*, vol. 25, no. 7, pp. 2567–2574, 2021, https://doi.org/10.1109/JBHI.2020.3043507.
33. M. H. Lee, S. K. Lee, R. J. Thomas, J. E. Yoon, C. H. Yun, and C. Shin, "Deep learning–based assessment of brain connectivity related to obstructive sleep apnea and daytime sleepiness," *Nat. Sci. Sleep*, vol. 13, pp. 1561–1572, 2021, https://doi.org/10.2147/NSS.S327110.
34. K. El Emam, S. Rodgers, and B. Malin, "Anonymising and sharing individual patient data," *BMJ (Online)*, vol. 350. 2015. https://doi.org/10.1136/bmj.h1139.
35. C. Heneghan, "St. Vincent's University Hospital / University College Dublin Sleep Apnea Database," 2011.
36. "MIT-BIH Arrhythmia Database v1.0.0." https://physionet.org/content/mitdb/1.0.0/ (accessed Jan. 14, 2021).
37. S. Khalighi, T. Sousa, J. M. Santos, and U. Nunes, "ISRUC-Sleep: A comprehensive public dataset for sleep researchers," *Comput. Methods Programs Biomed.*, vol. 124, no. November, pp. 180–192, 2016, https://doi.org/10.1016/j.cmpb.2015.10.013.
38. A. S. BaHammam and M. W. Chee, "Publicly Available Health Research Datasets: Opportunities and Responsibilities," *Nat. Sci. Sleep*, vol. Volume 14, no. September, pp. 1709–1712, 2022, https://doi.org/10.2147/nss.s390292.
39. D. A. Dean *et al.*, "Scaling up scientific discovery in sleep medicine: The national sleep research resource," *Sleep*, vol. 39, no. 5, pp. 1151–1164, 2016, https://doi.org/10.5665/sleep.5774.
40. (R24 HL114473), "National Heart, Lung, and Blood Institute," *Natl. sleep Res. Resour.*, 2022.
41. G. Q. Zhang *et al.*, "The National Sleep Research Resource: Towards a sleep data commons," *J. Am. Med. Informatics Assoc.*, vol. 25, no. 10, pp. 1351–1358, 2018, https://doi.org/10.1093/jamia/ocy064.

42. R. B. Berry, R. Brooks, C. E. Gamaldo, S. M. Harding, C. L. Marcus, and B. V. Vaughn, "The AASM Manual for the Scoring of Sleep and Associated Events," *Am. Acad. Sleep Med.*, vol. 53, no. 9, pp. 1689–1699, 2013.
43. M. A. Almarshad, M. S. Islam, S. Al-Ahmadi, and A. S. Bahammam, "Diagnostic Features and Potential Applications of PPG Signal in Healthcare: A Systematic Review," *Healthc.*, vol. 10, no. 3, pp. 1–28, 2022, https://doi.org/10.3390/healthcare10030547.
44. F. Peng, Z. Zhang, X. Gou, H. Liu, and W. Wang, "Motion artifact removal from photoplethysmographic signals by combining temporally constrained independent component analysis and adaptive filter," *Biomed. Eng. Online*, vol. 13, no. 1, 2014, https://doi.org/10.1186/1475-925X-13-50.
45. P. M. Pardalos, V. L. Boginski, and A. Vazacopoulos, *Data Mining in Biomedicine*. Springer, 2016.
46. R. Atri and M. Mohebbi, "Obstructive sleep apnea detection using spectrum and bispectrum analysis of single-lead ECG signal," *Physiol. Meas.*, vol. 36, no. 9, pp. 1963–1980, 2015, https://doi.org/10.1088/0967-3334/36/9/1963.
47. H. Yue and Y. Wu, "Deep Learning for Diagnosis and Classification of Obstructive Sleep Apnea: A Nasal Airflow-Based Multi-Resolution Residual Network," 2021.
48. S. M. I. Niroshana, X. Zhu, K. Nakamura, and W. Chen, "A fused-image-based approach to detect obstructive sleep apnea using a single-lead ECG and a 2D convolutional neural network," *PLoS One*, vol. 16, no. 4 April, pp. 1–22, 2021, https://doi.org/10.1371/journal.pone.0250618.
49. F. Rabbi, S. M. R. Islam, D. Kumar, S. M. R. Islam, and M. Ali, "SCNN: Scalogram-based convolutional neural network to detect obstructive sleep apnea using single-lead electrocardiogram signals," *Comput. Biol. Med.*, vol. 134, no. May, p. 104532, 2021, https://doi.org/10.1016/j.compbiomed.2021.104532.
50. Ian Goodfellow, Y. Bengio, and A. Courville, *Deep Learning*. MIT Press, 2016. [Online]. Available: http://www.deeplearningbook.org
51. A. Guillot and V. Thorey, "RobustSleepNet: Transfer Learning for Automated Sleep Staging at Scale," *IEEE Trans. Neural Syst. Rehabil. Eng.*, vol. 29, pp. 1441–1451, 2021, https://doi.org/10.1109/TNSRE.2021.3098968.
52. D. M. Roberts, M. M. Schade, G. M. Mathew, D. Gartenberg, and O. M. Buxton, "Detecting sleep using heart rate and motion data from multisensor consumer-grade wearables, relative to wrist actigraphy and polysomnography," *Sleep Res. Soc.*, no. March, pp. 1–19, 2020, https://doi.org/10.1093/sleep/zsaa045.
53. D. Bertoni, L. M. Sterni, K. D. Pereira, G. Das, and A. Isaiah, "Predicting polysomnographic severity thresholds in children using machine learning," *Pediatr. Res.*, vol. 88, no. 3, pp. 404–411, 2020, https://doi.org/10.1038/s41390-020-0944-0.
54. G. Allocca *et al.*, "Validation of 'somnivore', a machine learning algorithm for automated scoring and analysis of polysomnography data," *Front. Neurosci.*, vol. 13, no. March, pp. 1–18, 2019, https://doi.org/10.3389/fnins.2019.00207.
55. J. V. Stone, *Independent Component Analysis: A Tutorial Introduction*. The MIT Press, 2004. https://doi.org/10.7551/mitpress/4175.003.0003.
56. S. M. Isa, M. I. Fanany, W. Jatmiko, and A. M. Arymurthy, "Sleep apnea detection from ECG signal: Analysis on optimal features, principal components, and nonlinearity," *5th Int. Conf. Bioinforma. Biomed. Eng. iCBBE 2011*, no. June 2014, 2011, https://doi.org/10.1109/icbbe.2011.5780285.
57. E. Keogh, S. C. D. Hart, and M. Pazzani, "Segmenting Time Series: A Survey and Novel Approach," *Data Min. time Ser. databases*, vol. 36, no. 3, pp. 583–589, 2004.
58. M. Abreu, A. Fred, J. Valente, C. Wang, and H. Plácido, "Morphological autoencoders for apnea detection in respiratory gating radiotherapy," *Comput. Methods Programs Biomed.*, vol. 195, p. 105675, 2020, https://doi.org/10.1016/j.cmpb.2020.105675.

Sleep Stage Probabilities Derived from Neurological or Cardiorespiratory Signals by Means of Artificial Intelligence

Peter Anderer, Marco Ross, Andreas Cerny, and Pedro Fonseca

1 Introduction

Sleep is typically scored manually by visually identifying patterns in electroencephalogram (EEG), electrooculogram (EOG), and electromyogram (EMG) signals collected during polysomnography (PSG). These neurological signals provide the basic information requisite for visually differentiating wake from sleep, rapid eye-movement (REM), sleep from non-REM sleep, and for subclassifying non-REM sleep in three sleep stages N1, N2, and N3 in non-overlapping segments (so-called epochs) of 30 seconds, according to the rules defined in the Manual for the Scoring of Sleep and Associated Events (Version 2.6) published by the American Academy of Sleep Medicine (AASM) [1]. Visual scoring of a PSG is time-consuming, requires well-trained and experienced human scorers, and retains a degree of subjectivity which leads to rather limited interrater reliabilities [2–9]. Automatic scoring, with classification performance at least non-inferior to that of experienced humans, could alleviate the shortcomings of visual scoring.

P. Anderer (✉) · M. Ross
The Siesta Group, Vienna, Austria
e-mail: peter.anderer@thesiestagroup.com; marco.ross@thesiestagroup.com

A. Cerny
FH Technikum Wien, Vienna, Austria
e-mail: cerny@technikum-wien.at

P. Fonseca
Philips Sleep and Respiratory Care, Eindhoven, The Netherlands

Department of Electrical Engineering, Eindhoven University of Technology, Eindhoven, The Netherlands
e-mail: pedro.fonseca@philips.com; P.M.Ferreira@tue.nl

R. B. Berry et al. (eds.), *Handbook of AI and Data Sciences for Sleep Disorders*, Springer Optimization and Its Applications 216,
https://doi.org/10.1007/978-3-031-68263-6_3

Indeed, right after the first generally accepted manual for scoring of sleep was published in 1968 by Rechtschaffen and Kales [10], numerous attempts at a computer-assisted identification of sleep stages have been published. These had the initial goal to provide semi-automated scoring solutions that aimed at reducing scoring time and interrater variability [11–19]. After the first version of the AASM Manual for the Scoring of Sleep and Associated Events was published in 2007 [20], the scoring algorithms had to be adapted to the new rules and had to be tested again for validity in comparison with visual scoring. In 2010, we published an AASM version of the Somnolyzer algorithm [21] that was originally based on the R&K version [15]. The Somnolyzer scoring system consisted of a raw data quality check (including artifact minimization and identification as well as channel selection in case of backup channels), a feature extraction algorithm identifying the patterns that are used by humans to score sleep (density and intensity of sleep/wake-related patterns such as sleep spindles, delta waves, slow eye movements, and rapid eye movements), a classifier designed as an expert system and rule-based smoothing procedures for discriminating N1 and N2 and for determining the start and the end of stage REM. The validation of the semi-automated scoring solution was tested versus two independent manual scorings in a holdout dataset ($n = 72$). A comparison on an epoch-per-epoch basis between the manual and the semi-automated scorings revealed a Cohen's kappa coefficient of agreement with scorer 1 and 2 of 0.76 and 0.75, respectively. Since the Cohen's kappa between the two manual scorers was 0.76, this suggested equivalence between manual and the semi-automated Somnolyzer scoring [21]. In 2015, Punjabi et al. [22] compared Somnolyzer with manual expert scorings from 4 sites in 97 PSG studies and reported instead of kappa values pairwise intraclass correlation coefficients and Bland-Altman plots for the percentage of each sleep stage. Based on their analysis, the authors concluded that semi-automated analysis of PSGs using the Somnolyzer system provided results that are comparable to manual scoring for commonly used metrics in sleep medicine.

In contrast to PSG recordings where all neurological signals for sleep staging are available, home sleep apnea testing (HSAT) systems increasingly used in the diagnosis of sleep disordered breathing (SDB) typically do not include recordings of neurological signals. Consequently, manual sleep staging is not possible and instead of total sleep time, monitoring or recording time is used for calculating the number of respiratory events per hour. This may lead to reduced diagnostic sensitivity of SDB that is not easily quantifiable [23]. This limitation of HSATs motivated attempts to leverage the known expression of autonomic nervous system activity in sleep by analyzing cardiorespiratory signals which are in fact routinely recorded with these polygraphic systems: the non-REM progression from N1 to N3 is typically accompanied by an increase in cardiovagal drive and parasympathetic activity, which translates to a lower heart rate, more regular breathing, and an increased respiratory mediation of heart rate variability [24, 25]. REM sleep is characterized by a state of autonomic instability where sympathetic and parasympathetic nervous system activity fluctuate, producing abrupt changes in heart rate and irregular breathing [24, 25]. In the absence of neurological signals, these algorithms are typically limited to the estimation of the stages wake, light sleep (LS; comprising the combination of N1 and N2), deep sleep (DS; corresponding to N3), and REM sleep. The differentiation between N1 and N2 based on neurological signals requires not only the timing of arousals but also sleep spindles and k-complexes, neither of which are available with cardiorespiratory inputs. These algorithms can of course not mimic human scoring, since there are no rules, nor is it practically possible, to relate changes in heart rate and respiration to sleep stages. Most of the early algorithms that showed promise instead relied on manually engineered features carefully crafted to capture changes in autonomic nervous system activity during sleep, leveraging domain knowledge of sleep and cardiorespiratory physiology. In 2011, Hedner et al. [26] presented a sleep staging based on peripheral arterial tonometry (PAT) signals and reported a Cohen's kappa for the 4-stage comparison (wake, light sleep (LS), deep sleep (DS), and REM sleep) of 0.48 in 38 healthy subjects and 189 apnea patients. In 2015, Fonseca et al. [27] presented an algorithm to estimate sleep based on cardiorespiratory signals using manually engineered features and a linear discriminant classifier and reported a Cohen's kappa of 0.49 for the 4-stage comparison validated in 48 healthy subjects. By incorporating time information and replacing the classifier by a conditional random field, Cohen's kappa increased to 0.53 in 100 healthy subjects [28]. In 2017, Tataraidze et al. [29] reported a kappa of 0.56 based on respiratory inductance plethysmography (RIP) signals using an extreme gradient boosting classifier in 658 healthy subjects and Beattie et al. [30] reported a kappa of 0.52 based on photoplethysmography (PPG) and actigraphy signals using a linear discriminant classifier in 60 healthy controls.

In recent years, the field of AI has met significant advancements and now offers powerful tools for various classification tasks. An increased recognition of the possible relevance of AI in sleep medicine, and continuous improvements in the performance of machine learning algorithms, in particular with remarkable advances in the development and use of artificial neural networks, have fueled attention to the topic of automatic sleep scoring. This chapter starts with a review of interrater reliability studies of manual sleep scoring according to AASM to define benchmarks for autoscoring. It follows with a review of AI-based algorithms for sleep staging using neurological signals traditionally recorded with PSG and of AI-based algorithms for sleep staging based on cardiorespiratory signals such as ECG, PPG, airflow, or respiratory effort, with or without actigraphy. These advanced AI methods can often leverage, and even go beyond what humans can possibly encode. This is particularly true for cardiorespiratory sleep staging, since it requires the simultaneous observation of many cardiorespiratory characteristics and subtle changes over a context that might span far beyond each individual epoch. AI methods, can find relations in the data based on patterns that span entire recordings, simultaneously analyzing numerous characteristics of the various signals. In addition to the higher performance of recent AI-based scoring systems as compared to the aforementioned algorithms, these solutions offer additional benefits that could help interpreting sleep studies faster and more accurately. The last part of this chapter presents AI-based estimates of sleep stage probabilities per epoch (hypnodensity) using neurological or cardiorespiratory signals. It also gives examples of quantitative measures derived from the hypnodensity, such as sleep stage ambiguity and sleep stage epoch-to-epoch continuity which might be relevant for further clinical research and possible applications.

2 Defining Benchmarks for Autoscoring Solutions: Interrater Reliability of Manual Sleep Scoring

Autoscoring algorithms are usually trained and evaluated on manual sleep scoring. If the evaluation is based on a test set where all PSGs have been scored by one expert, the benchmark for the performance measure between autoscoring and manual scoring is set by the interscorer reliability between manual scorers. Thus, we reviewed interrater reliability studies with manual sleep scoring according to the AASM rules which reported kappa values between manual scorings for the 5-stage comparison (W, N1, N2, N3, R) as well as for each sleep stage separately. In total, 13 studies published between 2009 and 2022 have been identified and included in the review.

We summarized the major characteristics of these studies in Table 1, including author and publication year; the dataset (HC: healthy controls, PAT: patients with sleep disorders, OSA: patients with obstructive sleep apnea, Cohort: subjects from cohort studies); the number of scorers; the kappa values based on comparisons between the scorers and the applied statistics (Cohen's kappa or Fleiss' kappa). As can be seen in Table 1, there is a large difference in the size of the datasets (between 7 and 1066 PSGs) and the number of manual scorers (between 2 and 12). Note that in studies with more than 2 scorers either Fleiss' kappa [2, 31–33] or the mean Cohen's kappa values of all pairwise comparisons was reported [34, 35]. The kappa values for the 5-stage comparison ranged from 0.50 (in a small dataset with 8 PSGs comparing scorers from Berlin, Germany with scorers in Beijing, China [34]) to 0.87 (in a cohort with 40 PSGs comparing 5 Chinese scorers from the same sleep lab [33]). On average, Cohen's kappa value for the 5-stage comparison was 0.63. In all studies, Cohen's kappa values were low for N1 (on average 0.33), medium for N2 and N3 (on average 0.61 and 0.62), and highest for R and W (on average 0.79 and 0.76).

Considering the limited interscorer reliability, it would make sense to use a consensus based on multiple manual scorers to set the comparison standard [4]. All 586 PSGs of the Siesta database were scored independently by two experts from different sleep labs and a third expert from another sleep lab made, based on the two scorings, a consensus decision [36]. Alternatively, a consensus score can also be defined as the majority vote of multiple scorings. Different approaches are possible for dealing with epochs without a majority. If the consensus is based on an odd number of scorers, only a few epochs will not have a majority and thus these epochs can be excluded from the analysis. Alternatively, to avoid excluding any epochs, those without a majority may be set to the decision of the scorer with the highest agreement to all other scorers [37]. In yet another approach, Stephansen et al. [38]

Table 1 Review of interrater reliability studies reporting kappa values between manual scorers for all 5 AASM stages and per sleep stage

Author, year	Dataset	Scorers	All	N1	N2	N3	R	W	Statistic
Danker-Hopfe et al., 2009 [3]	Cohort: $N = 72$; SIESTA	26	0.78	0.46	0.72	0.73	0.91	0.86	Cohen's K
	Cohort: $N = 12$; SIESTA		0.72	0.50	0.70	0.50	0.93	0.88	Fleiss' K
Ruehland et al., 2011 [31]	Suspected OSA: $N = 10$	3	0.67	0.40	0.61	0.60	0.88	0.80	Fleiss' K
Magalang et al., 2013 [32]	Cohort: $N = 15$; SAGIC	9	0.63	0.31	0.60	0.67	0.78	0.78	Fleiss' K
Zhang et al., 2015 [34]	HC: $N = 8$	5	0.50	0.16	0.58	0.49	0.79	0.65	Cohen's K
	OSA: $N = 7$		0.58	0.19	0.50	0.64	0.69	0.76	
	Narcolepsy $N = 15$		0.54	0.30	0.55	0.68	0.66	0.58	
Deng et al., 2019 [33]	Cohort: $N = 40$	2[a]	0.75	0.45	0.72	0.79	0.87	0.89	Cohen's K
		5	0.87	0.69	0.85	0.90	0.94	0.94	Fleiss' K
Cesari et al., 2021 [8]	Cohort: $N = 1066$; SHIP	2	0.66	0.40	0.62	0.66	0.75	0.78	Cohen's K
Bakker et al., 2023 [35]	Cohort: $N = 70$; IS-RC	6	0.62	0.32	0.59	0.42	0.79	0.80	Cohen's K
	PAT: $N = 15$; SAGIC	9	0.62	0.33	0.60	0.65	0.80	0.76	
	PAT: $N = 10$; Somnoval	12	0.60	0.32	0.57	0.50	0.84	0.75	
Summary	**Dataset**	**Scorers**	**All**	**N1**	**N2**	**N3**	**R**	**W**	
Minimum	$\mathbf{N = 7}$	**2**	**0.50**	**0.16**	**0.50**	**0.42**	**0.66**	**0.58**	**Cohen's K**
Maximum	$\mathbf{N = 1066}$	**12**	**0.78**	**0.46**	**0.72**	**0.79**	**0.91**	**0.89**	**(9 studies)**
Mean ± SD			**0.63 ± 0.09**	**0.33 ± 0.10**	**0.61 ± 0.07**	**0.62 ± 0.12**	**0.79 ± 0.08**	**0.76 ± 0.10**	
Minimum	$\mathbf{N = 10}$	**3**	**0.63**	**0.31**	**0.60**	**0.50**	**0.78**	**0.78**	**Fleiss' K**
Maximum	$\mathbf{N = 40}$	**9**	**0.87**	**0.69**	**0.85**	**0.90**	**0.94**	**0.94**	**(4 studies)**
Mean ± SD			**0.72 ± 0.11**	**0.48 ± 0.16**	**0.69 ± 0.12**	**0.67 ± 0.17**	**0.88 ± 0.07**	**0.85 ± 0.07**	

Cohort cohort study, *HC* healthy controls, *PAT* patients with sleep disturbance, *OSA* patients with obstructive sleep apnea, *SIESTA* SIESTA sleep database, *IS-RC* Research study on sleep disordered breathing in women in midlife, University of Pennsylvania, Philadelphia, *SAGIC* Sleep Apnea Genetics International Consortium, The Ohio State University Medical Center, Columbus, *SHIP* Study of Health in Pomerania, *Somnoval* Somnolyzer validation study dataset

[a]Comparison between the consensus of 5 scorers from one lab to the consensus of 2 scorers from another lab

used a consensus based on a weighted majority vote, where the weight for each scorer is based on that scorer's kappa versus all other scorers. Thus, scorers with a higher consensus with the group are considered more reliable and their assessments are weighted more heavily than that of the other scorers. Using this approach, we defined consensus hypnograms for studies scored by 4, 5, 6, 9, or 12 scorers. In Table 2, we summarize Cohen's kappa values for these six studies comparing each scorer versus three different comparators: versus all other individual scorers (Single scorer), versus a consensus in which the assessed scorer was not included (Unbiased consensus), and versus a consensus in which all scorers have been included (Biased consensus). The agreement to the unbiased consensus scoring is in all six studies and for all stages higher than the averaged pairwise agreement between two scorers (*Difference (Unbiased-Single)*). The overestimation of the agreement caused by the inclusion of the assessed scorer in the consensus is, however, dependent on the sleep stage and on the number of scorers included in the consensus (*Difference (Biased-Unbiased)*). As can be seen, the highest overestimation occurs for stage N1 in the study with the lowest number of scorers. The overestimations of Cohen's kappa for stage N1 are 0.21, 0.13, 0.13, 0.11, and 0.07 for the studies with 4, 5, 6, 9, and 12 scorers. These differences suggest that when benchmarking the performance of autoscoring for datasets with multiple scorings, measures of agreement versus biased consensus should not be used.

Another challenge in evaluating and comparing automated approaches is that they should actually be evaluated on a common dataset, since performance can vary widely between datasets depending on various factors, such as age, diagnosis or severity of the disease. In 2020, Guillot et al. [37] presented open datasets intended for comparing autoscoring solutions. The datasets include PSGs from 25 healthy volunteers (DOD-H) and from 55 patients with OSA (DOD-O), all PSGs scored by 5 sleep technologists from different sleep centers. These datasets have been used since then in numerous validation studies [37, 39–41]. Note that Fiorillo et al. [40] presented the scorer performance of the DOD-H and DOD-O datasets by comparing the scorers versus the biased consensus, resulting in an average Cohen's kappa of 0.82 and 0.79 for DOD-H and DOD-O, respectively. In Table 2, we added for these two datasets the mean Cohen's kappa for the comparison to single scorers (0.70 and 0.68 for DOD-H and DOD-O) and for the comparison to the unbiased consensus (0.73 and 0.77 for DOD-H and DOD-O). Recently, the AASM has launched a 2-year pilot program for certification of autoscoring software that provides adult sleep stage scoring. The certification program's purpose is to independently verify the performance of autoscoring systems based on 100 PSGs (diagnostic and therapeutic) scored by seven "gold standard" scorers (i.e., scorers with at least 6 years of experience in scoring sleep studies who have demonstrated their quality in applying the AASM scoring rules during the application process).

Multi-scored datasets are, however, not only valuable for validation, but also in the training phase. Training against consensus scorings is not only more reliable, but it also additionally allows the actual sleep stage probabilities derived from the multiple scorings to be used as training targets (i.e., soft targets). Fiorillo et al. [40] showed, as compared to using hard targets, significant increases in performance

Table 2 Effect of the comparator on interrater reliability of manual sleep staging based on Cohen's kappa

Dataset	All	N1	N2	N3	R	W	Comparator
PAT: $N = 97$	0.67	0.29	0.64	0.48	0.87	0.80	Single scorer
Somnoval	0.71	0.34	0.70	0.53	0.89	0.83	Unbiased consensus
4 scorers	0.80	0.54	0.79	0.67	0.92	0.88	Biased consensus
	0.05	*0.05*	*0.06*	*0.05*	*0.02*	*0.03*	*Difference (unbiased-single)*
	0.09	*0.21*	*0.09*	*0.13*	*0.03*	*0.05*	*Difference (biased-unbiased)*
HC: $N = 25$	0.70	0.35	0.68	0.74	0.84	0.75	Single scorer
DOD-H	0.77	0.45	0.75	0.78	0.87	0.82	Unbiased consensus
5 scorers	0.82	0.58	0.81	0.84	0.90	0.86	Biased consensus
	0.06	*0.09*	*0.07*	*0.05*	*0.04*	*0.07*	*Difference (unbiased-single)*
	0.06	*0.13*	*0.06*	*0.06*	*0.03*	*0.04*	*Difference (biased-unbiased)*
OSA: $N = 55$	0.68	0.35	0.63	0.55	0.83	0.83	Single scorer
DOD-O	0.73	0.43	0.70	0.61	0.87	0.86	Unbiased consensus
5 scorers	0.79	0.56	0.78	0.73	0.90	0.90	Biased consensus
	0.05	*0.08*	*0.06*	*0.06*	*0.04*	*0.03*	*Difference (unbiased-single)*
	0.07	*0.13*	*0.08*	*0.11*	*0.03*	*0.04*	*Difference (biased-unbiased)*
Cohort: $N = 70$	0.62	0.32	0.59	0.42	0.79	0.80	Single scorer
IS-RC	0.69	0.42	0.68	0.51	0.83	0.85	Unbiased consensus
6 scorers	0.76	0.55	0.75	0.61	0.87	0.88	Biased consensus
	0.07	*0.10*	*0.09*	*0.09*	*0.04*	*0.05*	*Difference (unbiased-single)*
	0.06	*0.13*	*0.06*	*0.10*	*0.03*	*0.03*	*Difference (biased-unbiased)*
PAT: $N = 15$	0.62	0.33	0.60	0.65	0.80	0.76	Single scorer
SAGIC	0.69	0.42	0.67	0.72	0.85	0.82	Unbiased consensus
9 scorers	0.74	0.52	0.73	0.77	0.87	0.85	Biased consensus
	0.07	*0.09*	*0.07*	*0.07*	*0.05*	*0.06*	*Difference (unbiased-single)*
	0.05	*0.11*	*0.05*	*0.05*	*0.02*	*0.03*	*Difference (biased-unbiased)*
PAT: $N = 10$	0.60	0.32	0.57	0.50	0.84	0.75	Single scorer
Somnoval	0.69	0.44	0.66	0.59	0.88	0.82	Unbiased consensus
12 scorers	0.73	0.50	0.70	0.65	0.90	0.84	Biased consensus
	0.09	*0.12*	*0.09*	*0.09*	*0.04*	*0.07*	*Difference (unbiased-single)*
	0.04	*0.07*	*0.05*	*0.05*	*0.01*	*0.02*	*Difference (biased-unbiased)*

Single scorer: mean of all possible pairwise comparisons between two scorers. Unbiased consensus: mean of all scorers versus a consensus in which the assessed scorer is not included. Biased consensus: mean of all scorers versus a consensus in which all scorers (i.e., also the assessed scorer) are included

Cohort cohort study, *HC* healthy controls, *PAT* patients with sleep disturbance, *OSA* patients with obstructive sleep apnea, *Somnoval* Somnolyzer validation study dataset, *DOD-H* Dreem Open Dataset—Healthy Volunteers, *DOD-O* Dreem Open Dataset—Obstructive Sleep Apnea Patients, *IS-RC* Research study on sleep disordered breathing in women in midlife, University of Pennsylvania, Philadelphia, *SAGIC* Sleep Apnea Genetics International Consortium, The Ohio State University Medical Center, Columbus

measures by using targets with soft consensus label smoothing (i.e., weighted average of hard and soft targets with varying coefficients alpha that define the weight of the soft target). Our Somnolyzer scoring algorithm was trained directly on the sleep stage probabilities derived from multiple manual scorings corresponding to a soft consensus label smoothing with an alpha coefficient of 1 [35].

3 Review of AI-Based Algorithms Using Neurological Signals as Input

The review includes AI-based sleep scoring algorithms which used at least one EEG channel as input and reported Cohen's kappa for the 5-stage comparison (W, N1, N2, N3, R). In total, 33 studies published between 2017 and 2023 have been identified and included.

We summarized the major characteristics of these studies in Table 3, including author, publication year and, if appropriate, the name of the scoring system; the training dataset(s) (HC: healthy controls, PAT: patients with sleep disorders, OSA: patients with obstructive sleep apnea, PD: patients with Parkinson's disease; Cohort: subjects from cohort studies); the input channels and the feature extraction method (epoch encoder); the classifier (sequence encoder); the test dataset(s) and the testing approach (CV: cross-validation, HO: holdout validation, EXT: external test set); finally Cohen's kappa for the 5-stage comparison for internal testing (cross-validation or holdout dataset) or external testing (datasets completely unseen by the model during training and validation) [8, 35, 37–40, 42–66].

As can be seen in the last row of Table 3, there is a large difference in the size of the training data (between 10 and 15,684 PSGs) as well as in the size of the test data (between 10 and 2907). Cohen's kappa for the 45 internal test sets was significantly higher than Cohen's kappa for the 19 external test sets (0.78 ± 0.04 vs. 0.72 ± 0.06; $p < 0.001$ independent samples t-test). Interestingly, in all studies that reported Cohen's kappa for both, internal and external testing the kappa for the internal testing was always higher than for the external testing [39, 50, 51, 64]. Moreover, in studies reporting Cohen's kappa for patients and for healthy controls, the kappa was always highest for healthy controls [37, 39, 40, 44, 49, 61, 63]. In studies with internal testing the highest kappa (0.91) was reported in a test set with 8 healthy controls using a 20-fold epoch-wise cross-validation of all sleep stages [54]. In studies with external testing the highest kappa (0.80) was reported in a test set with 25 healthy controls [39]. These observations strongly suggest that the reported performance of these AI algorithms depends, to a certain extent, on the nature of the validation used. Efforts to carefully separate subjects between training and (holdout) validation might not be sufficient, as these algorithms probably remain vulnerable to factors such as selection bias, or even to scoring bias in case the same pool of annotators are used. Based on these findings, it is recommended that the performance of sleep scoring algorithms should be tested in datasets, which were completely unseen by the model both during training and validation, are representative of the population to be tested, and ideally collected in different centers and scored by different (pools of) humans.

The Somnolyzer version listed in Table 3 is still using sleep/wake-related features as described above in Anderer et al. [15, 21] for epoch encoding, while for sequence encoding the decision tree was replaced by a bidirectional long-short term memory recurrent neural network [35]. In the four recent external validation

Table 3 Review of AI sleep staging for PSG based on neurological signals (5-stages Cohen's Kappa: W, N1, N2, N3, R)

Author name, year	Training	Feature extraction/epoch encoder	Classifier/Sequence encoder	Test	Cohen's K	
					Internal	External
Supratak et al., 2017 [49] *DeepSleepNet*	Cohort: $N = 62$; MASS HC: $N = 20$; Sleep-EDF	Single-channel EEG (raw signal) + CNN	Bidirectional LSTMs with short-cut connection	Cohort: MASS HC: Sleep-EDF	0.80 (CV) 0.76 (CV)	
Sors et al., 2018 [47]	Cohort: $N = 5793$; SHHS	Single-channel EEG (raw signal) + CNN	Deep CNN	Cohort: $N = 1738$; SHHS	0.81 (HO)	
Biswal et al., 2018 [43]	PAT: $N = 9000$; MGH	2–6 EEG channels (spectrogram) + CNN	Unidirectional RNN	Cohort: $N = 580$; SHHS		0.73
Patanaik et al., 2018 [45]	HC: $N = 1330$; Duke-NUS	2 EEG & 2 EOG ch. (spectrogram)	Deep CNN	PAT: $N = 210$; SDU PD: $N = 77$; UCSD		0.74 0.60
Stephansen et al., 2018 [38] *Stanford-STAGES*	Cohort: $N = 2784$; 10 cohorts	EEG, EOG, EMG: Cross-correlation encoding + CNN	Unidirectional LSTM	Cohort: $N = 70$; IS-RC, 6 scorers		0.75
Anderer et al., JSR 2018 [42] *Somnolyzer*	Cohort: $N = 588$; SIESTA (7 sleep centers) 588 PSGs R&K, 3 scorers 72 PSGs AASM, 2–6 scorers	EEG, EOG, EMG (sleep/wake-related features) + MLP/CNN	Bidirectional LSTM (➔R&K) + CNN + unidirectional LSTM (➔AASM)	PAT (OSA): $N = 97$; Somnoval, 4 scorers		0.79

(continued)

Table 3 (continued)

Author name, year	Training	Feature extraction/epoch encoder	Classifier/Sequence encoder	Test	Cohen's K	
					Internal	External
Phan et al., 2019 [46] *SeqSleepNet*	Cohort: $N = 200$; MASS	EEG, EOG, EMG (power spectra) filterbank layers	Attention-based hierarchical bidirectional GRU	Cohort: MASS	0.82 (CV)	
Zhang et al., 2019 [64]	Cohort: $N = 5213$; SHHS	EEG, EOG, EMG (spectrogram) + CNN	Unidirectional LSTM	Cohort: $N = 580$; SHHS Cohort: $N = 461$; SOF Cohort: $N = 2907$; MrOS	0.82 (HO)	0.68 0.70
Sun et al., 2020 [48]	Cohort: $N = 147$; MASS	EEG, EOG, EMG (power spectra, energy, entropy, etc.) + CNN	Attention layer + bidirectional LSTM	Cohort: MASS	0.80 (CV)	
Guillot et al., 2020 [37] *Simple Sleep Net*	HC: $N = 25$; DOD-H, 5 scorers PAT (OSA): $N = 55$; DOD-O, 5 scorers	EEG, EOG, EMG (spectrogram) + bidirectional GRU + attention layer	Bidirectional GRU with short-cut connections	HC: DOD-H, 5 scorers PAT (OSA): DOD-O, 5 scorers	0.85 (CV) 0.82 (CV)	
Korkalainen et al., 2020 [44]	HC: $N = 153$; Sleep-EDF PAT (OSA): $N = 891$; Clinical DataSet	Single-channel EEG (& single-channel EOG) + CNN	Bidirectional LSTM	HC: Sleep-EDF PAT (OSA): Clinical DataSet	0.78 (CV) 0.78 (CV)	
Abou Jaoude et al., 2020 [50]	PAT: $N = 6341$; MGH	4 EEG channels (raw signal) + CNN	Unidirectional LSTM	PAT: $N = 791$; MGH HO PAT: $N = 243$; homePAP PAT: $N = 129$; ABC	0.74 (HO)	0.69 0.66

Alvares-Estevez & Rijsman, 2021 [51]	Cohort: $N = 443$; 6 datasets	EEG, EOG, EMG (raw signal) + CNN	Unidirectional LSTM	Cohort: $N = 88$ Cohort: $N = 20$–154; inter-cohort performance	0.80 (HO)	0.63
Cesari et al., 2021 [8] *Stanford-STAGES*	Cohort: $N = 2784$; 10 cohorts	EEG, EOG, EMG: Cross-correlation encoding + CNN	Unidirectional LSTM	Cohort: $N = 1066$; SHIP, 2 scorers		0.68
Olesen et al., 2021 [57]	Cohort: $N = 15{,}684$; 5 cohorts	EEG, EOG, EMG (raw signal) + CNN	Bidirectional GRU	Cohort: $N = 1584$	0.80 (HO)	
Vallat & Walker, 2021 [39] *YASA*	Cohort: $N = 3163$; 7 cohorts	EEG, EOG, EMG (time-domain features & spectrogram)	LightGBM	Cohort: $N = 585$; HO HC: $N = 25$; DOD-H, 5 scorers PAT(OSA): $N = 55$; DOD-O, 5 scorers	0.82 (HO)	0.80 0.77
Nasiri & Clifford, 2021 [56]	PAT: $N = 994$; PhysioNet	6 EEG channels (normalized raw signals and population subgrouping)	Deep CNN	PAT: Physio [40] Net	0.75 (CV)	
Fiorillo et al., 2021 [52] *DeepSleepNet-Lite*	HC: $N = 39$; Sleep-EDF 2013 HC: $N = 153$; Sleep-EDF 2018	Single-channel EEG (raw signal) + CNN	Deep CNN	HC: Sleep-EDF 2013 HC: Sleep-EDF 2018	0.78 (CV) 0.73 (CV)	

(continued)

Table 3 (continued)

Author name, year	Training	Feature extraction/epoch encoder	Classifier/Sequence encoder	Test	Cohen's K	
					Internal	External
Pathak et al., 2021	Cohort: $N = 5793$; SHHS PAT: $N = 1418$; Clinical	EEG, EOG, EMG (raw signals) + CNN	Bidirectional LSTM	Cohort: $N = 579$; SHHS PAT: $N = 142$; Clinical	0.79 (HO) 0.68 (HO)	
Jia et al., 2021 [53]	HC: $N = 10$; ISRUC-S3 HC: $N = 62$; MASS-SS3	EEG (6 channels ISRUC, 20 channels MASS) + MSTGCN	Deep CNN	HC: ISRUC HC: MASS	0.77 (CV) 0.84 (CV)	
Li T. et al., 2022 [55]	HC: $N = 61$; Sleep-EDF 2013 HC: $N = 197$; Sleep-EDF 2018	Single-channel EEG (raw signal) + CNN + attention module	Bidirectional LSTM	HC: Sleep-EDF 2013 HC: Sleep-EDF 2018	0.78 (CV) 0.74 (CV)	
Ji et al., 2022 [61]	HC: $N = 10$; ISRUC-S3 PAT: $N = 100$; ISRUC-S1	EEG, EOG, EMG, ECG (raw signals) + CNN	Jumping Knowledge Spatial-Temporal Graph Convolution (JK-STGCN)	HC: ISRUC-S3 PAT: ISRUC-S1	0.78 (CV) 0.77 (CV)	
Li C. et al., 2022 [54] *EEGS Net*	HC: $N = 8$; sleep-EDF-8 HC: $N = 39$; sleep-EDF-20 HC: $N = 153$; Sleep-EDF-78 Cohort: $N = 329$; SHHS	Single-channel EEG (spectrogram) + CNN	Bidirectional LSTM	HC: Sleep-EDF-8 HC: Sleep-EDF-20 HC: Sleep-EDF-78 Cohort: SHHS	0.91 (CV) 0.82 (CV) 0.77 (CV) 0.79 (CV)	
Sharma et al., 2022 [62]	Cohort: $N = 8455$; SHHS	EEG, EOG, EEG (filter-bank + entropy)	Ensemble bagged tree (EBT)	Cohort: $N = 580$; SHHS1 Cohort: $N = 2651$; SHHS2	0.77 (HO) 0.80 (HO)	

Cho et al., 2022 [60] *Stage Net*	PAT: $N = 530$; Clinical dataset	EEG, EOG, EMG (engineered features) + CNN	RNN	PAT: $N = 72$, Clinical dataset	0.84 (HO)	
Yubo et al., 2022 [63] *MMA Sleep Net*	HC: $N = 39$; Sleep-EDF-20 HC: $N = 153$; Sleep-EDF-78 HC: $N = 10$; ISRUC-Sleep3 PAT: $N = 100$; ISRUC-Sleep1	EEG, EOG, EMG (raw signals) attention-based feature fusing	Two linear fully connected layers	HC: Sleep-EDF-20 HC: Sleep-EDF-78 HC: ISRUC-Sleep3 PAT: ISRUC-Sleep1	0.83 (CV) 0.76 (CV) 0.77 (CV) 0.73 (CV)	
Anderer et al., 2022 [59] *Somnolyzer*	Cohort: $N = 588$; SIESTA (7 sleep centers) 2–6 scorers	EEG, EOG, EMG (sleep/wake-related features) + MLP/CNN	Bidirectional LSTM (➔R&K) + CNN + unidirectional LSTM (➔AASM)	Cohort: $N = 426$ ABC, homePAP, MESA		0.74
Bakker et al., 2023 [35] *Somnolyzer*	Cohort: $N = 588$; SIESTA (7 sleep centers) 2–6 scorers	EEG, EOG, EMG (sleep/wake-related features) + MLP/CNN	Bidirectional LSTM (➔R&K) + CNN + unidirectional LSTM (➔AASM)	Cohort: $N = 70$; IS-RC, 6 scorers PAT: $N = 15$; SAGIC, 9 scorers PAT: $N = 10$; Somnoval, 12 scorers		0.78 0.75 0.76
Cesari et al., 2022 [65] *Stanford-STAGES*	Cohort: $N = 2784$; 10 cohorts	EEG, EOG, EMG: Cross-correlation encoding + CNN	Unidirectional LSTM	PAT (hypersomnia): $N = 143$		0.75
Cesari et al., 2022 [65] *YASA*	Cohort: $N = 3163$; 7 cohorts	EEG, EOG, EMG (time-domain features & spectrogram)	Light GBM	PAT (hypersomnia): $N = 143$		0.76

(continued)

Table 3 (continued)

Author name, year	Training	Feature extraction/epoch encoder	Classifier/Sequence encoder	Test	Cohen's K	
					Internal	External
Brandmayr et al. 2022 [66] *ENGELBERT*	HC: $N = 20$; Sleep-EDF-20 HC: $N = 78$; Sleep-EDF-SC Cohort: $N = 62$; MASS-SS3	Single-channel EEG (raw signal) + CNN	Local MHSA on overlapping windows	HC: $N = 20$; Sleep-EDF-20 HC: $N = 78$; Sleep-EDF-SC Cohort: $N = 62$; MASS-SS3	0.82 (CV) 0.79 (CV) 0.80 (CV)	
Fiorillo et al., 2023 [40] *Deep Sleep Net-Light*	Cohort: $N = 70$; IS-RC, 6 scorers HC: $N = 25$; DOD-H, 5 scorers PAT (OSA): $N = 55$; DOD-O, 5 scorers	Single-channel EEG (raw signal) + CNN	Deep CNN (soft consensus label smoothing)	Cohort: $N = 70$; IS-RC, 6 scorers HC: $N = 25$; DOD-H, 5 scorers PAT (OSA): $N = 55$; DOD-O, 5 scorers	0.67 (CV) 0.76 (CV) 0.71 (CV)	
Fiorillo et al., 2023 [40] *Simple Sleep Net*	Cohort: $N = 70$; IS-RC, 6 scorers HC: $N = 25$; DOD-H, 5 scorers PAT (OSA): $N = 55$; DOD-O, 5 scorers	EEG, EOG, EMG (spectrogram) + bidirectional GRU + attention layer	Bidirectional GRU (soft consensus label smoothing)	Cohort: $N = 70$; IS-RC, 6 scorers HC: $N = 25$; DOD-H, 5 scorers PAT (OSA): $N = 55$; DOD-O, 5 scorers	0.73 (CV) 0.84 (CV) 0.80 (CV)	

Summary	Training data			Test data	Cohen's K	
					Internal	External
N-studies	33			64	45	19
Range: minimum	$N = 10$			$N = 10$	0.67	0.60
maximum	$N = 15{,}684$			$N = 2907$	0.91	0.80
Mean ± SD					0.78 ± 0.04	0.72 ± 0.06

Internal performance of holdout or cross-validation, *External* performance in datasets completely unseen by the model, *CV* cross-validation, *HO* holdout validation

Cohort cohort study, *HC* healthy controls, *PAT* patients with sleep disturbance, *OSA* patients with obstructive sleep apnea, *PD* Parkinson's Disease, *MASS* Montreal Archive of Sleep Studies, *Sleep-EDF* Sleep-EDF Database Expanded, *SHHS* Sleep Heart Health Study, *MGH* Massachusetts General Hospital, *Duke-NUS* Medical School, Singapore, *SDU* Sleep Disorders Unit, Singapore General Hospital, *UCSD* University of California, San Diego School of Medicine, *IS-RC* Research study on sleep disordered breathing in women in midlife, University of Pennsylvania, Philadelphia, *SIESTA* SIESTA sleep database, *Somnoval* Somnolyzer validation study dataset, *SOF* Study of Osteoporotic Fractures, *MrOS* Osteoporotic Fractures in Men study, *DOD-H* Dreem Open Dataset—Healthy Volunteers, *DOD-O* Dreem Open Dataset—Obstructive Sleep Apnea Patients, *homePAP* Home Positive Airway Pressure study, *ABC* Apnea, Bariatric surgery, and CPAP study, *SHIP* Study of Health in Pomerania, *PhysioNet* PhysioNet database resources, *ISRUC* ISRUC-SLEEP Dataset, *MESA* Multi-Ethnic Study of Atherosclerosis, *SAGIC* Sleep Apnea Genetics International Consortium, The Ohio State University Medical Center, Columbus *CNN* Convolutional neural network, *LSTM* long short-term memory, *RNN* Recurrent neural network, *MLP* multilayer perceptron, *GRU* gated recurrent unit, *LightGBM* decision tree-based gradient-boosting machine; decision tree, *MSTGCN* multi-view spatial-temporal graph convolutional network, *JK-STGCN* Jumping Knowledge Spatial-Temporal Graph Convolutional Network, *EBT* Ensemble bagged tree classifier, *MHSA* Multi-head self-attention studies, Somnolyzer achieved a kappa value of 0.74 versus a single scorer in 426 PSGs [59] and kappa values between 0.75 and 0.78 as compared to the consensus of multiple scorers in three clinical datasets [35]. These kappa values are well within the range of kappa values reported for external testing in Table 3. Most importantly, in the three studies with multiple scorers, the Somnolyzer autoscoring performance was compared to the interrater reliability between the manual scorers and the authors reported that within each dataset, agreement between autoscoring and unbiased manual consensus scoring was significantly higher than the mean agreement between individual manual scoring and unbiased manual consensus scoring (0.78 vs. 0.69; 0.74 vs. 0.67; and 0.75 vs. 0.67; all $p < 0.01$). Consequently, in contrast to the semi-automated scoring by the Somnolyzer version based on the decision tree [21], the AI-based Somnolyzer produced outputs ready for interpretation without the need for manual adjustment [35].

In addition to the overall accuracy, the performance of autoscoring systems should be evaluated per sleep stage. Table 4 gives an example of a confusion matrix for epoch-by-epoch sleep staging comparing Somnolyzer autoscoring with manual expert scoring in a NSRR (National Sleep Research Resource) dataset with 426 PSGs (see demographics in Table 5). As can be seen in Table 4, sensitivity (gray cells) and precision (equivalent to positive predictive value, PPV) was highest for stages W and R, intermediate for stages N2 and N3, and lowest for stage N1. The respective Cohen's kappa values indicated an almost perfect agreement for W and R (0.85 and 0.87), a substantial agreement for N2 and N3 (0.72 and 0.73) and still a moderate agreement for N1 (0.46) [59]. These Cohen's kappa values are close to the maximum values observed in the interrater reliability studies summarized in Table 1. Lee et al. [9] reported in their meta-analysis of interrater reliability of manual sleep stage scoring that the interrater reliabilities for stages W and R were substantial, those for stages N2 and N3 moderate, and that for stage N1 only fair.

Two noteworthy studies which scored sleep based on neurological signals were not included in the review in Table 3, since the authors did not report Cohen's kappa but rather $F1$ scores (i.e., harmonic mean of sensitivity and precision) [41, 67]. Both studies used a CNN-based encoder block (down scaling) for feature extraction and a CNN-based decoder block (up scaling). Applying this U-Net architecture, Perslev et al. [41] used 16 cohorts with 19,924 PSGs as training set and reported a $F1$ score of 0.79 in an external test set of 25 healthy controls and 0.76 in 55 patients with obstructive sleep apnea. Zhang et al. [67] used 1595 PSGs from 2 cohorts for training and reported a $F1$ score of 0.74 in a holdout test set with 199 PSGs. Perslev et al. [41] compared the performance of his algorithm (U-Sleep) with the performance obtained with the algorithms presented by Supratak et al. [49], Phan et al. [46], and Guillot et al. [37], and the results indicate similar performance of his methods with the algorithms listed in Table 3.

Table 4 Confusion matrix for epoch-by-epoch comparison between Somnolyzer sleep staging based on neurological signals and manual sleep staging (5-stages; $n = 426$)

		Manual staging				
		W	N1	N2	N3	R
Somnolyzer staging	W	87.1%	12.2%	1.2%	0.3%	2.6%
	N1	9.1%	61.7%	12.3%	0.3%	6.4%
	N2	1.9%	22.2%	81.5%	27.2%	4.2%
	N3	0.1%	0.1%	4.3%	72.2%	0.0%
	R	1.8%	3.9%	0.8%	0.0%	86.8%
	PPV	91.6%	46.0%	84.1%	78.9%	90.3%
Number of epochs[a]		114,645	46.756	160,432	36,146	55,626

Cohen's kappa (5-stages: W, N1, N2, N3, R): 0.739 (95%-CI 0.737–0.741); Accuracy: 80.7%
Cohen's kappa (4-stages: W, N1 + N2, N2, R): 0.812 (95%-CI 0.810–0.813); Accuracy: 88.0%
[a]Values indicate the number of manually scored epochs per sleep stage. Gray cells indicate the percentage of epochs within each manually defined sleep stage that were correctly identified by Somnolyzer (that is, sensitivity). The percentage values labeled as positive predictive value (PPV) represent the percentage of epochs within each Somnolyzer-defined sleep stage that was correct per manual staging (that is, precision)

4 Review of AI-Based Algorithms Using Cardiorespiratory Signals as Input

We included in the review AI-based sleep scoring algorithms which used cardio- and/or respiratory signals as input (such as those typically recorded in HSAT: respiratory flow/effort, PPG, ECG, actigraphy) and reported Cohen's kappa for the 4-stage comparison (wake, LS, DS, REM). In total, 10 studies published between 2018 and 2022 have been identified and included in the review.

We summarized the major characteristics of the studies based on cardiorespiratory signals in Table 6, including author, publication year and, if appropriate name of the scoring system; the training dataset(s) (HC: healthy controls, PAT: patients with sleep disorders, OSA: patients sleep obstructive sleep apnea, Cohort: subjects from cohort studies); the input channels and feature extraction method (epoch encoder); the classifier (sequence encoder); the test dataset(s) and the testing approach (CV: cross-validation, HO: holdout validation, EXT: external test set); finally Cohen's kappa for the 4-stage comparison for internal testing (cross-validation or in a

Table 5 Descriptive demographic and clinical information (Somnolyzer test study based on neurological signals; $n = 426$ PSGs)

Variable	MESA ($n = 224$)	HomePAP ($n = 178$)	ABC ($n = 24$)
Age (years)	69.8 ± 8.8	46.1 ± 12.1	50.5 ± 9.1
Gender (number; %)			
Female	110; 49.1%	89; 50.0%	14; 58.3%
Male	114; 50.9%	89; 50.0%	10; 41.7%
Ethnicity (number; %)	–		
Hispanic		14; 7.9%	2; 8.3%
Non-Hispanic		163; 91.6%	22; 91.7%
Unknown		1; 0.6%	–
Race (number; %)	–		
White		124; 69.7%	16; 66.7%
African American		44; 24.7%	4; 16.7%
Other		10; 5.6%	4; 16.7%
Ethnicity/race composite (number)		–	–
White/Caucasian	84; 37.5%		
Chinese-American	36; 16.1%		
African American	53; 23.7%		
Hispanic	51; 22.8%		
Other	–		
Body mass index (kg/m^2)	–	40.0 ± 9.2	38.6 ± 2.9
Neck circumference (cm)			
Systolic blood pressure (mmHg)	–	125.4 ± 12.9	–
Diastolic blood pressure (mmHg)	–	79.8 ± 9.0	–
AHI_{PSG} (events/hour)	28.0 ± 17.6 (range 1–88)	13.0 ± 16.7 (range 0–113)	50.5 ± 9.1 (range 15–115)
SDB severity (number; %)			
None	17; 7.6%	69; 38.8%	0; 0.0%
Mild	17; 7.6%	59; 33.1%	0; 0.0%
Moderate	107; 47.8%	31; 17.4%	4; 16.7%
Severe	83; 37.1%	19; 10.7%	20; 83.3%
Epworth Sleepiness Scale score (/24)	5.8 ± 3.9	14.2 ± 3.7	–
Total sleep time per PSG (hours)	5.9 ± 1.4	5.7 ± 1.1	7.0 ± 1.5
Recording time (hours)	10.6 ± 1.2	7.8 ± 1.1	8.4 ± 0.2

holdout dataset) or external testing (datasets completely unseen by the model during training and validation) [68–77].

As can be seen in the last row of Table 6, there is a large difference in the size of the training data (between 27 and 9338 PSGs) as well as in the size of the test data (between 9 and 1000). Like the algorithms using neurological signals, Cohen's kappa for the 11 internal test sets was higher than Cohen's kappa for the 10 external test sets (0.56 ± 0.12 vs. 0.47 ± 0.15). However, the difference was not significant due to the higher variance of the kappa values for the cardiorespiratory staging as compared to the variance of the kappa values for the neurological staging. The

Table 6 Review of AI sleep staging for HSAT based on cardiorespiratory signals (4-stages Cohen's Kappa: Wake, LS, DS, REM)

Author name, year	Training	Feature extraction/epoch encoder	Classifier/Sequence encoder	Test	Cohen's K	
					Internal	External
Li et al., 2018 [68]	PAT (OSA): $N = 18$ SLPDB Cohort: $N = 994$ PhysioNet CinC 2018 Cohort: $N = 5793$ SHHS	ECG (cardiorespiratory coupling spectrogram + CNN + engineered features)	SVM	PAT (OSA): SLPDB Cohort: PhysioNet CinC 2018 Cohort: SHHS	0.54 (CV) 0.31 (CV) 0.47 (CV)	
Radha et al., 2019 [69]	Cohort: $N = 584$; SIESTA (7 sleep centers) 2–6 scorers	ECG (IBI, engineered features)	MLP + bidirectional LSTM	Cohort: SIESTA	0.61 (CV)	
Wei et al., 2019 [74]	PAT: $N = 373$; Clinical	ECG (IBI, engineered features)	MLP + LSTM	PAT: $N = 75$; Clinical	0.55 (HO)	
Sun et al., 2020 [73]	PAT: $N = 8682$; MGH	ECG, respiratory effort (IBI, raw respiratory signals) + CNN	Bidirectional LSTM	PAT: MGH, Cohort: $N = 1000$; SHHS	0.59* (CV) *5 stages	0.53* *5 stages
Sridhar et al., 2020 [72]	Cohort: $N = 7499$ SHHS Cohort: $N = 1839$ MESA	ECG (IBI) + CNN	Dilated CNN	Cohort: $N = 794$; SHHS Cohort: $N = 220$; MESA Cohort: $N = 993$; PhysioNet CinC	0.66 (HO) 0.69 (HO)	0.55

(continued)

Table 6 (continued)

Author name, year	Training	Feature extraction/epoch encoder	Classifier/Sequence encoder	Test	Cohen's K	
					Internal	External
Fonseca et al., 2020 [71]	Cohort: $N = 584$; SIESTA (7 sleep centers) 2–6 scorers PAT: $N = 97$; Somnoval (3 sleep centers) 4 scorers	ECG, accelerometer (IBI, gross body movements, engineered features)	MLP + bidirectional LSTM	Clinical: $N = 389$; SOMNIA		0.60
Zhao & Sun, 2021 [75]	Cohort: $N = 27$; PhysioNet CAP	PPG (wavelet transform, engineered features)	LightGBM	Cohort: PhysioNet CAP	0.69 (CV)	
Huttunen et al., 2021 [76]	$N = 2149$; pre-training PAT (OSA): $N = 702$ clinical	Raw PPG signal + CNN	Bidirectional LSTM	PAT (OSA): $N = 175$; Clinical	0.64 (HO)	
Bakker et al., 2021 [70] *Somnolyzer-CReSS*	Cohort: $N = 588$ SIESTA (7 sleep centers), 2–6 scorers PAT: $N = 97$ Somnoval (3 sleep centers), 4 scorers	ECG or PPG, airflow, respiratory effort (IBI, raw respiratory signals), CNN + bidirectional LSTM	MLP + bidirectional LSTM	Cohort: $N = 296$; MESA Cohort: $N = 296$; SHHS		0.68 0.64

Garcia-Molina & Jiang, 2022 [77]	Cohort: $N = 700$ PhysioNet CinC	ECG (IBI) + CNN	LSTM	Cohort: $N = 294$; PhysioNet CinC HC: $N = 45$; Sleep Number smart bed, 3 scorers HC: $N = 16$; PhysioNet CAP INS: $N = 9$; PhysioNet CAP RBD: $N = 22$; PhysioNet CAP PLMD:$N = 10$;PhysioNetCAP	0.39 (HO)	0.44 0.31 0.39 0.24 0.36
Summary	**Training data**			**Test data**	**Cohen's K**	
					Internal	**External**
***N*-studies** **Range: minimum** **maximum** **Mean ± SD**	**10** $N = 27$ $N = 9338$			**21** $N = 9$ $N = 1000$	**11** **0.31** **0.69** **0.56 ± 0.12**	**10** **0.24** **0.68** **0.47 ± 0.15**

Internal performance of holdout or cross-validation, *External* performance in datasets completely unseen by the model, *CV* cross-validation, *HO* holdout validation

Cohort cohort study, *HC* healthy controls, *PAT* patients with sleep disturbance, *OSA* patients with obstructive sleep apnea, *INS* insomnia patients, *RBD* REM sleep behavior disorder, *PLMD* periodic limb movement disorder

SLPDB MIT-BIH Polysomnographic Database, *PhysioNet CinC* PhysioNet Computing in Cardiology Challenge database, *SHHS* Sleep Heart Health Study, *SIESTA* SIESTA sleep database, *MGH* Massachusetts General Hospital, *MESA* Multi-Ethnic Study of Atherosclerosis, *Somnoval* Somnolyzer validation study dataset, *SOMNIA* Sleep and OSA Monitoring with Non-Invasive Applications study, *PhysioNet CAP* PhysioNet CAP sleep database

CNN Convolutional neural network, *SVM* support vector machine, *MLP* multilayer perceptron, *LSTM* long short-term memory, *LightGBM* decision tree-based gradient-boosting machine

Somnolyzer-CReSS algorithm [70] achieved in a test set of 296 PSGs from the MESA study a kappa value of 0.68 and in a second test set of 296 PSGs from the SHHS a kappa value of 0.64, which are the two highest kappa values for external testing of cardiorespiratory sleep staging algorithms reported to date (Table 6).

The confusion matrix for epoch-by-epoch sleep staging comparing Somnolyzer-CReSS staging with manual sleep staging for each of the 4 sleep stages scored by CReSS (wake, LS, DS, REM) for 296 ambulatory PSGs from the MESA dataset is shown in Table 7 (see Table 8 for demographic and clinical information). As can be seen in Table 7, sensitivity (gray cells) and precision (PPV) is high for stages wake, LS, and REM sleep and lower for DS. As shown in Table 3, based on neurological signals, sensitivity and precision for detecting wake is 87.1% and 91.6%, respectively. Interestingly, sensitivity and precision for detecting wake based cardiorespiratory signals is not much worse (76.0% and 88.1%, Table 7). This indicates the good performance of the cardiorespiratory sleep staging for discriminating wake and sleep, which is important for the determination of the total sleep time and consequently for the determination of indices relating the number of respiratory or oxygen desaturation events to the hours of sleep. As compared to indices computed based on the duration of recording or monitoring time, the indices related to CReSS-determined total sleep time show a higher sensitivity, specifically in recordings with a significant amount of wake periods. To demonstrate the clinical relevance of CReSS, we determined the number of correctly diagnosed patients by HSAT as compared to the gold standard AHI in the 296 studies from the MESA dataset for a threshold of 15 events per hour. As can be seen in Table 9, using the CReSS-derived total sleep time (TST) instead of the recording time as denominator for the calculation of the indices reduced the false negative diagnosis from 33 patients (11.1%) to 5 patients (1.7%).

Concerning the detection of REM sleep, while Somnolyzer based on neurological signals achieved a sensitivity of 86.8% and a precision of 90.3% (Table 4), sensitivity and precision for detecting REM sleep based on cardiorespiratory signals is not much worse (85.3% and 79.6%, Table 7). This indicates the good performance of CReSS for discriminating REM sleep from Wake and NREM sleep. Thus, REM-related OSA can be detected based on CReSS-determined REM sleep with a clinically relevant accuracy. Using the definition for REM-related OSA by Mokhlesi and Punjabi [78] (i.e., an AHI_{NREM} of fewer than 5 events/h and an AHI_{REM} of at least 5 events/h with at least 30 minutes of REM sleep), we achieved a sensitivity of 91% and a specificity of 98% for detecting REM-related OSA by means of CReSS as compared to gold standard PSG scoring.

5 Summary of AI-Based Algorithms

Based on these reviews, there is now convincing evidence that AI-based sleep staging using neurological signals can achieve agreement with the "gold-standard" of manual scoring with accuracy comparable to interscorer reliability, suggesting

Table 7 Confusion matrix for epoch-by-epoch comparison between Somnolyzer sleep staging based on cardiorespiratory signals (CReSS) and manual sleep staging (4-stages; $n = 296$)

		Manual staging			
		W	N1 + N2	N3	R
Somnolyzer staging (CReSS)	Wake	76.0%	4.9%	0.5%	1.5%
	LS	20.2%	85.2%	49.5%	13.1%
	DS	0.2%	5.9%	49.6%	0.1%
	REM	3.5%	4.0%	0.3%	85.3%
	PPV	88.1%	79.4%	57.1%	79.6%
Number of epochs[a]		78,223	149,517	24,197	40,310

Cohen's kappa (4-stages): 0.680 (95%-CI 0.678–0.682); Accuracy: 79.8%

[a]Values indicate the number of manually scored epochs per sleep stage. Gray cells indicate the percentage of epochs within each manually defined sleep stage that were correctly identified by CReSS (that is, sensitivity). The percentage values labeled as positive predictive value (PPV) represent the percentage of epochs within each CReSS-defined sleep stage that was correct per manual staging (that is, precision)

that these algorithms are valid alternatives to manual scoring. It is also clear that AI-based sleep staging using cardiorespiratory signals can provide valuable estimates of wake and REM sleep as well as light and deep sleep in HSATs where typically no neurological signals are recorded.

In addition, these AI-based autoscoring systems offer several advantages to visual scoring. They provide a valid alternative to the rather expensive, time-consuming, and difficult visual scoring task that can be performed only by well-trained and experienced human scorers while attaining consistent scoring results. Furthermore, they enable proposition of added value such as scoring in real-time, and the estimation of sleep stage probabilities per epoch (hypnodensity). The remainder of this chapter will deal with this concept, and its possible applications in clinical research, and eventually, in clinical practice.

Table 8 Descriptive demographic and clinical information (Somnolyzer-CReSS test study based on cardiorespiratory signals; $n = 296$ PSGs)

	MESA ($n = 296$)
Age (years)	69.4 ± 8.8
Gender (number; %)	
Female	154; 52.0%
Male	142; 48.0%
Race/ethnicity (number)	
White/Caucasian	117; 39.5%
Chinese-American	31; 10.5%
African American	76; 25.7%
Hispanic	72; 24.3%
Other	–
AHI (events/hour)	22.9 ± 21.1 (median 16.9; Q1 5.7; Q3 34.5) (range 0–88)
SDB severity per AHI (number; %)[a]	
None	63; 21.3%
Mild	76; 25.7%
Moderate	73; 24.7%
Severe	84; 28.4%
Epworth sleepiness scale (/24)	6.2 ± 4.2
Total sleep time per PSG (hours)	6.0 ± 1.4
Recording time (hours)	10.6 ± 1.3

Data are provided as mean ± standard deviation unless otherwise indicated
[a]PSGs were selected for inclusion based on the AHI variable available in the NSRR metadata

Table 9 Confusion matrices comparing the diagnostic performance of HSAT with and without CReSS to gold standard PSG ($n = 296$)

		AHI_{PSG}	
		<15 events/hour	≥15 events/hour
REI_{RT}	<15 events/hour	**139 (47.0%)**	33 (11.1%)
	≥15 events/hour	0 (0.0%)	**124 (41.9%)**
AHI_{CReSS}	<15 events/hour	**139 (47.0%)**	5 (1.7%)
	≥15 events/hour	0 (0.0%)	**152 (51.4%)**

AHI_{PSG}: Apnea-hypopnea index based on PSG-determined total sleep time
REI_{RT}: Respiratory event index based on recording time (RT)
AHI_{CReSS}: Apnea-hypopnea index based on CReSS-determined total sleep time

6 Estimating Sleep Stage Probabilities per Epoch (Hypnodensity)

The primary output of AI-based sleep staging algorithms is usually sleep stage probabilities per 30-s epoch which can be translated into a traditional, discrete hypnogram using a simple rule-based approach. However, the probabilities can also be plotted in pseudo color graphs which have been referred to as hypnodensity by

Stephansen et al. [38]. If multiple human scorings are available, a hypnodensity graph can also be derived from these scorings to visualize ambiguous epochs. Van Gorp et al. [79] recently introduced a framework to analyze uncertainty in sleep staging differentiating aleatoric uncertainty that arises from biological factors (such as age, drugs, pathologies, or local sleep) or measurement factors (such as placing of electrodes or interferences and artifacts) and epistemic uncertainty that arises from a lack of knowledge about the data or the optimal model.

Twelve hypnograms as scored independently by 12 technologists are displayed in Fig. 1 (Manual-1 to Manual-12). In addition, the hypnogram based on manual consensus scoring using a majority vote (Manual) and the hypnogram based on Somnolyzer autoscoring (Somnolyzer) are shown. Cohen's kappa based on the epoch-by-epoch comparison between the Somnolyzer and manual consensus scoring is 0.852, while Cohen's kappa comparing the manual scorers with the unbiased consensus scoring (i.e., consensus scoring without the assessed scorer included in the consensus) ranged between 0.654 (Manual-1) and 0.824 (Manual-7). Superimposed on the two latter hypnograms are the hypnodensity graphs based on the sleep stage probabilities derived from the 12 manual scorings and on the sleep stage probabilities derived from Somnolyzer. The intraclass correlation coefficient (ICC) for absolute agreement (ICC (1, 2) according to Shroud and Fleiss [80]) was used to determine the agreement between the two sets of sleep stage probabilities. For the example in Fig. 1, the ICCs were for stage W: 0.96, for N1: 0.80, for N2: 0.93, for N3: 0.97, for R: 0.96, across all 5 stages: 0.94. In Fig. 2, the hypnodensity charts based on manual scoring and based on Somnolyzer autoscoring are compared for the 10 studies where 12 independent expert scorings were available (i.e., dataset C in Bakker et al. [35]). As can be seen, the ICCs between manually derived probabilities and autoscoring-derived probabilities ranged from 0.82 to 0.98 (mean: 0.91 ± 0.05), indicating almost perfect agreement between the probability curves. While we have shown in previous sections that AI-based neurological scoring can achieve a high level of agreement with manual scorings, we showed here that the AI-derived hypnodensity accurately reflects the epoch-by-epoch ambiguity resulting from multiple manual scorings. This ambiguity reflects the uncertainty of manual scorers for assigning the sleep stages, despite following the same rules.

The AI-based classifier using the cardiorespiratory signals (CReSS) can also output sleep stage probabilities per 30-s epoch for stages Wake, LS, DS, and REM sleep. The CReSS-derived probability curves can be directly compared to the probabilities derived from multiple manual scorings using neurological signals as input (Fig. 3). Note that the probabilities for N1 and N2 are summed up for the manual scorings to correspond to the light sleep probability of the CReSS autoscoring. As can be seen, the ICCs between manually derived probabilities and CReSS-derived probabilities range from 0.81 to 0.95 (mean: 0.88 ± 0.05), indicating good agreement between the probability curves. Consequently, also the CReSS-derived hypnodensity reflects a good estimate of the epoch-by-epoch ambiguity of manual scorings. The fact that very similar probabilities are derived from cardiorespiratory signals and neurological signals suggests that many of these uncertainties between sleep stages manifest in both, the central and the autonomic

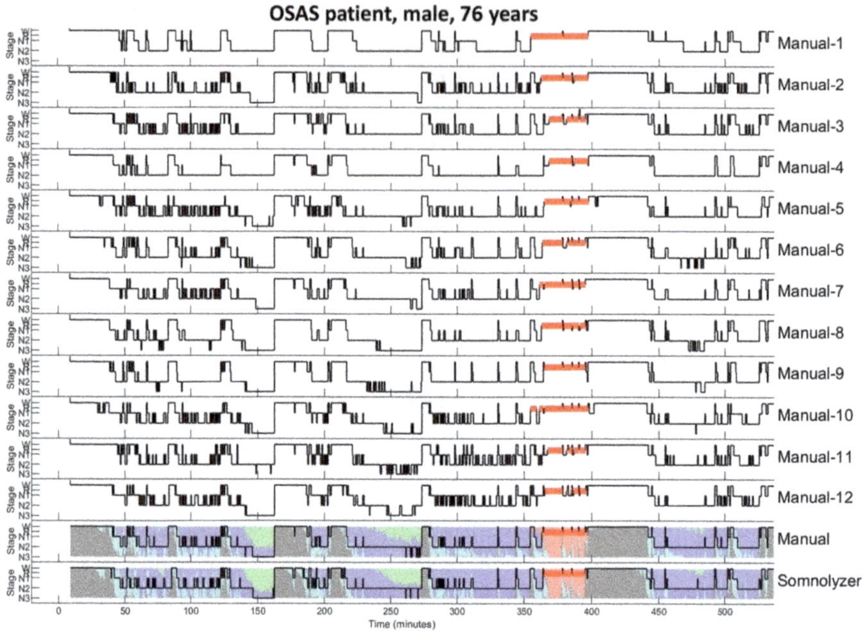

Fig. 1 A representative example of 12 manually scored hypnograms, the derived manual consensus hypnogram superimposed on the hypnodensity chart based on manual scorings, and the Somnolyzer autoscored hypnogram superimposed on the hypnodensity based on Somnolyzer scoring for a single PSG (OSAS patient, male, 76 years). This PSG was scored by 12 technologists and by Somnolyzer. Individual hypnograms are presented in *Manual-1* to *Manual-12*. *Manual* depicts the hypnogram based on manual consensus scoring and the hypnodensity chart based on sleep stage probabilities derived from the 12 manual scorings. *Somnolyzer* depicts the hypnogram and the hypnodensity chart based on autoscoring. Color codes for the hypnodensity chart are W: gray; N1: cyan; N2: blue; N3: green; R: red

nervous system activity. This supports the view that states in-between two sleep stages are normal physiological states and that much of the uncertainty observed in sleep scorings is of an aleatoric nature, limiting the potential for further increases in interscorer agreement by means of improved scoring rules, training, or models.

All sleep scoring parameters usually reported in PSG studies according to the AASM manual (total sleep time, sleep efficiency, time and percentage in each sleep stage, sleep and REM latency, and wake after sleep onset), can be derived directly from the hypnodensity in two different ways. The traditional way is to determine a single hypnogram from the hypnodensity (e.g., based on multiple manual scorings, one can obtain the majority vote per epoch) and compute all parameters based on this hypnogram. Alternatively, the parameters can be computed directly from the sleep stage probabilities by calculating the area under the probability curves of the respective stages. If the hypnodensity is based on multiple manual scorers, the hypnodensity-derived sleep parameters correspond to the mean of the sleep parameters calculated from each manually scored hypnogram. Note that these mean

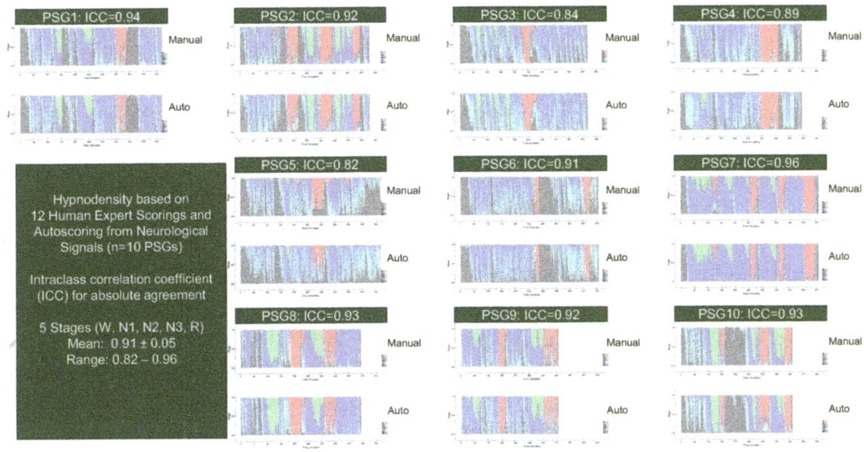

Fig. 2 Comparison between the hypnodensity chart obtained from 12 manual scorings and from Somnolyzer autoscoring based on neurological signals ($n = 10$). For each of the 10 studies from the Somnoval dataset, the hypnodensity graph based on the 12 manual scorings (*Manual*) is compared to the hypnodensity graph based on the Somnolyzer autoscoring (*Auto*). In addition, the intraclass correlation coefficient (ICC) for absolute agreement between the manual and the autoscored probability traces are given. Color codes for the hypnodensity chart are W: gray; N1: cyan; N2: blue; N3: green; R: red

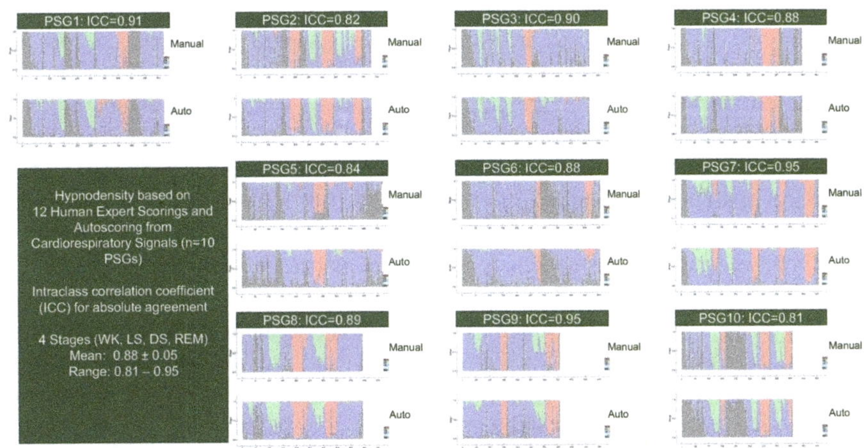

Fig. 3 Comparison between the hypnodensity chart obtained from 12 manual scorings based on neurological signals and from Somnolyzer autoscoring based on cardiorespiratory signals (CReSS) ($n = 10$). For each of the 10 studies from the Somnoval dataset, the hypnodensity graph based on the 12 manual scorings (*Manual*) is compared to the hypnodensity graph based on the Somnolyzer-CReSS autoscoring (*Auto*). In addition, the intraclass correlation coefficient (ICC) for absolute agreement between the manual and the autoscored probability traces are given. Color codes for the hypnodensity chart are W: gray; N1 + N2 (LS): blue; N3 (DS): green; R: red

values are not necessarily equal to the parameters computed from a majority vote hypnogram. Table 10 summarizes the sleep parameters for the study shown in Fig. 1. Note the high variability of the parameters derived from each manually scored hypnogram (for instance 23.5–134 minutes N1 or 0–67 minutes N3). While the time in N1 and N3 are—based on the majority vote hypnogram—66 and 17.5 minutes, respectively, the time in N1 averaged over the 12 scorers is 78 minutes and the time in N3 27 minutes. As shown in Figs. 2 and 3, the sleep stage probabilities derived from autoscoring are in good agreement with the sleep stage probabilities derived from multiple human scorers. Thus, parameters computed directly from the autoscored hypnodensity also mimic well the average of the parameters obtained from multiple manually scored hypnograms (see Table 10).

In Table 11, we compare total sleep time (TST), sleep latency (SL), REM latency (REML), sleep efficiency (SEFF), wake after sleep onset (WASO), and the time in N1, N2, N3, and R derived from the autoscored *hypnogram*, to the parameters derived from the autoscored *hypnodensity* for young (20–<40 years), middle-aged (40–<60 years), and older (60–95 years) healthy controls from the Siesta database (n = 195, 93 males and 102 females aged 20–95 years) [36]. In the last column of Table 11, the correlation coefficients between age and the respective parameters are given. Overall, the hypnogram-derived and the hypnodensity-derived parameters show very similar age-related changes. However, the correlation coefficients based on the hypnodensity-derived parameters were slightly higher than the coefficients derived traditionally from the hypnogram (see also Fig. 4).

Moreover, as can be seen in Table 11, the standard deviations are, for all parameters and age groups slightly, yet consistently smaller for the hypnodensity-derived parameters than for the hypnogram-derived parameters, indicating that the hypnodensity-derived parameters are more robust estimates of the sleep stage distributions. Note that sleep and REM latency are identical for both approaches, since the first epoch automatically scored as sleep or REM is also the first epoch with a wake probability below 0.5 or a REM probability above 0.5, respectively.

Moreover, since the hypnodensity reflects the uncertainty of manual experts for assigning a sleep stage to each epoch, $100 * (1 - p(i)_{\mathrm{MAX}})$ is a quantitative measure of sleep stage ambiguity in percent, where $p(i)_{\mathrm{MAX}}$ is the highest probability for epoch i. In case of no ambiguity, $p(i)_{\mathrm{MAX}}$ is 1 and thus the ambiguity for that epoch is 0%. As can be clearly seen in Fig. 2 for both manually determined and Somnolyzer-determined sleep stage probabilities, the vast majority of epochs have a $p(i)_{\mathrm{MAX}} < 1.0$, indicating some amount of ambiguity. The mean ambiguity for epochs assigned as sleep (TST), wake after sleep onset (WASO), N1, N2, N3, and R are listed for each age group in Table 11 and plotted in Fig. 5.

The highest ambiguity (34%) is seen in epochs scored as N1. This was to be expected given the low agreement of manual scorers on scoring N1. Interestingly, with a non-significant correlation of 0.02, this high ambiguity of N1 seems independent of age. In contrast, the highest correlation with age was found in the increase of ambiguity of the epochs scored as sleep from young to older subjects (11.5% and 16.5%, respectively) with a Pearson correlation coefficient of 0.62, higher than the correlation coefficient found with any of the other standard sleep

Table 10 Sleep parameters derived from individual manual scorings, from multiple manual scorings, and from Somnolyzer autoscoring (OSAS patient, male, 76 years)

Scorer	TST (min)	N1 (min)	N2 (min)	N3 (min)	R (min)
Manual-1	356.5	83	231.5	0	42
Manual-2	381.5	74.5	253	21	33
Manual-3	357.5	88	247	0	22.5
Manual-4	387	48	311.5	0	27.5
Manual-5	408	94.5	264	18.5	31
Manual-6	360	53.5	245.5	33.5	27.5
Manual-7	382	83.5	248	19.5	31
Manual-8	370.5	45	228.5	67	30
Manual-9	370.5	23.5	255.5	62.5	29
Manual-10	399	115.5	200	45	38.5
Manual-11	348	96	217	13	22
Manual-12	375.5	134	180	39	22.5
Manual-mean = Manual-hypnodensity	374.7	78.3	240.1	26.6	29.7
Manual-consensus hypnogram	372.5	62	259	20.5	31
Somnolyzer-hypnodensity	389.0	88.5	243.9	31.0	25.6
Somnolyzer-hypnogram	385	68	270.5	17	29.5

Manual-1 to Manual-12: parameters derived from the twelve individual manual scorings
Manual-Mean: mean value of the 12 parameters, which is equal to parameters derived from the hypnodensity based on the manual scorings. *Manuel-Consensus Hypnogram*: parameters derived from the manual consensus hypnogram. *Somnolyzer-Hypnodensity:* parameters derived from the Somnolyzer-based hypnodensity. *Somnolyzer-Hypnogram:* parameters derived from Somnolyzer-scored hypnogram
Light and dark ocher cells indicate per parameter the lowest and highest value, respectively; gray cells indicate parameters based on multiple manual scorers; blue cells indicate parameters based on Somnolyzer autoscoring

Table 11 Age-related changes in Somnolyzer autoscored hypnogram (HG)- and hypnodensity (HD)-derived parameters in healthy controls ($n = 195$)

		Young ($n = 61$) Mean ± SD	Middle-aged ($n = 59$) Mean ± SD	Older ($n = 75$) Mean ± SD	Correlation ($n = 195$)r (p)
TST	HG (min)	418.1 ± 39.6	403.1 ± 39.0	372.3 ± 49.0	−0.39 (0.001)
	HD (min)	419.6 ± 38.7	402.7 ± 37.6	373.0 ± 47.7	−0.44 (0.001)
	HD-ambiguity (%)	11.5 ± 2.3	13.6 ± 2.6	16.5 ± 3.7	+0.62 (0.001)
	HD-continuity (%)	95.1 ± 0.9	94.5 ± 1.2	93.4 ± 1.5	−0.52 (0.001)
SL	HG, HD (min)	19.3 ± 20.3	20.2 ± 18.6	16.8 ± 11.9	−0.05 (0.456)
REML	HG, HD (min)	83.4 ± 32.2	88.1 ± 37.6	82.8 ± 44.6	−0.02 (0.771)
SEFF	HG (%)	88.1 ± 7.4	84.5 ± 6.6	77.9 ± 9.6	−0.47 (0.001)
	HD (%)	88.4 ± 7.2	84.5 ± 6.2	78.1 ± 9.3	−0.49(0.001)
WASO	HG (min)	37.7 ± 30.3	53.5 ± 26.4	88.7 ± 43.5	+0.53 (0.001)
	HD (min)	37.4 ± 28.9	55.3 ± 25.7	89.3 ± 42.4	+0.55 (0.001)
	HD-ambiguity (%)	15.3 ± 5.4	13.0 ± 4.7	11.1 ± 4.6	−0.33 (0.001)
	HD-continuity (%)	90.4 ± 5.1	91.9 ± 3.9	93.9 ± 3.2	+0.35 (0.001)
N1	HG (min)	32.2 ± 15.4	43.3 ± 17.1	58.3 ± 35.1	+0.40 (0.001)
	HD (min)	38.6 ± 13.6	48.3 ± 15.7	62.0 ± 27.7	+0.44 (0.001)
	HD-ambiguity (%)	34.2 ± 3.6	34.3 ± 4.0	34.2 ± 5.3	0.02 (0.770)
	HD-continuity (%)	86.5 ± 2.4	86.1 ± 2.4	86.2 ± 2.3	−0.06 (0.390)
N2	HG (min)	217.1 ± 35.2	223.6 ± 39.7	200.1 ± 43.0	−0.16 (0.024)
	HD (min)	213.2 ± 33.6	217.3 ± 35.2	193.7 ± 39.2	−0.20 (0.004)
	HD-ambiguity (%)	8.4 ± 2.0	9.8 ± 2.4	12.8 ± 3.7	+0.56 (0.001)
	HD-continuity (%)	95.3 ± 1.0	95.2 ± 1.2	93.8 ± 1.8	−0.42 (0.001)
N3	HG (min)	71.6 ± 21.4	46.9 ± 25.7	42.9 ± 31.5	−0.39 (0.001)
	HD (min)	77.5 ± 20.0	54.5 ± 24.0	51.5 ± 31.1	−0.37 (0.001)
	HD-ambiguity (%)	11.9 ± 6.9	20.1 ± 9.4	22.3 ± 9.3	+0.48 (0.001)
	HD-continuity (%)	97.3 ± 1.1	96.3 ± 1.2	96.0 ± 1.2	−0.46 (0.001)
R	HG (min)	97.2 ± 23.7	89.2 ± 21.8	70.9 ± 25.4	−0.42 (0.001)
	HD (min)	90.4 ± 20.0	82.6 ± 20.8	65.8 ± 22.9	−0.44 (0.001)
	HD-ambiguity (%)	10.4 ± 2.6	10.6 ± 3.5	11.7 ± 6.1	+0.15 (0.031)
	HD-continuity (%)	93.8 ± 1.8	93.5 ± 2.8	93.0 ± 3.2	−0.15 (0.038)

parameters (see Fig. 4). Figure 6 shows the scatter plot between age and the ambiguity of sleep epochs with separate regression lines for males and females. As can be seen, the age-related changes are similar for males and females. Males, however, show, independently of age, higher ambiguity values ($t = 2.33$; df = 193; $p = 0.021$). Univariate ANOVA reveals a significant effect of age ($F = 2.60$; df = 64.90; $p < 0.001$) and sex ($F = 12.39$; df = 1.90; $p < 0.001$), while the interaction between age and sex is not significant ($F = 0.97$; df = 39.90; $p = 0.524$).

The increase in ambiguity over age is specifically seen in N2 sleep. Note that in young and middle-aged subjects, N2 sleep shows the lowest ambiguity of all stages (8.4% and 9.8%, respectively). The ambiguity of N3 sleep is also rather

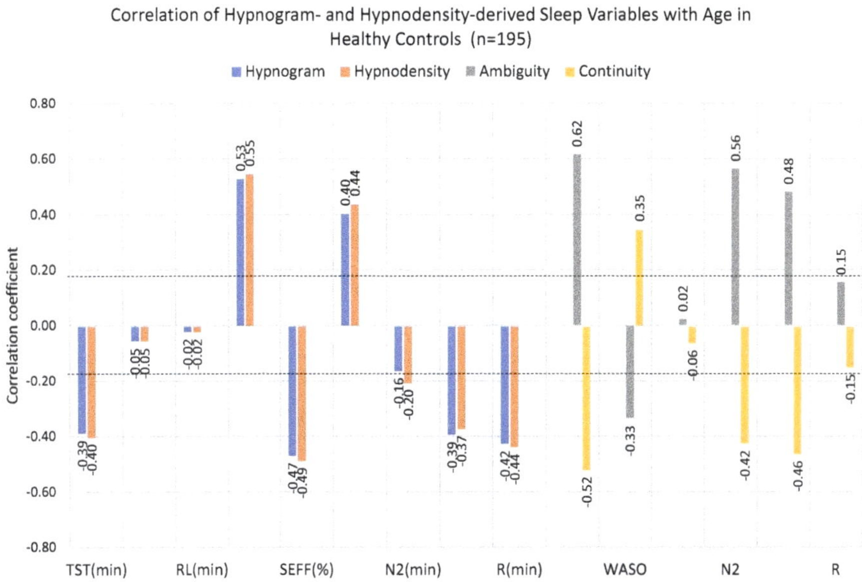

Fig. 4 Correlation between auto-scored hypnogram- and hypnodensity-derived parameters and age in healthy controls ($n = 195$). The figure depicts the Pearson correlation coefficients of various sleep parameters with age for the healthy subjects from the SIESTA sleep database (93 males and 102 females aged 20–95 years): Blue bars: sleep parameters derived from hypnogram; Orange bars: sleep parameters derived from hypnodensity; Gray bars: sleep stage ambiguity derived from hypnodensity; Yellow bars: epoch-to-epoch sleep stage continuity derived from hypnodensity; TST total sleep time, SL sleep latency, RL REM latency, WASO wake after sleep onset; The dotted lines indicate the $p < 0.01$ significance thresholds for the correlation coefficients

low in young subjects (11.9%) but increases significantly to middle-aged subjects (20.1%) and older subjects (22.3%). Finally, REM sleep ambiguity is, at about 11%, independent of the age group. In contrast to the increase in ambiguity during sleep, the ambiguity of epochs scored as wake after sleep onset decreases over age from 15.3% in young subjects to 11.1% in old subjects ($r = -0.33$).

In addition, we computed for each epoch i a measure of sleep stage continuity in percent: $100 * (1 - \text{abs}(p(i)_{\text{MAX}} - p(i + 1)_{\text{MAX}}))$, after excluding transition epochs (i.e., epoch with a change in the assigned sleep stage in the following epoch), thereby excluding the influence of sleep fragmentation due to stage shifts on the sleep stage continuity measure. In case of only small changes in the hypnodensity between two adjacent epochs, the continuity measure is close to 100%. Consequently, the continuity measure will decrease when the change in the hypnodensity between two adjacent epochs increases. The mean continuity for epochs assigned as sleep (TST), wake after sleep onset (WASO), N1, N2, N3, and R are listed for each age group in Table 11 and plotted in Fig. 7. The lowest continuity measure is seen in N1 (86%, independent of the age group), which corresponds to the fact that N1 sleep is typically an instable sleep state. While the hypnodensity-

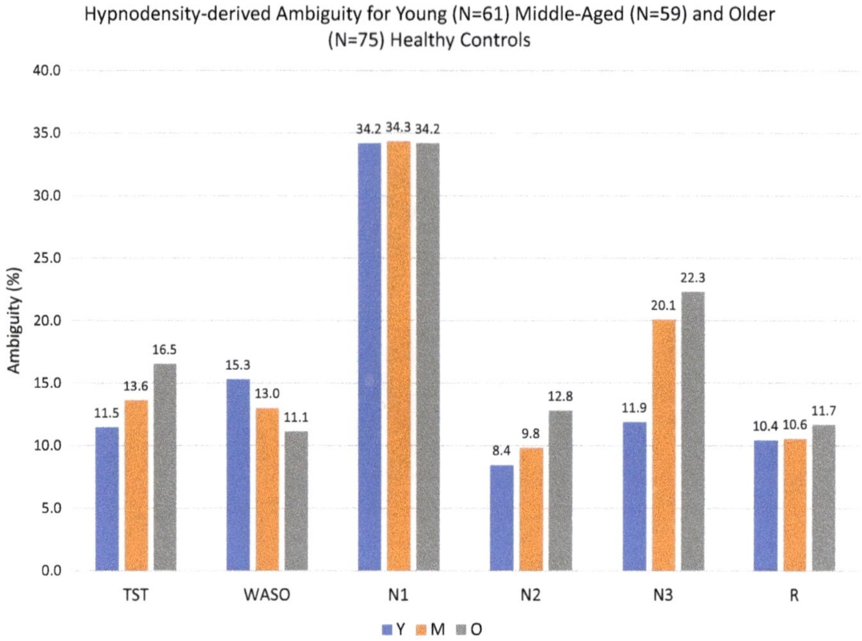

Fig. 5 Hypnodensity-derived sleep stage ambiguity in young ($n = 61$), middle-aged ($n = 59$), and older ($n = 75$) healthy controls. The figure depicts sleep stage ambiguity in percent averaged over epochs scored as sleep (TST), wake after sleep onset (WASO), N1, N2, N3, or R for young (20–<40 years), middle-aged (40–<60 years), and older (60–95 years) healthy controls from the Siesta database

derived continuity in epochs scored as wake after sleep onset increased with age ($r = 0.35$), the continuity of epochs scored as sleep decreased significantly with age ($r = -0.52$). This decrease in continuity was seen in both N2 ($r = -0.42$) and N3 ($r = -0.46$), while the continuity measure in stages N1 and R did not change significantly with age.

Partial correlation coefficients (controlling for the effect of age) are compared in Fig. 8 between sleep parameters derived from hypnogram and hypnodensity with the arousal index in the 195 healthy controls. As for the correlation with age, the hypnogram-derived and the hypnodensity-derived parameters show similar correlations with the arousal index (ArI). And again, the parameters determined directly from the area under the sleep stage probability curves showed higher correlations than the parameters derived from the majority vote hypnogram, further supporting the higher robustness of the hypnodensity-derived parameters. While the correlation with the time in N1 and the ArI is 0.46 for the hypnogram-derived parameter, the correlation is 0.59 for the time in N1 derived directly from the hypnodensity. The highest correlation with ArI is seen for the continuity in epochs scored as sleep indicating that the higher the ArI, the lower is the sleep stage continuity as measured by changes in epoch-to-epoch sleep stage probability ($r = -0.75$).

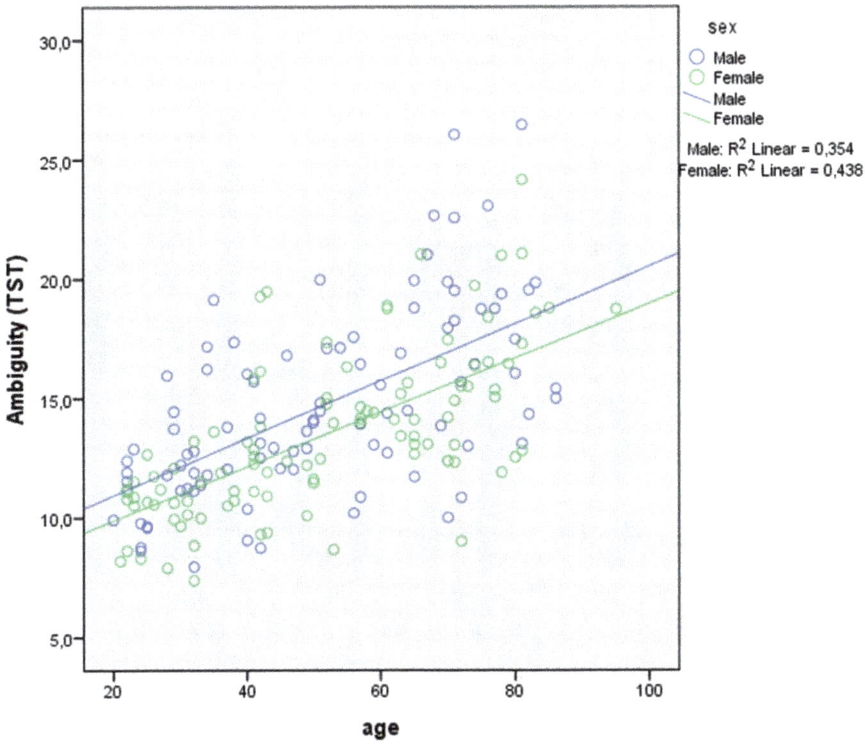

Fig. 6 Relationship between sleep stage ambiguity and age in healthy controls ($n = 195$). The scatterplot shows the increase of sleep stage ambiguity (%) as a function of age. The blue circles represent males ($n = 93$), the green circles females ($n = 102$). The blue line represents the regression line for males, the green line for females

7 Discussion and Conclusion

In summary, there is now convincing evidence that AI-based sleep staging using neurological signals can achieve agreement with the "gold-standard" of manual scoring, with accuracy comparable to the inter-scorer reliability across scorers, suggesting that these algorithms are valid alternatives to manual scoring while having the advantages of efficiency and consistency. This consistency of an automated scoring process can be beneficial in both clinical and research settings by minimizing inter- and intra-scorer variability. In an earlier study with 426 PSGs, we showed that Somnolyzer achieved an agreement with manual expert scoring that clearly exceeded the pre-defined performance targets which were based on published interscorer reliability studies [59]. We thus concluded that the variability between Somnolyzer and human scoring was no higher than the variability observed across experts. A key strength of this study was the inclusion of a large, ethnically/racially diverse sample, which supports the generalizability

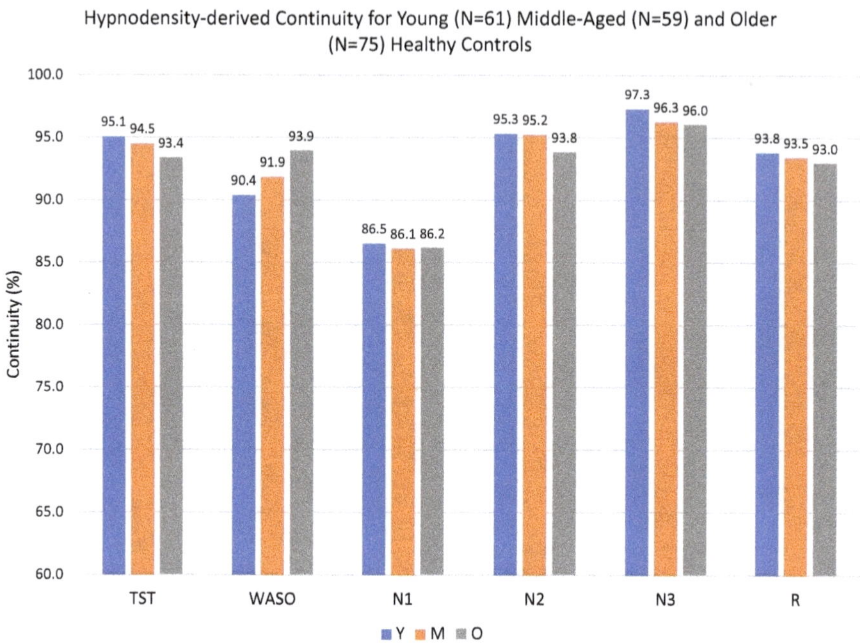

Fig. 7 Hypnodensity-derived epoch-to-epoch sleep stage continuity in young ($n = 61$), middle-aged ($n = 59$), and older ($n = 75$) healthy controls. The figure depicts sleep stage continuity in percent averaged over epochs scored as sleep (TST), wake after sleep onset (WASO), N1, N2, N3, or R for young (20–<40 years), middle-aged (40–<60 years), and older (60–95 years) healthy controls from the Siesta database

of algorithm performance, as well as the fact that the PSGs were collected in a range of clinical and research settings using various data collection platforms and montages. This selection criteria ensured that the performance of Somnolyzer was assessed across the full range of disease severity. An important limitation, however, was the fact that each PSG was scored only by a single technologist. Given the aforementioned variability across scorers, single expert scoring may not represent the true "gold standard" of manual scoring [4]. Note, however, that numerous different technologists scored the 426 PSGs and thus that the variability across scorers is reflected in the manual scorings used as the comparator in this study. In that respect, the comparator reflects standard practice in most clinical settings in which a single technologist is responsible for scoring each sleep study. In further studies, Bakker et al. [35] evaluated Somnolyzer in three external datasets with multiple scorers per study. Compared to consensus manual scoring, sleep staging derived from autoscoring was, for each individual PSG, non-inferior to manual scoring, suggesting that the output of Somnolyzer is ready for clinical interpretation without the need for manual adjustment. Based on these studies, the Somnolyzer 4.1 automatic scoring solution (an optional component of the Sleepware G3 software; Philips Respironics, Pittsburgh, PA) was cleared by the FDA (K202142) to be

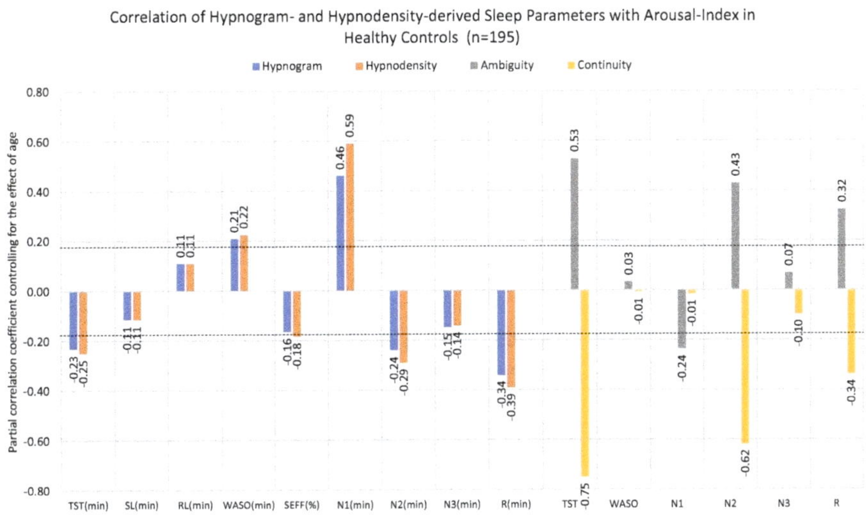

Fig. 8 Correlation between auto-scored hypnogram- and hypnodensity-derived parameters and the arousal index in healthy controls ($n = 195$). The figure depicts the partial correlation coefficients controlling for the effect of age of various sleep parameters with arousal index for the healthy subjects from the SIESTA sleep database (93 males and 102 females aged 20–95 years): Blue bars: sleep parameters derived from hypnogram; Orange bars: sleep parameters derived from hypnodensity; Gray bars: sleep stage ambiguity derived from hypnodensity; Yellow bars: epoch-to-epoch sleep stage continuity derived from hypnodensity; TST total sleep time, SL sleep latency, RL REM latency, WASO wake after sleep onset. The dotted lines indicate the $p < 0.01$ significance thresholds for the correlation coefficients

used in adults (18 and older) to generate an output that is ready for review and interpretation by a physician.

AI-based sleep staging using cardiorespiratory signals provide valuable estimates of wake and REM sleep as well as light and deep sleep in HSATs where typically no neurological signals are recorded, thereby increasing the sensitivity of diagnosing SDB [70]. This is particularly important in patients with low sleep efficiency, a hallmark of sleep disruptions and comorbid insomnia, which is very prevalent in patients with OSA [81]. Moreover, using cardiorespiratory sleep staging allows the detection of REM-related OSA. Note that patients with a relatively low overall AHI may be experiencing severe OSA during REM, which is particularly important given that events taking place during REM are longer, and are associated with more pronounced hypoxemia, higher sympathetic activation, and greater surges in blood pressure and heart rate [82–84]. Consequently, REM-related OSA is associated with adverse cardiovascular, metabolic, and neurocognitive outcomes. For a comprehensive review on risks for adverse health outcomes and on novel treatments of REM-related OSA, see Varga and Mokhlesi [85].

On the other hand, cardiorespiratory sleep staging does not achieve a performance comparable to sleep staging based on neurological signals. Cardiorespiratory signals are a surrogate measurement of sleep, while the clinical standard for quantitatively measuring sleep will remain a scoring based on neurological signals acquired with PSG. Note that the kappa values for cardiorespiratory sleep staging as presented in Table 6 (external kappa: 0.47 ± 0.15) are in average far below the kappa values for neurological sleep staging as presented in Table 3 (external kappa: 0.72 ± 0.06), even though the neurological signal-based kappa values are for 5-stage comparison, while those for the cardiorespiratory sleep staging are for 4-stage comparison. Indeed, as shown in Table 4, the Somnolyzer analysis based on the neurological signals combining N1 and N2 increases Cohen's kappa from 0.74 to 0.81 in the NSRR dataset ($n = 426$).

As discussed in the review of AI-based sleep staging algorithms, it is strongly recommended that the performance of sleep scoring algorithms is tested in datasets which were completely unseen by the model both during training and validation and are representative of the population to be tested. In fact, the AASM has announced in August 2022, that an AI/Autoscoring Pilot Certification is coming soon. They stated that "*modern sleep disorders center is seeing a shift in how day-to-day tasks are being performed. Artificial intelligence technology has opened the door for highly accurate auto-scoring solutions that will likely play a bigger role in AASM-accredited facilities in the future. While the U.S. Food and Drug Administration has oversight over many of these solutions, FDA requirements for scoring accuracy is not very stringent. Additionally, sleep medicine professionals may not feel confident with available solutions since they are radically different than the status quo of manual scoring. To help usher in auto-scoring solutions, the AASM board of directors approved a plan to create a two-year pilot certification program for software that has auto-scoring functionality. The pilot certification is limited to sleep stage scoring. The purpose of the certification program is to independently verify the performance of auto-scoring systems. To obtain certification, software must demonstrate accuracy that is equivalent or better than human scorers.*" As mentioned in the section on manual scoring, the AASM has launched a program for certification of autoscoring software that provides adult sleep stage scoring. The program guarantees testing of the various scoring solutions to one and the same external dataset with 100 representative recordings versus seven manual expert scorers. This will allow a direct comparison of the performance of the published algorithms and will give the sleep centers an objective measure for deciding which algorithm to use.

Concerning the features derived from the hypnodensity, our results suggest more robust estimates of sleep architecture by computing the recommended sleep parameters by integrating over the probabilities per sleep stage over the night. Indeed, for all age groups, the standard deviations of all parameters were smaller using the hypnodensity-derived values as compared to the traditionally hypnogram-derived values. Moreover, also the correlations with age as well as with the arousal index (ArI) was higher for the hypnodensity-derived as compared to the hypnogram-derived parameters.

In addition, parameters not determinable from the hypnogram, such as sleep stage ambiguity—reflecting the uncertainty of manual expert scorers—as well as sleep stage continuity—reflecting epoch-to-epoch changes of these uncertainties—

may give valuable additional information. Interestingly, sleep stage ambiguity and continuity show opposite changes with age for epochs scored as sleep as compared to epochs scored as wake. In wake, ambiguity decreases, and continuity increases with age. Together with the significant increase in WASO with age, this means that with increasing age subjects are longer wake and these wake periods are more definite and stable. On the other hand, during sleep, ambiguity increases, and continuity decreases over age, indicating more uncertainty and less sleep stability with increasing age. Interestingly, the highest correlation with age was the increase in ambiguity of epochs scored as sleep (Fig. 4) and the highest partial correlation with the ArI (controlling for the effect of age) was the decrease in sleep continuity with increasing ArI (Fig. 8).

Future studies should investigate further applications of the hypnodensity and other AI-derived measures for describing human sleep. AI-based approaches can identify complex patterns in empirical data and can take (spatio)-temporal context into account, which allows a direct application of deep-learning algorithms to raw data. Deep-learning algorithms can be trained on targets such as manually scored sleep stages (supervised deep learning), but also hypothesis-free without targets (unsupervised deep learning) based on large datasets (Big Data), which preferably contain also clinical outcome data. Such datasets could also be used to identify physiological biomarkers based on the recorded PSG signals to complement the usual biomarkers taken from clinical chemistry. Penzel et al. [86] suggest that such physiological biomarkers might be more appropriate to characterize functional characteristics, as seen in the variety of sleep disorders. An example for a successful construction and evaluation of a narcolepsy biomarker including variables derived from hypnodensity can be found in Stephansen et al. [38]. They created a biomarker for narcolepsy that achieved with a specificity of 96% and a sensitivity of 91% similar performance to the current clinical gold standard, the multiple sleep latency test (MSLT), but only requires a single sleep study. One of the key features that their system identified, was the uncertainty between different stages (particularly between REM sleep, light sleep, and wake) at the beginning of the night. Quantification of this uncertainty would have been unattainable with traditional hypnogram scoring by one expert. Moreover, they showed that addition of human leukocyte antigen (HLA) or other genetic typing in the model can increase the specificity above 99% without loss of sensitivity. Steiger et al. [87] presented a review on sleep EEG biomarkers for the diagnosis, treatment, and prognosis of depression. The authors concluded that sleep EEG variables are among the biomarkers that should be included in the classification of mood disorders and reported that in patients with depression disturbed sleep continuity, REM sleep disinhibition and impaired non-REM sleep were the characteristic findings. In summary, the large number of successfully applied machine learning approaches for scoring sleep confirms impressively the potential of AI applications for sleep diagnostics. AI could not only facilitate the routine monitoring of patients, but in addition, it could help uncover biomarkers derived from ambiguity and continuity measures which are not traditionally capturable with standard manual scoring.

Disclosure Statement Peter Anderer, Marco Ross, Andreas Cerny, and Pedro Fonseca are part- or full-time employees of Philips. Peter Anderer is in addition a freelancer and shareholder of The Siesta Group.

References

1. Berry RB, Albertario CL, Harding SM. *The AASM manual for the Scoring of Sleep and Associated Events: Rules, Terminology and Technical Specifications. Version 2.6*. American Academy of Sleep Medicine; 2020.
2. Danker-Hopfe H, Kunz D, Gruber G, et al. Interrater reliability between scorers from eight European sleep laboratories in subjects with different sleep disorders. *J Sleep Res*. Mar 2004;13(1):63–9. https://doi.org/10.1046/j.1365-2869.2003.00375.x
3. Danker-Hopfe H, Anderer P, Zeitlhofer J, et al. Interrater reliability for sleep scoring according to the Rechtschaffen & Kales and the new AASM standard. *J Sleep Res*. Mar 2009;18(1):74–84. https://doi.org/10.1111/j.1365-2869.2008.00700.x
4. Penzel T, Zhang X, Fietze I. Inter-scorer reliability between sleep centers can teach us what to improve in the scoring rules. *J Clin Sleep Med*. Jan 15 2013;9(1):89–91. https://doi.org/10.5664/jcsm.2352
5. Rosenberg RS, Van Hout S. The American Academy of Sleep Medicine inter-scorer reliability program: sleep stage scoring. *J Clin Sleep Med*. Jan 15 2013;9(1):81–7. https://doi.org/10.5664/jcsm.2350
6. Younes M, Kuna ST, Pack AI, et al. Reliability of the American Academy of Sleep Medicine Rules for Assessing Sleep Depth in Clinical Practice. *J Clin Sleep Med*. Feb 15 2018;14(2):205–213. https://doi.org/10.5664/jcsm.6934
7. Younes M, Raneri J, Hanly P. Staging Sleep in Polysomnograms: Analysis of Inter-Scorer Variability. *J Clin Sleep Med*. Jun 15 2016;12(6):885–94. https://doi.org/10.5664/jcsm.5894
8. Cesari M, Stefani A, Penzel T, et al. Interrater sleep stage scoring reliability between manual scoring from two European sleep centers and automatic scoring performed by the artificial intelligence-based Stanford-STAGES algorithm. *J Clin Sleep Med*. Jun 1 2021;17(6):1237–1247. https://doi.org/10.5664/jcsm.9174
9. Lee YJ, Lee JY, Cho JH, Choi JH. Interrater reliability of sleep stage scoring: a meta-analysis. *J Clin Sleep Med*. Jan 1 2022;18(1):193–202. https://doi.org/10.5664/jcsm.9538
10. Rechtschaffen A, Kales A. A manual of standardized terminology, techniques, and scoring systems for sleep stages of human subjects. *UCLA Brain Information Service/Brain Research Institute, Los Angeles*. 1968
11. Itil TM, Shapiro DM, Fink M, Kassebaum D. Digital computer classifications of EEG sleep stages. *Electroencephalogr Clin Neurophysiol*. Jul 1969;27(1):76–83. https://doi.org/10.1016/0013-4694(69)90112-6
12. Larsen LE, Walter DO. On automatic methods of sleep staging by EEG spectra. *Electroencephalogr Clin Neurophysiol*. May 1970;28(5):459–67. https://doi.org/10.1016/0013-4694(70)90271-3
13. Smith JR, Karacan I. EEG sleep stage scoring by an automatic hybrid system. *Electroencephalogr Clin Neurophysiol*. Sep 1971;31(3):231–7. https://doi.org/10.1016/0013-4694(71)90092-7
14. Martin WB, Johnson LC, Viglione SS, Naitoh P, Joseph RD, Moses JD. Pattern recognition of EEG-EOG as a technique for all-night sleep stage scoring. *Electroencephalogr Clin Neurophysiol*. Apr 1972;32(4):417–27. https://doi.org/10.1016/0013-4694(72)90009-0
15. Anderer P, Gruber G, Parapatics S, et al. An E-health solution for automatic sleep classification according to Rechtschaffen and Kales: validation study of the Somnolyzer 24 x 7 utilizing the Siesta database. *Neuropsychobiology*. 2005;51(3):115–33. https://doi.org/10.1159/000085205
16. Gaillard JM, Tissot R. Principles of automatic analysis of sleep records with a hybrid system. *Comput Biomed Res*. Feb 1973;6(1):1–13. https://doi.org/10.1016/0010-4809(73)90059-1

17. Hoffmann R, Moffitt A, Wells R, Sussman P, Pigeau R, Shearer J. Quantitative description of sleep stage electrophysiology using digital period analytic techniques. *Sleep*. 1984;7(4):356–64. https://doi.org/10.1093/sleep/7.4.356
18. Kubicki S, Holler L, Berg I, Pastelak-Price C, Dorow R. Sleep EEG evaluation: a comparison of results obtained by visual scoring and automatic analysis with the Oxford sleep stager. *Sleep*. Apr 1989;12(2):140–9. https://doi.org/10.1093/sleep/12.2.140
19. Schwaibold M, Schochlin J, Bolz A. Automated sleep stage detection with a classical and a neural learning algorithm–methodological aspects. *Biomed Tech (Berl)*. 2002;47 Suppl 1 Pt 1:318–20. https://doi.org/10.1515/bmte.2002.47.s1a.318
20. Iber C, Ancoli-Israel S, Chesson A, Quan S. *The AASM manual for the scoring of sleep and associated events*. American Academy of Sleep Medicine; 2007:59.
21. Anderer P, Moreau A, Woertz M, et al. Computer-assisted sleep classification according to the standard of the American Academy of Sleep Medicine: validation study of the AASM version of the Somnolyzer 24 x 7. *Neuropsychobiology*. 2010;62(4):250–64. https://doi.org/10.1159/000320864
22. Punjabi NM, Shifa N, Dorffner G, Patil S, Pien G, Aurora RN. Computer-Assisted Automated Scoring of Polysomnograms Using the Somnolyzer System. *Sleep*. Oct 1 2015;38(10):1555–66. https://doi.org/10.5665/sleep.5046
23. Bianchi MT, Goparaju B. Potential Underestimation of Sleep Apnea Severity by At-Home Kits: Rescoring In-Laboratory Polysomnography Without Sleep Staging. *J Clin Sleep Med*. Apr 15 2017;13(4):551–555. https://doi.org/10.5664/jcsm.6540
24. Lanfranchi PA, Pépin, J.-L., & Somers, V. K. Cardiovascular Physiology: Autonomic Control in Health and in Sleep Disorders. In: M. Kryger TR, & W. C. Dement, ed. *Principles and Practice of Sleep Medicine*. 6th ed. Elsevier; 2016:142–154.
25. Eckert DJ, Butler, J. E. Respiratory Physiology: Understanding the Control of Ventilation. In: M. Kryger TR, & W. C. Dement ed. *Principles and Practice of Sleep Medicine*. 6th ed. Elsevier; 2016:167–173.
26. Hedner J, White DP, Malhotra A, et al. Sleep staging based on autonomic signals: a multi-center validation study. *J Clin Sleep Med*. Jun 15 2011;7(3):301–6. https://doi.org/10.5664/JCSM.1078
27. Fonseca P, Long X, Radha M, Haakma R, Aarts RM, Rolink J. Sleep stage classification with ECG and respiratory effort. *Physiol Meas*. Oct 2015;36(10):2027–40. https://doi.org/10.1088/0967-3334/36/10/2027
28. Fonseca P, den Teuling N, Long X, Aarts RM. A comparison of probabilistic classifiers for sleep stage classification. *Physiol Meas*. May 15 2018;39(5):055001. https://doi.org/10.1088/1361-6579/aabbc2
29. Tataraidze A, Anishchenko L, Korostovtseva L, Bochkarev M, Sviryaev Y, Ivashov S. Estimation of a priori probabilities of sleep stages: A cycle-based approach. *Annu Int Conf IEEE Eng Med Biol Soc*. Jul 2017;2017:3745–3748. https://doi.org/10.1109/EMBC.2017.8037671
30. Beattie Z, Oyang Y, Statan A, et al. Estimation of sleep stages in a healthy adult population from optical plethysmography and accelerometer signals. *Physiol Meas*. Oct 31 2017;38(11):1968–1979. https://doi.org/10.1088/1361-6579/aa9047
31. Ruehland WR, O'Donoghue FJ, Pierce RJ, et al. The 2007 AASM recommendations for EEG electrode placement in polysomnography: impact on sleep and cortical arousal scoring. *Sleep*. Jan 1 2011;34(1):73–81. https://doi.org/10.1093/sleep/34.1.73
32. Magalang UJ, Chen NH, Cistulli PA, et al. Agreement in the scoring of respiratory events and sleep among international sleep centers. *Sleep*. Apr 1 2013;36(4):591–6. https://doi.org/10.5665/sleep.2552
33. Deng S, Zhang X, Zhang Y, et al. Interrater agreement between American and Chinese sleep centers according to the 2014 AASM standard. *Sleep Breath*. Jun 2019;23(2):719–728. https://doi.org/10.1007/s11325-019-01801-x
34. Zhang X, Dong X, Kantelhardt JW, et al. Process and outcome for international reliability in sleep scoring. *Sleep Breath*. Mar 2015;19(1):191–5. https://doi.org/10.1007/s11325-014-0990-0

35. Bakker JP, Ross M, Cerny A, et al. Scoring sleep with artificial intelligence enables quantification of sleep stage ambiguity: Hypnodensity based on multiple expert scorers and auto-scoring. *Sleep*. Feb 8 2023;46(2). https://doi.org/10.1093/sleep/zsac154
36. Klosch G, Kemp B, Penzel T, et al. The SIESTA project polygraphic and clinical database. *IEEE Eng Med Biol Mag*. May-Jun 2001;20(3):51–7. https://doi.org/10.1109/51.932725
37. Guillot A, Sauvet F, During EH, Thorey V. Dreem Open Datasets: Multi-Scored Sleep Datasets to Compare Human and Automated Sleep Staging. *IEEE Trans Neural Syst Rehabil Eng*. Sep 2020;28(9):1955–1965. https://doi.org/10.1109/TNSRE.2020.3011181
38. Stephansen JB, Olesen AN, Olsen M, et al. Neural network analysis of sleep stages enables efficient diagnosis of narcolepsy. *Nat Commun*. Dec 6 2018;9(1):5229. https://doi.org/10.1038/s41467-018-07229-3
39. Vallat R, Walker MP. An open-source, high-performance tool for automated sleep staging. *Elife*. Oct 14 2021;10https://doi.org/10.7554/eLife.70092
40. Fiorillo L, Pedroncelli D, Agostini V, Favaro P, Faraci FD. Multi-Scored Sleep Databases: How to Exploit the Multiple-Labels in Automated Sleep Scoring. *Sleep*. Feb 10 2023;https://doi.org/10.1093/sleep/zsad028
41. Perslev M, Darkner S, Kempfner L, Nikolic M, Jennum PJ, Igel C. U-Sleep: resilient high-frequency sleep staging. *NPJ Digit Med*. Apr 15 2021;4(1):72. https://doi.org/10.1038/s41746-021-00440-5
42. Anderer P, Ross M, Cerny A, Moreau A. Scoring sleep with artificial intelligence enables quantification of sleep stage ambiguity. *J Sleep Res*. 2018;27 Supplement 1 (SI):O025.
43. Biswal S, Sun H, Goparaju B, Westover MB, Sun J, Bianchi MT. Expert-level sleep scoring with deep neural networks. *J Am Med Inform Assoc*. Dec 1 2018;25(12):1643–1650. https://doi.org/10.1093/jamia/ocy131
44. Korkalainen H, Aakko J, Nikkonen S, et al. Accurate Deep Learning-Based Sleep Staging in a Clinical Population With Suspected Obstructive Sleep Apnea. *IEEE J Biomed Health Inform*. Jul 2020;24(7):2073–2081. https://doi.org/10.1109/JBHI.2019.2951346
45. Patanaik A, Ong JL, Gooley JJ, Ancoli-Israel S, Chee MWL. An end-to-end framework for real-time automatic sleep stage classification. *Sleep*. May 1 2018;41(5). https://doi.org/10.1093/sleep/zsy041
46. Phan H, Andreotti F, Cooray N, Chen OY, De Vos M. SeqSleepNet: End-to-End Hierarchical Recurrent Neural Network for Sequence-to-Sequence Automatic Sleep Staging. *IEEE Trans Neural Syst Rehabil Eng*. Mar 2019;27(3):400–410. https://doi.org/10.1109/TNSRE.2019.2896659
47. Sors, A; Bonnet, S.; Mirek, S.; Vercueil, L.; Payen, J-F. A convolutional neural network for sleep stage scoring from raw single-channel EEG. *Biomedical Signal Processing and Control*. 2018;42:107–114.
48. Sun C, Chen C, Li W, Fan J, Chen W. A Hierarchical Neural Network for Sleep Stage Classification Based on Comprehensive Feature Learning and Multi-Flow Sequence Learning. *IEEE J Biomed Health Inform*. May 2020;24(5):1351–1366. https://doi.org/10.1109/JBHI.2019.2937558
49. Supratak A, Dong H, Wu C, Guo Y. DeepSleepNet: A Model for Automatic Sleep Stage Scoring Based on Raw Single-Channel EEG. *IEEE Trans Neural Syst Rehabil Eng*. Nov 2017;25(11):1998–2008. https://doi.org/10.1109/TNSRE.2017.2721116
50. Abou Jaoude M, Sun H, Pellerin KR, et al. Expert-level automated sleep staging of long-term scalp electroencephalography recordings using deep learning. *Sleep*. Nov 12 2020;43(11). https://doi.org/10.1093/sleep/zsaa112
51. Alvarez-Estevez D, Rijsman RM. Inter-database validation of a deep learning approach for automatic sleep scoring. *PLoS One*. 2021;16(8):e0256111. https://doi.org/10.1371/journal.pone.0256111
52. Fiorillo L, Favaro P, Faraci FD. DeepSleepNet-Lite: A Simplified Automatic Sleep Stage Scoring Model With Uncertainty Estimates. *IEEE Trans Neural Syst Rehabil Eng*. 2021;29:2076–2085. https://doi.org/10.1109/TNSRE.2021.3117970

53. Jia Z, Lin Y, Wang J, et al. Multi-View Spatial-Temporal Graph Convolutional Networks With Domain Generalization for Sleep Stage Classification. *IEEE Trans Neural Syst Rehabil Eng*. 2021;29:1977–1986. https://doi.org/10.1109/TNSRE.2021.3110665
54. Li C, Qi Y, Ding X, Zhao J, Sang T, Lee M. A Deep Learning Method Approach for Sleep Stage Classification with EEG Spectrogram. *Int J Environ Res Public Health*. May 23 2022;19(10). https://doi.org/10.3390/ijerph19106322
55. Li T, Zhang B, Lv H, Hu S, Xu Z, Tuergong Y. CAttSleepNet: Automatic End-to-End Sleep Staging Using Attention-Based Deep Neural Networks on Single-Channel EEG. *Int J Environ Res Public Health*. Apr 25 2022;19(9). https://doi.org/10.3390/ijerph19095199
56. Nasiri S, Clifford GD. Boosting automated sleep staging performance in big datasets using population subgrouping. *Sleep*. Jul 9 2021;44(7). https://doi.org/10.1093/sleep/zsab027
57. Olesen AN, Jorgen Jennum P, Mignot E, Sorensen HBD. Automatic sleep stage classification with deep residual networks in a mixed-cohort setting. *Sleep*. Jan 21 2021;44(1). https://doi.org/10.1093/sleep/zsaa161
58. Pathak S, Lu C, Nagaraj SB, van Putten M, Seifert C. STQS: Interpretable multi-modal Spatial-Temporal-seQuential model for automatic Sleep scoring. *Artif Intell Med*. Apr 2021;114:102038. https://doi.org/10.1016/j.artmed.2021.102038
59. Anderer P, Ross M, Cerny A, Shaw E. Automated Scoring of Sleep and Associated Events. *Adv Exp Med Biol*. 2022;1384:107–130. https://doi.org/10.1007/978-3-031-06413-5_7
60. Cho JH, Choi JH, Moon JE, Lee YJ, Lee HD, Ha TK. Validation Study on Automated Sleep Stage Scoring Using a Deep Learning Algorithm. *Medicina (Kaunas)*. Jun 9 2022;58(6). https://doi.org/10.3390/medicina58060779
61. Ji X, Li Y, Wen P. Jumping Knowledge Based Spatial-Temporal Graph Convolutional Networks for Automatic Sleep Stage Classification. *IEEE Trans Neural Syst Rehabil Eng*. 2022;30:1464–1472. https://doi.org/10.1109/TNSRE.2022.3176004
62. Sharma M, Yadav A, Tiwari J, Karabatak M, Yildirim O, Acharya UR. An Automated Wavelet-Based Sleep Scoring Model Using EEG, EMG, and EOG Signals with More Than 8000 Subjects. *Int J Environ Res Public Health*. Jun 11 2022;19(12). https://doi.org/10.3390/ijerph19127176
63. Yubo Z, Yingying L, Bing Z, Lin Z, Lei L. MMASleepNet: A multimodal attention network based on electrophysiological signals for automatic sleep staging. *Front Neurosci*. 2022;16:973761. https://doi.org/10.3389/fnins.2022.973761
64. Zhang LD, Fabbri D, Upender R, Kent D. Automated sleep stage scoring of the Sleep Heart Health Study using deep neural networks. *Sleep*. Nov 2019;42(11). https://doi.org/10.1093/sleep/zsz159
65. Cesari M, Egger K, Stefani A, et al. Differentiation of central disorders of hypersomnolence with manual and artificial-intelligence-derived polysomnographic measures. *Sleep*. Dec 2 2022;https://doi.org/10.1093/sleep/zsac288
66. Brandmayr G, Hartmann M, Furbass F, et al. Relational local electroencephalography representations for sleep scoring. *Neural Netw*. Oct 2022;154:310–322. https://doi.org/10.1016/j.neunet.2022.07.020
67. Zhang H, Wang X, Li H, Mehendale S, Guan Y. Auto-annotating sleep stages based on polysomnographic data. *Patterns (N Y)*. Jan 14 2022;3(1):100371. https://doi.org/10.1016/j.patter.2021.100371
68. Li Q, Li Q, Liu C, Shashikumar SP, Nemati S, Clifford GD. Deep learning in the cross-time frequency domain for sleep staging from a single-lead electrocardiogram. *Physiol Meas*. Dec 21 2018;39(12):124005. https://doi.org/10.1088/1361-6579/aaf339
69. Radha M, Fonseca P, Moreau A, et al. Sleep stage classification from heart-rate variability using long short-term memory neural networks. *Sci Rep*. Oct 2 2019;9(1):14149. https://doi.org/10.1038/s41598-019-49703-y
70. Bakker JP, Ross M, Vasko R, et al. Estimating sleep stages using cardiorespiratory signals: validation of a novel algorithm across a wide range of sleep-disordered breathing severity. *J Clin Sleep Med*. Mar 4 2021; https://doi.org/10.5664/jcsm.9192

71. Fonseca P, van Gilst MM, Radha M, et al. Automatic sleep staging using heart rate variability, body movements, and recurrent neural networks in a sleep disordered population. *Sleep*. Apr 6 2020; https://doi.org/10.1093/sleep/zsaa048
72. Sridhar N, Shoeb A, Stephens P, et al. Deep learning for automated sleep staging using instantaneous heart rate. *NPJ Digit Med.* 2020;3:106. https://doi.org/10.1038/s41746-020-0291-x
73. Sun H, Ganglberger W, Panneerselvam E, et al. Sleep staging from electrocardiography and respiration with deep learning. *Sleep*. Jul 13 2020;43(7). https://doi.org/10.1093/sleep/zsz306
74. Wei, Y; Qi, X.; Wang, H.; Liu, Z.; Wang, G.; Yan, X. A Multi-Class Automatic Sleep Staging Method Based on Long Short-Term Memory Network Using Single-Lead Electrocardiogram Signals. *IEEE Access*. 2019;7:85959–85970. https://doi.org/10.1109/ACCESS.2019.2924980
75. Zhao X, Sun G. A Multi-Class Automatic Sleep Staging Method Based on Photoplethysmography Signals. *Entropy (Basel)*. Jan 18 2021;23(1). https://doi.org/10.3390/e23010116
76. Huttunen R, Leppanen T, Duce B, et al. Assessment of obstructive sleep apnea-related sleep fragmentation utilizing deep learning-based sleep staging from photoplethysmography. *Sleep*. Oct 11 2021;44(10). https://doi.org/10.1093/sleep/zsab142
77. Garcia-Molina G, Jiang J. Interbeat interval-based sleep staging: work in progress toward real-time implementation. *Physiol Meas*. Mar 17 2022;43(2). https://doi.org/10.1088/1361-6579/ac5a78
78. Mokhlesi B, Punjabi NM. "REM-related" obstructive sleep apnea: an epiphenomenon or a clinically important entity? *Sleep*. Jan 1 2012;35(1):5–7. https://doi.org/10.5665/sleep.1570
79. van Gorp H, Huijben IAM, Fonseca P, van Sloun RJG, Overeem S, van Gilst MM. Certainty about uncertainty in sleep staging: a theoretical framework. *Sleep*. Aug 11 2022;45(8). https://doi.org/10.1093/sleep/zsac134
80. Shrout PE, Fleiss JL. Intraclass correlations: uses in assessing rater reliability. *Psychol Bull.* Mar 1979;86(2):420–8. https://doi.org/10.1037//0033-2909.86.2.420
81. Lechat B, Loffler KA, Wallace DM, et al. All-Cause Mortality in People with Co-Occurring Insomnia Symptoms and Sleep Apnea: Analysis of the Wisconsin Sleep Cohort. *Nat Sci Sleep*. 2022;14:1817–1828. https://doi.org/10.2147/NSS.S379252
82. Findley LJ, Wilhoit SC, Suratt PM. Apnea duration and hypoxemia during REM sleep in patients with obstructive sleep apnea. *Chest*. Apr 1985;87(4):432–6. https://doi.org/10.1378/chest.87.4.432
83. Peppard PE, Ward NR, Morrell MJ. The impact of obesity on oxygen desaturation during sleep-disordered breathing. *Am J Respir Crit Care Med*. Oct 15 2009;180(8):788–93. https://doi.org/10.1164/rccm.200905-0773OC
84. Somers VK, Dyken ME, Clary MP, Abboud FM. Sympathetic neural mechanisms in obstructive sleep apnea. *J Clin Invest*. Oct 1995;96(4):1897–904. https://doi.org/10.1172/JCI118235
85. Varga AW, Mokhlesi B. REM obstructive sleep apnea: risk for adverse health outcomes and novel treatments. *Sleep Breath*. Jun 2019;23(2):413–423. https://doi.org/10.1007/s11325-018-1727-2
86. Penzel T, Fietze I, Veauthier C. The Need for a Reliable Sleep EEG Biomarker. *J Clin Sleep Med*. Jun 15 2017;13(6):771–772. https://doi.org/10.5664/jcsm.6608
87. Steiger A, Pawlowski M. Depression and Sleep. *Int J Mol Sci*. Jan 31 2019;20(3). https://doi.org/10.3390/ijms20030607

From Screening at Clinic to Diagnosis at Home: How AI/ML/DL Algorithms Are Transforming Sleep Apnea Detection

Pei-Lin Lee, Wenbo Gu, Wen-Chi Huang, and Ambrose A. Chiang

Abbreviations

AASM	American Academy of Sleep Medicine
AHI	Apnea-hypopnea index
AI	Artificial intelligence
ANN	Artificial neural network
ASSS	Automatic sleep staging systems
AUROC	Area under receiver operating characteristic
Bi-LSTM	Bi-directional long short-term memory

P.-L. Lee (✉)
Center of Sleep Disorder, National Taiwan University Hospital, Taipei, Taiwan

School of Medicine, National Taiwan University, Taipei, Taiwan
e-mail: leepeilin@ntu.edu.tw

W. Gu
Department of Computer Science, National Yang Ming Chiao Tung University, Hsinchu, Taiwan
e-mail: wendygu.cs08g@nctu.edu.tw

W.-C. Huang
FTSE International Taiwan Ltd, Taipei, Taiwan
e-mail: d03922025@ntu.edu.tw

A. A. Chiang
Sleep Medicine Section, Louis Stokes Cleveland VA Medical Center, Cleveland, OH, USA
e-mail: Ambrose.chiang@va.gov

Division of Pulmonary, Critical Care, and Sleep Medicine, University Hospitals Cleveland Medical Center, Cleveland, OH, USA
e-mail: Ambrose.chiang@va.gov

Department of Medicine, Case Western Reserve University, Cleveland, OH, USA
e-mail: Ambrose.chiang@va.gov

R. B. Berry et al. (eds.), *Handbook of AI and Data Sciences for Sleep Disorders*, Springer Optimization and Its Applications 216,
https://doi.org/10.1007/978-3-031-68263-6_4

BMI	Body mass index
BQ	Berlin Questionnaire
CNN	Convolutional neural network
DL	Deep learning
EBE	Epoch-by-epoch
ECG	Electrocardiography
EEG	Electroencephalogram
EMG	Electromyography
EMR	Electronic medical record
EOG	Electrooculogram
ESS	Epworth Sleepiness Scale
FDA	U.S. Food and Drug Administration
FSFS	Forward stepwise feature selection
GMLP	Good Machine Learning Practice
HRV	Heart rate viability
HSAT	Home sleep apnea testing
LLM	Large language model
LR	Logistic regression
LSTM	Long short-term memory
MESA	Multi-Ethnic Study of Atherosclerosis
ML	Machine learning
ODI	Oxygen desaturation index
OSA	Obstructive sleep apnea
PAT	Peripheral arterial tonometry
PLMI	Periodic limb movement index
PPG	Photoplethysmography
PPV	Positive predictive value
PRV	Pulse rate variability
PSG	Polysomnography
RDI	Respiratory disturbance index
RF	Random Forest
RNN	Recurrent neural network
SaMD	Software as a Medical Device
SCOPER	Sleep, cardiovascular, oximetry, position, effort and respiratory parameters
SE	Sleep efficiency
SHHS	Sleep Heart Health Study
SLIM	Supersparse linear integer models
SOL	Sleep onset latency
SOMNIA	Sleep and Obstructive Sleep Apnea Monitoring with Non-Invasive Applications project
SpO2	Oxygen saturation
STAGES	Stanford Technological Analytics and Genomics in Sleep Study
SVM	Support vector machine
TBI	Traumatic Brain Injury Study
TCN	Temporal convolutional network

1 Introduction

Obstructive sleep apnea (OSA) represents a prevalent sleep disorder, affecting 9–38% of individuals with an apnea-hypopnea index (AHI) ≥5/h and 6–17% at AHI ≥15/h within community settings [1, 2]. Despite its common occurrence, OSA often goes unnoticed and remains undiagnosed and untreated [3]. Research indicates that untreated OSA is associated with many adverse health outcomes, including diminished quality of life, depression, diabetes, metabolic syndrome, various cardiovascular diseases such as hypertension, atrial fibrillation, coronary artery disease, heart failure, and stroke, as well as increased motor vehicle accidents [2, 4–9]. Also, in comparison to snorers and those with mild or moderate OSA, patients with untreated severe OSA face a two to three fold increased risk of all-cause mortality and major adverse cardiac and cerebrovascular events over 5–10 years [10–12]. Hence, early diagnosis and intervention for OSA can potentially mitigate the health care burden.

In recent years, the landscape of clinical sleep medicine has undergone significant transformation, driven by the rapid evolution of sleep technologies [13–19]. In this chapter, we discuss how OSA detection, from screening at the clinic to diagnosis at home, has been drastically changed by AI/ML/DL algorithms. We aim to (1) grasp the fundamentals of OSA and its clinical assessment, encompassing both screening and diagnostic methodologies; (2) develop proficiency in constructing AI/ML/DL models that leverage clinical features for OSA screening; (3) navigate the current landscape of innovative AI/ML/DL models employing photoplethysmography (PPG) and accelerometry for at-home OSA diagnosis; and (4) critically evaluate the key considerations involved in developing and validating robust AI/ML/DL algorithms for OSA detection. It is noteworthy that Sect. 3 of this chapter deliberately restricts its scope to PPG and accelerometry-based wearables. Exploration of AI applications in non-PPG-based modalities, such as in acoustic or respiratory effort-based devices, is addressed in separate chapters.

1.1 Pathophysiology and Clinical Presentation

OSA is characterized by recurrent upper airway collapse during sleep, leading to airflow cessation, paradoxical movements of the chest and abdomen, cortical arousal, and oxygen desaturation. These alterations can further instigate pathophysiological abnormalities, including chronic intermittent hypoxia, increased sympathetic activation, sleep fragmentation, and increased intrathoracic pressure swings [8, 20, 21].

Clinically, patients with OSA frequently present with symptoms such as habitual snoring, witnessed apneas, choking and gasping during sleep, frequent awakenings, unrefreshing sleep, tiredness, excessive daytime sleepiness, morning headaches, and nocturia [8, 20, 21]. Risk factors contributing to OSA encompass advancing age, male gender, obesity, non-white race/ethnicity, certain craniofacial features, and post-menopause in women [8, 20, 22].

1.2 OSA Assessment and the Use of Screening Tools

The assessment of OSA commences with a comprehensive review of sleep history and a thorough upper airway examination. This includes inquiries into the frequency of witnessed apneas, occurrences of choking and gasping episodes in sleep, frequency of sleep disruptions, and the extent of daytime sleepiness and fatigue [8, 20, 21]. Moreover, screening tools, such as questionnaire instruments, prediction equations, and consumer or medical-grade devices including smartphone applications (Apps) may be employed to early identify patients with OSA. An emerging technology in this domain involves the utilization of large language models (LLMs) for home screening of various medical conditions, including OSA [23, 24].

1.2.1 Questionnaire Instruments

Questionnaires commonly employed to assess the risk of OSA and excessive sleepiness include the STOP-Bang [25, 26], NoSAS [27, 28], Berlin Questionnaire (BQ) [29], and Epworth Sleepiness Scale (ESS) [30]. A meta-analysis comparing the diagnostic performance of the STOP-Bang, BQ, and ESS at three different AHI cutoffs (≥5/h, ≥15/h, ≥30/h) indicated that STOP-Bang exhibited the highest sensitivity, while ESS displayed the lowest sensitivity across all three cutoffs (Table 1) [31]. Another recent meta-analysis on the use of STOP-Bang for OSA screening across geographic regions revealed that a STOP-Bang score of ≥3 had an overall good sensitivity (95%) but low specificity (28%) in detecting moderate-severe OSA in sleep clinic populations [32]. Notably, patients with cardiovascular disease often manifest less daytime sleepiness and reduced snoring, thereby diminishing the discriminative capability of these questionnaires in identifying moderate-severe OSA [8, 33–36].

1.2.2 Prediction Models

Over the years, many OSA prediction models have been developed, relying on symptoms, physical findings, or physiological measurements. These models typically prioritize heightened sensitivity and reduced specificity to facilitate the early detection of moderate-to-severe OSA. However, this emphasis on sensitivity may contribute to an elevated false-positive rate, potentially resulting in excessive prescriptions for sleep testing [37–43]. The details of these prediction models are discussed in Sect. 2.

Table 1 Questionnaire to assess OSA risk (A) parameters of questionnaire (B) OSA discriminative ability

(A)

Questionnaire title	Description of questionnaire	Scoring method
STOP-Bang [26]	Eight-item questionnaire comprising snoring characteristics, tiredness, witnessed apnea, high blood pressure, BMI, age, neck circumference, and man	Score 0–2: Low risk of OSA Score 3–4: Intermediate risk of OSA Score 5–8: High risk of OSA STOP ≥2 + male or BMI > 35 kg/m^2 or neck> 40 cm: High risk of OSA
NoSAS [27]	Five-item questionnaire that includes neck circumference, BMI, snoring, age, and sex	4 points allotted for neck circumference >40 cm, 3 for BMI 25–30 kg/m^2, 5 for BMI ≥ 30 kg/m^2, 2 for snoring, 4 for >55 y/o and 2 for male sex. A total score ≥8 indicates a high risk for OSA
Berlin Questionnaire [29]	Three categories, namely, snoring, fatigue, and hypertension, with each category including 2–5 questions for a total of 11 questions	Positive responses to two or more categories indicate a high risk for OSA
Epworth Sleepiness Scale [30]	Eight-item questionnaire that asks respondents to rate their usual chances of dozing off or falling asleep during eight activities	An ESS score ≥ 10 was defined as excessive daytime sleepiness

(B)

AHI cutoff	Performance	STOP-Bang [31]	Berlin Questionnaire [31]	NoSAS [28]	Epworth Sleepiness Scale [31]
≥5 (/h)	Sensitivity (%)	88 (83–91)	76 (71–81)	80 (75–83)	54 (45–63)
	Specificity (%)	42 (35–50)	59 (48–66)	58 (51–65)	65 (57–72)
≥15 (/h)	Sensitivity (%)	90 (86–93)	77 (73–81)	NA	47 (35–59)
	Specificity (%)	36 (29–44)	44 (38–51)	NA	62 (56–68)
≥30 (/h)	Sensitivity (%)	93 (89–95)	84 (79–88)	NA	58 (48–67)
	Specificity (%)	35 (28–44)	38 (31–56)	NA	60 (53–68)

Adapted under a CC BY 4.0 license from Lee and Wu et al. [8]
Data are presented as the mean (95% confidence interval)
Abbreviations: *AHI* apnea-hypopnea index, *BMI* body mass index, *ESS* Epworth Sleepiness Scale, *NA* not available, *OSA* obstructive sleep apnea

1.2.3 Smartphone Apps, Nearables, and Wearables

Consumer OSA-detecting wearables, nearables, and smartphone apps each possess unique advantages and drawbacks when used for OSA screening. While some nearables show promise, they require further validation, especially in scenarios involving bed partners, children, or pets in the same bed. One notable shortcoming of nearables, smartphone apps, and non-PPG-based wearables lies in the absence of pulse oximetry, which inevitably constrains the accuracy of OSA detection. In recent years, acoustic-based smartphone apps and wearable devices have emerged as early OSA detection tools. Drowzle (Resonea, Scottsdale, Arizona), SleepCheck Rx (ResApp Health, Brisbane, Queensland, Australia), and AcuPebble SA100 (Acurable, London, UK) exemplify this trend, having received clearance by the U.S. Food and Drug Administration (FDA) for OSA screening at home [44–46]. These devices leverage acoustic signals to analyze the breathing pattern in sleep and assess the risk of OSA. A detailed discussion of nearables and sound-based technologies extends beyond the scope of this chapter.

1.2.4 Large Language Model

Recent studies have investigated the accuracy of ChatGPT responses to questions regarding OSA for patient education [23, 24]. Overall, ChatGPT delivers appropriate responses to most OSA inquiries, exhibiting a 70% agreement with experts [23, 24]. Given the rapid advancements in this domain, LLM holds promise as a tool for OSA home screening. Nevertheless, further research is warranted in this realm.

1.3 OSA Diagnostic Tools

Traditionally, the diagnostic testing can be attended in-laboratory polysomnography (PSG), unattended PSG, or home sleep apnea testing (HSAT). These tests should be conducted within the context of a comprehensive sleep evaluation and subsequent follow-up [47]. Diagnostic testing is recommended for individuals exhibiting OSA symptoms or in circumstances requiring mandatory screening, such as in pilots or commercial drivers, as well as in those with substantial comorbidities, such as cardiovascular disease and diabetes [47]. In contrast, sleep testing is not recommended for asymptomatic patients within the general population due to the absence of clear benefits [20, 48].

1.3.1 Polysomnography

PSG serves as the benchmark for assessing sleep/wake status, respiratory variables, oxygen saturation, and cardiac variables (Table 2) [49]. Standard overnight PSG incorporates channels monitoring six electroencephalogram (EEG) leads (F4-M1, C4-M1, O2-M1, F3-M2, C3-M2, O1-M2), two electrooculography (EOG) leads (E1-M2, E2-M2), three submental electromyography (EMG) leads, two leg EMG leads, electrocardiography (ECG), nasal pressure, thermistor, pulse oximetry, and thoracic and abdominal respiratory effort. Parameters collected through the night encompass total recording time, total sleep time (TST), time spent in each sleep

Table 2 Diagnostic testing to confirm OSA

	Physiological signal/channel	Diagnostic criteria	AHI cutoff for OSA severity	Accuracy in a high-risk population [47]
PSG	Sleep/wake status: EEG, EOG, chin EMG Air flows: nasal pressure, thermistor Respiratory effort: thoracic and abdominal Oxygen saturation: pulse oximetry Cardiac variable: pulse oximetry, ECG Others: body position, leg movement, snoring	AHI RDI (including RERA) ODI (3% or 4%)	Mild: 5/h $\leq$ AHI < 15/h Moderate: 15/h $\leq$ AHI <30/h Severe: $\geq$30/h	Gold standard
HSAT	Type II–IV portable monitor Type II: unattended polysomnography ($\geq$7 channels); Type III: limited cardiopulmonary parameters (4–7 channels), including respiratory variables, oxygen saturation, and cardiac variables; Type IV: 1–2 parameters, including oximetry or ECG SCOPER[a]	REI	Presence of OSA: $\geq$5/h Moderate–severe: $\geq$15/h Severe: $\geq$30/h	Type II: AHI $\geq$5/h, 84–91%; AHI $\geq$15/h: 88% Type III: AHI $\geq$5/h, 84–91%; AHI $\geq$15/h: 65–91%; AHI $\geq$30/h, 88% Type IV (oximetry): AHI $\geq$5/h, 73% (95% CI, 68–78%); AHI $\geq$15/h: 86% (95% CI, 83–91%); AHI $\geq$30/h, 74% (95% CI, 71–76%)

Abbreviations: *AHI* apnea-hypopnea index, *CI* confidence interval, *ECG* electrocardiogram, *EEG* electroencephalography, *EMG* electromyography, *EOG* electrooculography, *HSAT* home sleep apnea test, *ODI* oxygen desaturation index, *OSA* obstructive sleep apnea, *PSG* polysomnography, *RDI* respiratory disturbance index, *REI* respiratory event index, *RERA* respiratory effort-related arousal

[a]SCOPER: Sleep, cardiovascular, oximetry, position, effort, and respiratory parameters

stage (wake, N1, N2, N3, and REM), AHI, oxygen desaturation index (ODI), percentage of total sleep time with oxygen saturation (SpO2) <90% (%TST-SpO2 <90%), arousal index, and periodic limb movement index (PLMI). Sleep onset latency (SOL) is defined as the time from lights out to the first epoch of sleep, while sleep efficiency (SE) is calculated as the percentage of TST divided by total record time.

Currently, the diagnostic criteria for OSA by the International Classification of Sleep Disorders, Third Edition (ICSD-3) entail either a Respiratory Disturbance Index (RDI) (AHI plus respiratory effort-related arousal index) of ≥5/h accompanied by OSA-related symptoms or an RDI ≥15/h irrespective of symptoms [50]. The severity of OSA is determined by the AHI or RDI, with cutoffs for mild OSA (5/h ≤ AHI < 15/h), moderate OSA (15/h ≤ AHI < 30/h), and severe OSA (AHI ≥ 30/h) [47, 51]. Several limitations hinder the widespread utilization of PSG for OSA diagnosis. Apart from the high demand for trained personnel, limited accessibility, and high costs, PSG often restricts patients to the supine position and precludes longitudinal monitoring and frequent follow-ups. Moreover, in-lab PSG is associated with the first-night effect or reverse first-night effect, especially among those with low SE [52]. Despite many limitations, it is also necessary to use the results of PSG as a reference benchmark for model training and validation when developing OSA diagnosis tools.

1.3.2 Home Sleep Apnea Testing

HSAT is generally considered an adequate substitute for PSG in patients with a high pretest probability for moderate-severe OSA and without significant comorbidities (notable cardiopulmonary disease, neuromuscular disease, stroke, opiate usage, central hypersomnia, parasomnia, sleep-related movement disorder, severe insomnia, and circadian rhythm disorders) [47]. While HSAT offers advantages such as lower cost, increased accessibility, and reduced complexity compared to PSG, it may lack the capability to assess TST, potentially leading to an underestimation of AHI. Consequently, if a single HSAT yields negative, inconclusive, or technically inadequate results, PSG should be arranged for further assessment [47]. Notably, HSAT should be administered by an accredited sleep center under the supervision of board-certified or board-eligible sleep physicians.

1.3.2.1 Classification and Technique

Portable monitoring devices can be classified using two distinct systems: the American Academy of Sleep Medicine (AASM) portable monitor classification (Type I–IV) based on study location and number of channels and the SCOPER categorization based on sensor types (sleep, cardiovascular, oximetry, position, effort, and respiratory) (Table 2) [47, 53, 54]. The AASM portable monitor classification is as follows: type I denotes attended polysomnography; type II represents unattended PSG (≥7 channels); type III encompasses limited cardiopulmonary parameters (4–7 channels), such as respiratory variables, oxygen saturation, and cardiac variables; while type IV involves 1–2 parameters including oximetry or ECG [54, 55]. The respiratory event index (REI = (apnea + hypopnea)/total sleep time or total recording time) is used to define OSA severity for HSAT. A technically adequate diagnostic test comprises the acquisition of ≥4 h of technically adequate oximetry and airflow data obtained during a recording attempt within the habitual sleep period. The SCOPER categorization system consisted of sleep, cardiovascular, oximetry, position, effort, and respiratory [53]. Each category was leveled and numbered from 1 to 5 based on the type of sensor measurement used in that category. The devices are judged on whether or not they can produce a positive likelihood ratio of ≥5 and sensitivity of ≥0.825 at in-lab PSG AHI ≥5/h in patients with a high pre-test probability of having OSA. Overall, either Type III HSAT incorporating nasal pressure, chest and abdominal effort, and oximetry or peripheral arterial tonometry (PAT) device are deemed acceptable HSAT devices [47, 53].

1.3.2.2 Incorporation of Sleep Information to Type III HSAT

The primary limitation of Type III HSAT lies in its inability to provide sleep stage information and TST necessary for accurate calculation of REI. This deficiency can be addressed by integrating one or more EEG leads, which not only offer insights into sleep-wake outcomes and sleep stage classification but also enhance concordance with PSG in assessing OSA severity [56].

In recent years, various automatic sleep staging systems (ASSS) utilizing frontal EEG have emerged to incorporate sleep staging into self-administered Type III HSAT [56–60]. While the agreement on an epoch-by-epoch (EBE) basis with expert scoring of in-lab PSG was generally satisfactory, consistency in the agreement of whole-night sleep transition variables, such as SOL and wake after sleep onset (WASO), varied across studies [56–60]. Lee et al. recently devised a four stage (wake/light sleep/deep sleep/REM) ASSS based on a single-channel frontal EEG (F4-M1), exhibiting good overall EBE validity and good-excellent for whole-night SOL, WASO, TST, and SE [49]. Moreover, to enable real-time and long-term sleep monitoring, Chang et al. proposed a low-power dual-mode ASSS processor utilizing a neural network-based decision tree classifier [61].

1.3.3 Emerging OSA-Detecting Sleep Technology

Among the emerging sleep technologies, including wearables, nearables (such as under-mattress devices and radar-based “airable” solutions), and smartphone apps, wearables equipped with PPG and accelerometer are at the forefront. Consumer wearable sleep trackers commonly rely on accelerometry to determine sleep-wake states and employ PPG to capture SpO2 data and derive sleep stages through AI/ML/DL algorithms. Although numerous consumer wearables offer sleep-wake information and sleep staging, only a select few have backed their claims with peer-reviewed articles from the industry [16, 62, 63].

Between 2019 and February 2024, a total of ten novel wearable devices or software as a medical device (SaMD) employing various sensors and mechanisms have received FDA clearance for at-home OSA diagnosis. While some rely on rule-based algorithms, the majority of these devices integrate AI/ML/DL algorithms. These emerging devices can be classified into four groups based on their sensors and mechanisms: (1) PAT-based; (2) PPG-based; (3) effort-based; and (4) sound-based [64]. Further details about these devices and their AI/ML/DL algorithms will be discussed in Sect. 3.

2 AI/ML/DL Algorithms Using Clinical Features for OSA Screening: The Clinic Setting

As outlined in Sects. 1.2.1 and 1.2.2, conventional tools like questionnaire instruments and OSA prediction equations using clinical features have historically been advocated for OSA screening [25–28, 31]. In contemporary times, there appears to be a discernible momentum toward embracing novel screening methodologies that leverage AI/ML/DL algorithms and various device-dependent sleep technologies have been proposed [44–46]. In the upcoming section, we will explore the alternative "device-less" screening approach, involving sole utilization of clinical features including demographic information, patient-reported symptoms, sleep history, comorbidities, and anthropometric measurements to forecast the presence of OSA through the application of AI/ML/DL [17, 27, 37, 39–43, 65–79].

2.1 Introduction of AI/ML/DL Algorithms Utilizing Clinical Features

Many AI/ML/DL algorithms are adept at scrutinizing diverse datasets and discerning patterns. A diverse array of algorithms, each possessing unique strengths and weaknesses, have been employed in various AI models for this purpose. Before further depicting our approach for OSA screening in this section, we will first discuss several commonly used ML and DL algorithms, including logistic regression, decision tree and Random Forest, Gradient Boosting, support vector machine, and, briefly, on neural network.

1. *Logistic Regression*: Logistic regression (LR) stands out for its simplicity and ease of interpretation, making it a favorable choice for the development of OSA screening tools using clinical features in earlier studies. Logistic regression

assumes a linear relationship between features and the log odds of the outcome, which may not always hold true. Additionally, logistic regression is sensitive to outliers and multicollinearity among features, potentially impacting model performance. Consequently, logistic regression may encounter challenges in capturing complex nonlinear relationships within datasets. It is also not adept at handling nonlinear decision boundaries or effectively capturing interactions between features. Overall, despite its simplicity, logistic regression may be limited in scenarios where linear relationship is violated or when dealing with highly intricate data structures [80].

2. *Decision Tree and Random Forests*: Decision trees and Random Forests (RF) are renowned for their capability to manage complex datasets, thereby enhancing the accuracy of OSA predictions. Random Forests, integrating insights from multiple decision trees, yield a more reliable outcome by mitigating variance and employing a consensus-based approach. These methods are invaluable for navigating intricate data and offering nuanced insights into the likelihood of OSA by utilizing entropy and event probability. Notably, decision trees and Random Forests are prone to overfitting (especially decision trees) and can be computationally expensive due to their complexity. Also, while decision trees offer interpretability, Random Forests, being ensembles, are more complex. They may exhibit bias toward majority classes in imbalanced datasets. Consequently, proper tuning of hyperparameters is crucial, as suboptimal choices can degrade performance. Lastly, these models tend to struggle with extrapolation and depend heavily on the quality of the input data [81].
3. *Gradient Boosting*: Gradient Boosting is mostly celebrated for its precision and ability to manage diverse datasets. This technique iteratively rectifies errors made by preceding models, continuously refining its predictions. Its methodological sophistication allows for a highly accurate approach to OSA screening, highlighting the potential of advanced algorithms in enhancing diagnostic accuracy. However, Gradient Boosting may be prone to overfitting, particularly with complex models or noisy data, necessitating meticulous tuning of hyperparameters. Training can be computationally expensive due to its sequential nature, making it less suitable for large datasets or real-time applications. Moreover, Gradient Boosting struggles with handling categorical variables, requiring encoding techniques. The interpretation of individual trees within the ensemble can also be challenging, restricting its transparency [82].
4. *Support Vector Machines*: Support Vector Machines (SVMs) excel in analyzing high-dimensional data, rendering them powerful tools for really complex classification tasks. By delineating the optimal boundary that segregates individuals with and without OSA, SVMs exhibit a high level of sophistication in diagnostic modeling, offering a robust solution to the challenges of accurately classifying OSA. SVMs can be computationally intensive, particularly for large datasets, diminishing their efficiency for big data applications. Their performance is highly dependent on the selection of the kernel function, and identifying the

optimal kernel parameters can be challenging. Moreover, SVMs can encounter difficulties with handling multiple-class classification, necessitating strategies like one-vs-one or one-vs-all, which can amplify complexity. Additionally, SVMs are less interpretable than some other models, as the decision function may not be readily understandable without a profound comprehension of the kernel space [83, 84].

5. *Neural Networks*: Neural networks, renowned for their sophisticated learning capabilities, represent the forefront of pattern recognition within extensive datasets. They demonstrate exceptional proficiency in directly analyzing raw data to discern subtle indicators of OSA, underscoring the revolutionary impact of AI in medical diagnostics. Their complex nature requires substantial amounts of data, such as PSG or PPG signals, and computational resources. They may not consistently offer the interpretability required in medical contexts [85, 86]. The application of neural networks will be further elaborated in detail in Sect. 3.1. Table 3 illustrates five different types of AI/ML/DL models with the strengths and weaknesses of their features.

2.2 *AI/ML/DL Model Development*

Algorithm development unfolds through meticulously refined, iterative cycles to ensure a robust and generalizable model. This process starts with data aggregation and preprocessing. At this stage, raw data is actively collected and undergoes preparation to ensure its quality and suitability for modeling. The dataset is then strategically divided into training datasets used to build the model and internal validation datasets for performance optimization. After selecting the most effective model, internal parameters are adjusted to further optimize its performance and minimize the risk of overfitting or underfitting. The thoroughly optimized model is then rigorously tested on an independent external validation to guarantee its generalizability to unseen data [43]. This iterative process of refinement ensures a robust performance. However, potential sources of error may still arise from issues concerning dataset selection, coding/labeling, model design, overfitting, or underfitting.

2.2.1 Clinical Features

The selection of AI/ML/DL algorithms for OSA screening using clinical features hinges on factors such as the size and features of the collected data, the required computational efficiency, and the balance between interpretability and predictive performance. The characteristics of the data primarily fall into the following categories: demographic information, OSA symptoms, sleep history, comorbidities, anthropometric data, and craniofacial anatomic risk factors (tonsil size,

Table 3 Five common machine learning algorithms used for OSA screening

Feature	Logistic regression	Decision tree and Random Forests	Gradient Boosting	Support vector machines	Neural networks
Ease of interpretation	High	High for decision trees, low for random forests	Low	Low	Low
Ability to handle complex datasets	Low	High	High	High	High
Risk of overfitting	Low	High (especially for random forests)	High	Depends on regularization and kernel choice	High
Computational efficiency	High	Low (computationally expensive)	Low (computationally expensive, especially for large datasets)	Low (especially for large datasets)	Low (requires substantial computational resources)
Handling nonlinear relationships	Poor	Good	Good	Good	Excellent
Sensitivity to outliers and multicollinearity	High	Moderate	Low	Moderate	Low
Suitability for large datasets	Moderate	Moderate	Low	Low	Moderate to high (depending on architecture)
Dependency on quality of input data	High	High	Moderate	Moderate	High
Interactions between features	Poorly captures	Good at capturing	Good at capturing	Can capture depending on kernel	Excellent at capturing
Tuning required	Low	High	High	High	High
Handling of categorical variables	Directly handles	Requires encoding techniques	Requires encoding techniques	Requires encoding techniques	Requires preprocessing

mandibular) (Table 4) [27, 37, 39–42, 65–76, 78, 79]. Continuous variables within these categories can be either directly used in the analysis or transformed into categorical variables for specific modeling techniques. A holistic data collection facilitates a thorough and accessible screening process, improving the ability to assess OSA across diverse populations [17, 43]. The majority of the features, such as demographic information, OSA symptoms, sleep history, and co-morbidities, can be integrated into questionnaires administered during clinic visits. Standardized questionnaires such as ESS, STOP-Bang, and insomnia severity index, among others, can also be used to aid data collection. Most of the OSA-associated information, including anthropometric data like body mass index (BMI), neck size, and waist size, is typically captured from the electronic medical record (EMR) or during clinic visits. Notably, OSA symptoms may suffer from low repeatability, while measurements of craniofacial anatomical risk factors lack standardization.

2.2.2 AI/ML/DL Algorithm: Summary of Selection in the Literature

Tables 4 and 5 summarize studies of various OSA prediction models [27, 37, 39–42, 65–76, 78]. Table 4 outlines the proposed training algorithms and specific clinical features used in each model, including the original features considered and those ultimately incorporated. Overall, logistic regression is the most prevalent modeling approach, but algorithms like SVM, RF, and artificial neural network (ANN) have emerged in recent years and can outperform LR with fewer features. Table 5 displays the performances of these models in the test datasets. Notably, there are significant variations in the source of participants, number of subjects, age, male-female ratio of the participants, race/ethnicity, features selected and incorporated, AHI cutoffs, and prevalence of different OSA severity across studies.

Also worth noting is that recent research often explores constructing and validating multiple machine learning algorithms within a single study, allowing comparison of model performance and the identification of the algorithm with the highest discriminative ability. For instance, Holfinger et al. developed four AI models, including LR, ANN, RF, and Kernel support vector machine using a large sleep clinic retrospective dataset from the international Sleep Apnea Global Interdisciplinary Consortium (SAGIC) [41]. The models were further externally validated utilizing two separate datasets: the prospectively collected SAGIC dataset and the Sleep Heart Health Study (SHHS), a community-based dataset. The researchers compared the performance of these models to the STOP-Bang questionnaire. Their results showed that a specific symptomless ANN model, using only age, sex, BMI, and race, achieved performance similar to STOP-Bang in both clinical and community settings. However, it's important to note that while the sensitivity of the ANN was comparable to STOP-Bang, its specificity remained low.

Table 4 Proposed algorithm and selected features of OSA prediction model with clinical features

Author/year	Algorithm	Feature no. included	Feature no. in the final model	Feature detail in the final model
Kirby 1999 [65]	GRNN	23	23	Age, gender, frequent awakening, witnessed apnea, observed chocking, excessive daytime sleepiness, ESS, HTN, alcohol consumption, smoking (pack-year), height, weight, BMI, SBP $\geq$ 140, DBP $\geq$ 90, tonsillar enlargement, soft palate enlargement, crowding of the oral pharynx, sum of the clinical score for the binary categorical values
Caffo 2010 [42]	Boosting	53	10	Neck circumference, BMI, age, snoring frequency, waist circumference, snoring loudness, gender, SOL, response to "What is the chance that you would doze off or fall asleep while sitting and reading?", and presence or absence of a heart attack.
Bouloukaki 2011 [66]	LR	11	4	Neck circumference, ESS, BMI, gender
Zou 2013 [67]	LR	5^a	5^a	Age, BMI, waist circumference, ESS score, and gender
		4^b	4^b	Age, waist circumference, ESS score, and minimum oxygen saturation (SaO2)
Marti-Soler 2016 [27]	LR		5	Neck circumference, BMI, snoring, age, and gender
Shah 2016 [68]	LR		4	Gender, age, BMI, and snoring frequency
Ustun 2016 [40]	SLIM	31	4^c	Age, BMI, HTN, and gender
			6^d	Age, HTN, BMI, diabetes, smoker, and gender
Wang 2016 [69]	SMOTE+FDT, LR, AN SVM	18	8	Waist circumference, height, hip circumference, age, Berlin_sum, IRLSSG, Forehead circumference, PS_DPB
Liu 2017 [39]	SVM		4	BMI, neck circumference, waist circumference, and age
Shin 2017 [70]	LR		14	Gender, BMI, ASA score, age, dyslipidemia, chronic pulmonary disease, liver disease, HTN, CHF, pulmonary HTN, AF, diabetes, CAD, and hemiplegia/paraplegia
Traxdorf 2017 [71]	LR	10	5	ESS score, age, gasping, cardiovascular risk factors (e.g., CHF, CAD, myocardial infarction, AF, stroke) or difficulty in adjusting high blood pressure, and witnessed apneas
Duarte 2018 [72]	LR		2	Neck circumference, and age

(continued)

Table 4 (continued)

Author/year	Algorithm	Feature no. included	Feature no. in the final model	Feature detail in the final model
Huang 2020 [37]	SVM, LR, NN, RF, GBT	32	2[e]	Waist circumference, and age
			6[f]	Waist circumference, age, neck circumference, snoring, witnessed apnea, and SOL < 30 min
Kim 2021 [73]	SVM, LR, RF, XGBoost		8	Waist circumference, loudness of snoring from BQ, FSS total score, subnasale to stomion, falling sleep from the BQ, HTN, snoring from the BQ
Keshavarz 2021 [74]	NB, LR, NN, KNN, SVM, RF	49	8	Severe snore, nocturia, awakening due to the sound of snoring, witnessed snore, witnessed apnea, back pain, restless sleep, and BMI
Zhang 2021 [75]	SVM		7	Sex, age, BMI, maximum interincisal distance, ratio of height to thyro-sternum distance, neck circumference and waist circumference
Holfinger 2022 [41]	LR, ANN, RF, KSVM		4	Age, gender, BMI, and race
Casal-Guisande 2023 [76]	ANFIS (multiple algorithms)		41	Gender, age, BMI, neck circumference, smoking habits, cigarettes per day, years as a smoker, pack year index, drinking habits, grams of alcohol, HTN, resistant HTN, ACVA, ACVA in less than a year, DM, Ischemic heart disease, COPD, home oxygen therapy, rhinitis, depression, AF, HF, Antidepressants, Antihistamines, Benzodiazepines, Morphics, Neuroleptics, Tranquilizers/Hypnotics, hours of sleep, minutes until falling asleep, prolonged intra-sleep awakenings, feeling of unrefreshing sleep, daytime tiredness, morning dullness, unjustified multiple awakenings, nocturia, breathless awakenings, reported apneas, snorer, high intensity snorer, and snore related awakenings

Han 2023 [79]	XGBoost, LightGBM, CatBoost, and RF	19	9[g]	Hip circumference, head circumference, age, neck circumference (sitting position), weight, BMI, abdominal circumference
			8[h]	Age, abdominal circumference, PSQI total score, BMI, weight, hip circumference, SSS total score, head circumference, height
			8[i]	Sex, hours of sleep, abdominal circumference, weight, hip circumference, SSS total score, head circumference, height
Huo 2023 [78]	LR, SVC, KNN, DT, ET, AB, GNB, RF	23	6	BMI, gender, neck girth, snoring loudness, hypertension, and age

Abbreviations: *AB* Ada boost, *ANFIS* Adaptive Neuro-fuzzy Inference System, *ANN* artificial neural network, *ASA* American Society of Anesthesiologists, *AF* atrial fibrillation, *BMI* body mass index, *BQ* Berlin Questionnaire, *CAD* coronary artery disease, *CHF* congestive heart failure, *DBP* diastolic blood pressure, *DT* decision tree, *EDS* excessive daytime sleepiness, *ESS* Epworth Sleepiness Scale, *ET* extra tree, *FDT* Fuzzy decision tree, *FSS* Fatigue Severity Scale, *GBT* Gradient Boosting Tree, *GNB* Gaussian Naïve Bayes, *GRNN* generalized regression neural network, *HTN* hypertension, *IRLSSG* task force of the International RLS Study Group, *KNN* k-nearest neighbors, *KSVM* kernel support vector machine, *LR* logistic regression, *NB* Naïve Bayes, *NN* neural network, *RF* Random Forest, *SBP* systolic blood pressure, *SLIM* supersparse linear integer model, *SOL* sleep onset latency, *SOMTE* synthetic minority oversampling technique, *SVC* support vector classifier, *SVM* support vector machine, *XGBoost* Extreme Gradient Boosting

[a]$\text{Prediction1} = 1/[1+\exp(0.0486 \times \text{age} + 0.1356 \times \text{BMI} + 0.0616\ \text{WC} + 0.1626 \times \text{ESS} + 0.4546 \times \text{sex} - 10.535)]$

[b]$\text{Prediction2} = 1/[1+\exp(0.0296 \times \text{age} + 0.0596 \times \text{WC} + 0.1116 \times \text{ESS} - 0.3596 \times \text{minimum SaO2} + 26.202)]$

[c]Size 5, false positive rate goal of 20%

[d]Size 10, false positive rate goal of 20%

[e]SVM predict AHI $\geq$ 5/h

[f]SVM predict AHI $\geq$ 15/h and $\geq$30/h

[g]AHI $\geq$ 5/h

[h]AHI $\geq$ 15/h

[i]AHI $\geq$ 30/h

Table 5 Data profile and performance of OSA prediction models with clinical features

Author/year	Source	Subject no.	Age (y/o)	Male (%)	AHI cutoff (/h)	Preva (%)	Algorithm	AUROC	Accu (%)	Sen (%)	Spec (%)	PPV (%)	NPV (%)
Kirby 1999 [65]	S	150	51	66	≥10	65.00	GRNN	0.94	91.3	98.90	80.00	88.10	98.00
Caffo 2010 [42]	C	1383	65.0	47.3	≥7[a]	37.80	LR	0.75	N/A	66.00	70.00	57.00	77.21
Bouloukaki 2011 [66]	S	2690	50.7	79.0	≥15	79.00	LR	0.78	N/A	70.00	73.10	81.00	62.00
Zou 2013 [67]	S	784	41.0	83.2	≥5	83.80	LR	1. 0.84[b]	N/A	1. 86.91	1. 74.80	1.94.69	1. 52.49
								2. 0.98[c]	N/A	2. 94.22	2. 85.83	2. 97.17	2. 74.15
Marti-Soler 2016 [27]	C	1042	42.0	45.0	>20	11.52	LR	0.74	N/A	85.00	77.00	33.0	98.0
Shah 2016 [68]	C	12,158	48.1	39.4	≥15	9.02	LR	0.83	N/A	77.00	75.00	23.39	97.05
Ustun 2016 [40]	S	1922	50.2	58.7	>5 or >10[a]	76.90	SLIM	1. 0.77[d]	N/A	1. 82.80	1. 56.20	1. 86.29	1. 49.53
								2. 0.79[e]	N/A	2. 83.20	2. 58.90	2. 87.08	2. 51.29
Wang 2016 [69]	S	3343	N/A	N/A	<5, 5–15, 15–30, >30	85.68	SMOTE+FDT	N/A	81.82	N/A	N/A	N/A	N/A
Liu 2017 [39]	S	1154	47.4	70.7	1. ≥15	1. 61.87	SVM	N/A[f]	N/A[f]	1. 68.35	1. 82.55	1. 86.40	1. 61.65
					2. ≥30	2. 44.04		N/A		2. 68.32	2. 79.85	2. 64.99	2. 77.45
Shin 2017 [70]	SW	108,781	54.4	44.4	>5	2.08	LR	0.82	N/A	72.30	76.20	6.06	99.23
Traxdorf 2017 [71]	S	100	48.1	76.0	1. ≥5	1. 70.00	LR	N/A	N/A	1. 94.30	1. 50.00	1. 81.50	1. 78.90
					2. ≥15	2. 55.50		N/A	N/A	2. 92.70	2. 33.30	2. 62.90	2. 78.90
					3. ≥30	3. 26.00		N/A	N/A	3. 92.30	3. 22.90	3. 29.60	3. 89.50
Duarte 2018 [72]	S	2035	44.0	53.2	1. ≥5	1. 76.40	LR	1. 0.78	1.77.20	1.83.10	2.58.20	1. 86.50	1. 51.60
					2. ≥15	2. 54.70		2. 0.76	2.69.00	2. 88.70	2. 45.30	2. 66.20	2. 76.80
					3. ≥30	3. 35.80		3. 0.75	3.56.40	3. 91.50	3. 36.80	3. 44.60	3. 88.60
Huang 2020 [37]	S	6875	47.8	76.0	1. ≥5	1. 82.45	SVM	1. 0.82	1.74.24	1. 74.14	1. 74.71	1. 93.23	1. 38.15
					2. ≥15	2. 61.25		2. 0.80	2.72.68	2. 75.18	2. 68.73	2. 79.32	2. 64.03
					3. ≥30	3. 40.60		3. 0.78	3.70.28	3. 70.26	3. 70.30	3. 61.97	3. 77.86

Kim 2021 [73]	S	279	45.4[g]	83.9	≥5	76.3	SVM	0.87	83.33	80.33	86.96	88.52	69.57
Keshavarz 2021 [74]	S	250	N/A	61.9	≥15	65.8	NB	0.768	72.3	78.95	59.49	N/A	N/A
Zhang 2021 [75]	S	481	47.3	67.6	≥15	35.55	SVM	0.83	N/A	92	75	N/A	N/A
Holfinger 2022 [41]	S	17,448	32.7	48.0	≥15	53.22	ANN	0.68	N/A	74	51	0.63	0.64
Casal-Guisande 2023 [76]	S	5000	55.1	63.7	1. ≥10	1. 72.59	ANFIS	1. 0.88	N/A	1. 89	1. 67	N/A	N/A
					2. ≥15	2. 61.46		2. 0.88	N/A	2. 87	2. 74	N/A	N/A
					3. ≥20	3. 51.30		3. 0.83	N/A	3. 87	3. 65	N/A	N/A
					4. ≥25	4. 43.41		4. 0.83	N/A	4. 70	4. 81	N/A	N/A
					5. ≥30	5. 36.80		5. 0.86	N/A	5. 76	5. 80	N/A	N/A
Han 2023 [79]	S	803	54	68.7	1. ≥5	1. 22.42	LightGBM	1. 0.82	1. 87.82	1. 97.85	N/A	1. 88.56	N/A
					2. ≥15	2. 24.16		2. 0.95	2. 87.84	2. 92.65	N/A	2. 89.27	N/A
					3. ≥30	3. 35.87		3. 0.95	3. 91.06	3. 70.19	N/A	3. 90.87	N/A
Huo 2023 [78]	C	1237	60.2	50.8	≥15	54.81	LR	0.78	N/A	77	68	N/A	N/A

Abbreviations: *Acc* accuracy, *AHI* apnea-hypopnea index, *ANN* artificial neural network, *ANFIS* Adaptive Neuro-fuzzy Inference System, *AUROC* area under receiver operating characteristic, *Accu* accuracy, *C* community, *FDT* Fuzzy decision tree, *GRNN* generalized regression neural network, *LR* logistic regression, *N/A* not available, *NB* Naïve Bayes, *NPV* negative predictive value, *PPV* positive predictive value, *Preva* prevalence, *S* sleep clinic, *Sen* sensitivity, *SLIM* supersparse linear integer model, *Spec* specificity, *SOMTE* synthetic minority oversampling technique, *SVM* support vector machine, *SW* surgical ward

[a] Respiratory disturbance index (RDI)

[b] Prediction1 = 1/[1+ exp (0.0486 × age +0.1356 BMI +0.0616 × WC +0.1626 ESS +0.4546 × sex −10.535)]

[c] Prediction2 = 1/[1+ exp (0.0296 × age +0.0596 × WC +0.1116 × ESS −0.3596 × minimum SaO2 +26.202)]

[d] Size 5, false positive rate goal of 20%

[e] Size 10, false positive rate goal of 20%

[f] No whole-group data available

[g] OSA

2.3 Case Study: Development of an OSA Prediction Model Using Clinical Features

Here we present a case study for developing an ML model to predict OSA using clinical features. We utilize the 2020 article by Huang et al. as a reference [37]. This investigation stands as one of the recent efforts to build an OSA screening model upon SVM, leveraging a large clinical dataset obtained from a single sleep center.

This study addressed two key limitations in recent OSA screening models. First, it tackled the class imbalance issue between sensitivity and specificity, which often leads to over-prediction of OSA, resulting in unnecessary PSG testing for patients who do not actually have the condition. Second, it designed a two-stage feature selection process with three AHI cutoffs. The first stage allowed the categorical features and continuous features to be selected separately, and the second stage allowed priorities of features to change with different AHI cutoffs. In this following section, we offer insights concerning the dataset characteristics, algorithm selection rationale, feature selection process, SVM model training procedure, results, and a discussion of the study's strengths and limitations.

2.3.1 Dataset

The dataset for the OSA screening model training was collected from 7830 adult patients who underwent overnight PSG for the first time in the Center of Sleep Disorder of National Taiwan University Hospital between Jan. 2009 and Dec. 2016. For data mining, only patients who had any following conditions were excluded: non-Chinese ($n = 11$), total recording time <240 min ($n = 7$), and missing data ($n = 936$). A total of 6875 patients, with 5223 men and 1652 women (5985 <65 y/o and 890 ≥65 y/o) were included. The data included 32 features, encompassing subject basic information, anthropometrics, comorbidities, and sleep history (Table 6).

Overnight PSG was performed on subjects as previously reported [31]. Sleep stages and respiratory events were scored according to the 2007 AASM scoring rule [32]. Apnea was defined as ≥90% decrease in airflow for ≥10 s, while hypopnea was ≥30% decrease in airflow for ≥10 s associated with ≥4% reduction in arterial oxygen saturation. The PSG parameters collected included SE, percentage of slow-wave sleep and rapid eye movement, AHI, ODI, percentage of total sleep time with SpO2 <90% (%TST-SpO2 <90%), and arousal index.

2.3.2 Algorithm Selection

The performance of eight different algorithms was assessed and compared, including SVM with radial basis function (RBF) kernel, SVM with polynomial (Poly) kernel, LR, neural network, RF, RF combined with LR, Gradient Boosting Tree,

Table 6 Thirty-two input features and category

Demographics	Anthropometric	Co-morbidities	Sleep history	Symptoms suggestive of OSA
Age	BMI	Hypertension	SOL (min)	Snore
Gender	Neck circumference	Diabetes	SOL <30 min	Witnessed apnea
Alcohol consumption	Waist circumference	CAD	Sleep duration, <6, 6–8, and ≥8 h	Frequency of nocturia (time/night)
Current smoking		CHF	Unrefreshed sleep	Nocturia ≥2 times/night
Hypnotics		CVA	Frequency of awakening at sleep (time/night)	Witnessed leg jerks in sleep
		CKD	Awakening at sleep ≥3 times/night	Morning headache
		COPD	ESS score	Dry throat at waking up
		Asthma	EDS (ESS score ≥10)	
		Hypothyroidism		

Adapted under a CC BY-NC 4.0 license from Huang and Lee et al. [37]
Abbreviations: *BMI* body mass index, *circum.* circumference, *CAD* coronary artery disease, *CHF* congestive heart failure, *CVA* cerebrovascular accident, *CKD* chronic kidney disease, *COPD* chronic obstructive pulmonary disease, *ESS* Epworth Sleepiness Scale, *EDS* excessive daytime sleepiness, *SOL* sleep onset latency

and Gradient Boosting Tree integrated with LR. These algorithms were utilized to develop models using 32 features across three AHI thresholds. The effectiveness of these models was determined using their area under the receiver operating characteristics (AUROC) scores, with the SVM achieving the highest AUROC. Figure 1 illustrates the AUROC score comparison among the eight algorithms. Following this evaluation, SVM model was further refined through feature selection to improve the model's generalizability and potential for real-world application.

2.3.3 Feature Selection

Figure 2 depicts the flowchart outlining the SVM prediction model's development. The training procedure of the proposed prediction model includes data input, data exclusion, two-stage feature selection, and model training with optimization. Recognizing the distinct mathematical characteristics of continuous and categorical features, this study implemented a two-stage feature selection procedure. This safeguards against the selection process being unduly influenced by a singular feature type during model training. In the first stage, both the continuous and categorical features underwent filtering based on the median of AUROC and Matthews correlation coefficient, respectively. This filtering aimed to mitigate the influence

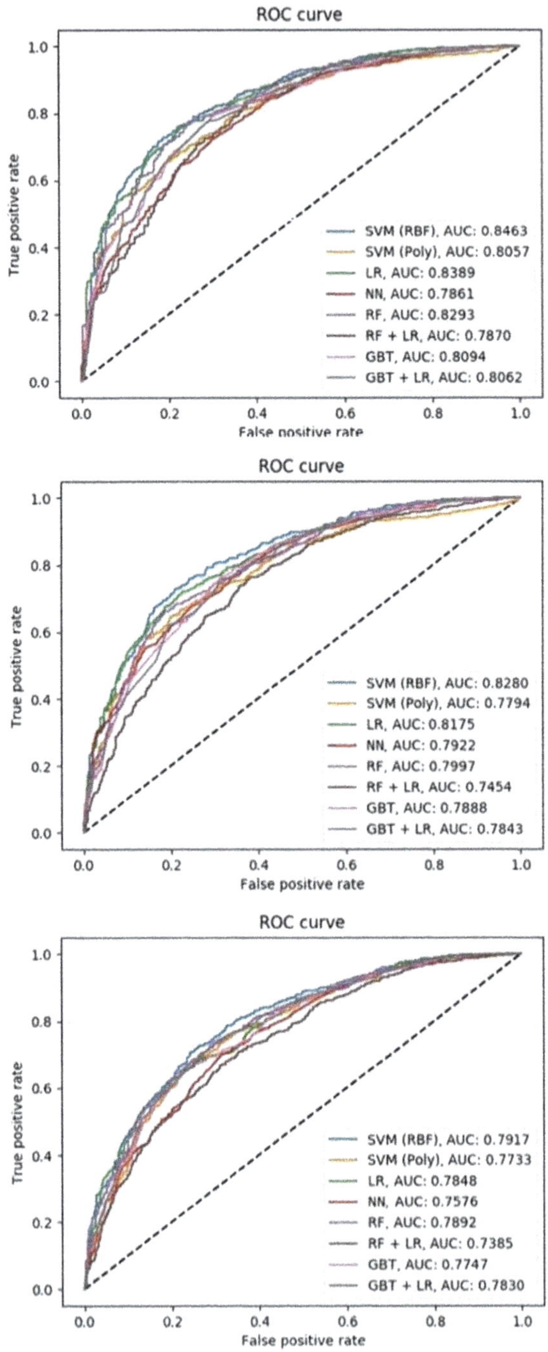

Fig. 1 ROC curves and AUROC comparison of eight algorithms. From top to bottom, the AHI cutoff for classification is 5/h, 15/h, and 30/h, respectively. Abbreviation: SVM (RBF), SVM with radial basis function kernel; SVM (Poly), SVM with polynomial kernel

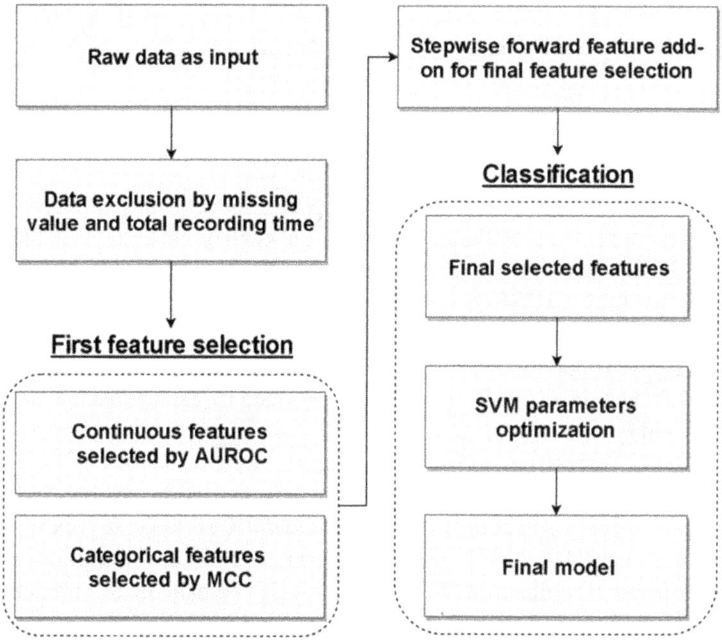

Fig. 2 The flow chart of developing an SVM prediction model. Non-Chinese ($n = 11$), total recording time < 240 min ($n = 7$), and any missing data ($n = 936$) were excluded. In the first feature selection stage, we observed that the top half of AUROC and MCC feature ranks were similar in all three different AHI cutoffs suggesting the robustness of these features. Therefore, only features with AUROC or MCC higher than median remained in the model. In forward stepwise feature selection stage, the fewest features were selected to keep AUROC $\geq$ 0.80. Abbreviations: AUROC, area under receiver operating characteristic curve; MCC, Matthew correlation coefficient. (Adapted under a CC BY-NC 4.0 license from Huang and Lee et al. [37])

of redundant features. Subsequently, forward stepwise feature selection (FSFS) was leveraged in the second stage of feature selection. Finally, the meticulously chosen features were employed to train and optimize the SVM models.

During the first feature selection stage, we observed that the top half of AUROC and MCC feature ranks were similar in all three different AHI cutoffs, suggesting the robustness of these features. This means only features exceeding the median AUROC or MCC score were retained. In the FSFS stage, we defined two key criteria to guide the feature selection process: (1) minimizing the total number of selected features, and (2) ensuring an AUROC value $\geq$0.80.

To further optimize classification performance, Youden's index was employed to identify the optimal threshold of SVM posterior probability in assigning categories. In addition, the fivefold cross-validation was randomly repeated five times to verify the reliability of the model. The average AUROC for each of the three AHI cutoffs was calculated using the fivefold cross-validation. Notably, the training of the prediction model leveraged a sleep lab-based dataset encompassing these three aforementioned AHI cutoffs, which suggests the models based on the three AHI cutoffs were fairly trained and internally validated.

2.3.4 Data Analysis

The discriminative ability of the proposed SVM model was evaluated using an average of fivefold cross-validation approach. For each of the three AHI cutoffs (5/h, 15/h, and 30/h), the following performance metrics were calculated and averaged across the five folds: AUROC, accuracy, sensitivity, specificity, positive predictive value (PPV), and negative predictive value (NPV). The cutoff of AUROC value was identified using Youden's index. The model's discriminative ability was evaluated for the whole data set and four subgroups categorized by gender and age (<65 versus ≥65 years old [y/o]).

For logistic regression, 67% of participants were randomly selected as the training set, while the remaining 33% were selected as the testing set. Logistic models with forward selection were used to identify suitable factors to establish the prediction model for AHI ≥5/h, ≥15/h, and ≥30/h in the training set. Each factor has to be significant at the 0.0001 level to remain in the model. All the remaining variables were listed with odds ratio and 95% confidence interval. The model's ability to predict each AHI cutoff was evaluated using AUROC.

The performance of the SVM model was compared to logistic regression, BQ, NoSAS score, and supersparse linear integer model (SLIM) scoring system.

2.3.5 Model Discriminative Ability

The results of this study indicated that higher AHI cutoffs required more features to achieve AUROC ≥0.80. For the three AHI cutoffs, 2, 6, and 6 features were needed, respectively. The classifiers were tested with 6875 subject data by fivefold cross-validation. Table 7 shows features selected by SVM and logistic regression. The discriminative ability of SVM, logistic regression, BQ, NoSAS score, and SLIM scoring systems for three AHI cutoffs is shown in Table 8. In the SVM model, when employing 2, 6, and 6 features for AHI cutoffs of 5/h, 15/h, and 30/h, the model achieved the following performance: AUROC (0.82, 0.8, 0.78), accuracy (74.24%, 72.68%, and 70.28%), sensitivity (74.14%, 75.18%, and 70.26%), specificity (74.71%, 68.73%, and 70.30%), PPV (93.23%, 79.32%, 61.93%), and NPV (38.15%, 64.03%, 77.86%). The discriminative ability was best for males <65 y/o and modest for females ≥65 y/o. The learning curve showed no evidence of overfitting (Fig. 3).

Compared to logistic regression, this SVM model offers a simple and accurate modality with only two to six features routinely collected at clinic visits. It exhibits non-inferior discriminative ability and balanced sensitivity and specificity. Overall, the SVM model outperformed the BQ, NoSAS score, and SLIM scoring system. However, limitations exist. Significantly, the dataset originated from a Chinese sleep

Table 7 The features selected with forward stepwise feature selection of SVM model and logistic regression for three AHI cutoffs

Method	Order	AHI ≥ 5/h	AHI ≥ 15/h	AHI ≥ 30/h
SVM	1	Waist circumference	Waist circumference	Waist circumference
	2	Age	Age	Witnessed apnea
	3		Neck circumference	Age
	4		Snoring	Neck circumference
	5		Witnessed apnea	Snoring
	6		SOL < 30 min	SOL < 30 min
Logistic regression	N/A	Snoring	Snoring	Witnessed apnea
		Gender	Witnessed apnea	Gender
		Age	Dry throat	Snoring
		Neck circumference	Gender	Hypertension
		SOL	Hypnotic	Dry throat
		BMI	Age	Waist circumference
		Waist circumference	Waist circumference	Age
			Neck circumference	Neck circumference
			SOL	BMI
			BMI	SOL

In SVM model, the minimal feature set was selected to achieve the target criteria in the AUROC. When AHI cutoffs were 5/h and 15/h, the target AUROC was set as 0.8. While AHI cutoff was 30/h, the experiment showed that the maximum AUROC was 0.78, so the minimum features were selected to achieve the performance
Abbreviations: *AHI* apnea-hypopnea index, *BMI* body mass index, *N/A* not applicable, *SVM* support vector machine, *SOL* sleep onset latency

clinic cohort with high OSA prevalence. Further external validation is needed in the community setting with lower OSA prevalence and diverse racial/ethnic groups.

2.3.6 Considerations Concerning Modeling

Several critical issues should be taken into consideration in the modeling process.

Data imbalance: The prevalence of OSA can potentially impact the model's sensitivity and positive predictive value. It is essential to note that sleep clinic datasets tend to be skewed toward moderate-to-severe OSA cases compared to community datasets. This imbalance can lead to an overestimation of the model's ability to distinguish between different OSA severity levels [37, 69].

Continuous versus categorical features: Feature selection is usually based on the algorithm's preference. Some algorithms like SVMs often favor continuous variables. To ensure all relevant information is utilized, the process of feature selection for SVM models might require stratification to prevent overlooking valuable categorical variables [37].

Table 8 The performance of SVM, logistic regression, Berlin Questionnaire, NoSAS score, and SLIM scoring system at three AHI cutoffs

Model	AHI cutoff (/h)	Feature no.	AUROC	Accuracy (%)	Sensitivity (%)	Specificity (%)	PPV (%)	NPV (%)
SVM	≥5	2	0.82 (0.79–0.85)	74.24 (71.59–76.89)	74.14 (71.33–76.95)	74.71 (70.88–78.54)	93.23 (92.17–94.29)	38.15 (34.79–41.52)
	≥15	6	0.80 (0.79–0.81)	72.68 (70.52–74.84)	75.18 (67.61–82.76)	68.73 (61.72–75.75)	79.32 (76.84–81.80)	64.03 (59.75–68.31)
	≥30	6	0.78 (0.77–0.80)	70.28 (68.68–71.88)	70.26 (60.21–80.31)	70.30 (64.18–76.43)	61.93 (59.21–64.35)	77.86 (73.68–82.03)
LR	≥5	7	0.84 (0.83–0.86)	73.77	94.41	37.87	72.55	79.56
	≥15	10	0.81 (0.80–0.82)	72.14	79.94	62.69	72.21	72.03
	≥30	10	0.79 (0.78–0.81)	72.83	65.01	78.77	69.94	74.77
BQ	≥5	–	0.54 (0.52–0.56)	67.58	74.95	32.91	84.01	21.89
	≥15	–	0.53 (0.52–0.55)	58.39	76.09	30.41	63.34	44.58
	≥30	–	0.53 (0.51–0.54)	48.09	76.68	28.55	42.31	64.17
NoSAS score	≥5	4	0.70 (0.68–0.71)	57.25	50.62	88.39	95.31	27.58
	≥15	4	0.68 (0.67–0.70)	66.01	57.99	78.67	81.13	54.23
	≥30	4	0.68 (0.67–0.69)	68.30	64.88	70.64	60.16	74.64

Adapted under a CC BY-NC 4.0 license from Huang and Lee et al. [37]
The data were presented as mean (95% confidence interval)
Abbreviations: *AHI* apnea-hypopnea index, *AUROC* area under receiver operating characteristic, *BQ* Berlin Questionnaire, *LR* logistic regression, *NPV* negative predictive value, *PPV* positive predictive value, *SVM* support vector machines

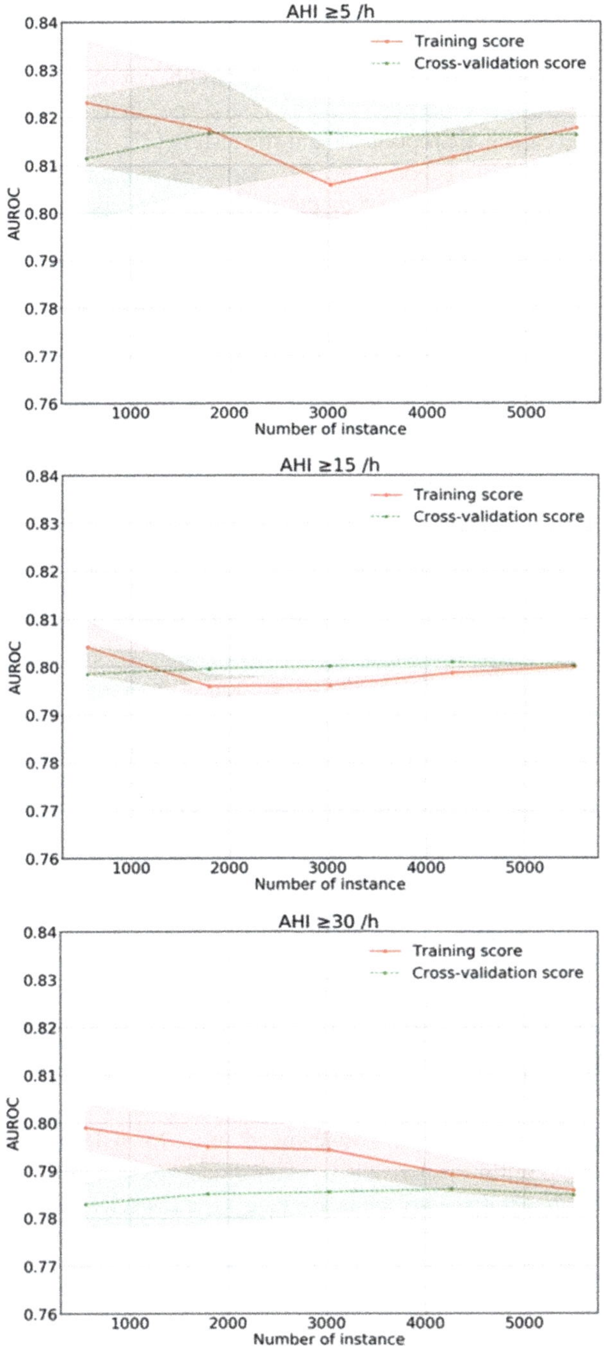

Fig. 3 Learning curve of the prediction model with two, six, and six features for prediction of AHI ≥5/h, ≥15/h, and ≥30/h. The red line indicates the training score, and the green line indicates the cross-validation score. The colored area represents the 95% confidence interval (CI). The training and testing curves showed similar results, and they converged in the end. The 95% CI also showed the convergence of training and testing curves as the training data increased

Sensitivity versus specificity tradeoff: Many prediction models tend to prioritize high sensitivity at the expense of low specificity. This approach can lead to over-prescription of sleep studies for individuals who might not actually have OSA. It is crucial to strike a balance between sensitivity and specificity to optimize resource allocation and to ensure appropriate diagnostic testing [37, 41, 87].

Generalizability: All AI models need to be tested utilizing a separate external dataset to ensure the robustness of model performance, especially for those built with small datasets, lacking diverse ethnicities and races, or using data from a single institution [41, 43, 77, 78, 87]. Beyond performance, the feasibility of deploying the model in various clinical settings should also be considered. Overall, the more clinical features a model incorporates, the more challenging its implementation might be. Relying on fewer features readily available during clinic visits, as opposed to utilizing long questionnaires, can potentially enhance the adoption of the model for OSA screening at clinics [37, 41, 43, 77].

2.3.7 Future Implication

AI/ML/DL models built on clinical features are poised to revolutionize OSA screening in clinics. These models can become invaluable assets for busy family physicians or non-sleep specialists swamped by managing a multitude of chronic illnesses. Particularly promising is the integration of these prediction models with existing questionnaire instruments and EMR. Imagine an advanced system that can proactively flag high-risk patients for moderate or severe OSA during routine visits, thereby prompting clinicians of the need for further diagnostic testing and therapeutic interventions [17, 43]. Marrying this AI-powered screening approach with the compact, user-friendly, novel OSA-detecting wearables discussed in Sect. 3 has the potential to transform how we identify and manage OSA in the years to come, redefining the landscape of clinical sleep medicine.

3 AI/ML/DL Algorithms Using Physiological Signals for OSA Diagnosis: The Home Setting

In this segment, we explore the advancements in AI/ML/DL algorithms for OSA diagnosis at home settings across three major dimensions: (1) FDA-cleared SaMD and algorithms integrated into medical-grade wearables for OSA diagnosis; (2) algorithms incorporated in consumer wearables that are capable for OSA detection; and (3) published standalone algorithms without any devices. As nearables and sound-based technologies are discussed in other chapters, we limit our discussions to the algorithms utilizing PPG and/or accelerometry signals in this section.

It is crucial to recognize that our discourse surrounding these algorithms, whether device-integrated or standalone, is often constrained due to their commercial and proprietary nature. Additionally, "transitional devices" (those transitioning from consumer to medical-grade) with the potential for future regulatory approval often have limited publicly available technical details regarding their algorithms. Consequently, our primary objective here is to provide a comparative overview of the different AI/ML/DL model architectures and their reported performance, rather than explore the intricacies of model development processes.

It is also important to note that the information presented in this section draws from FDA 510(k) notifications, peer-reviewed publications, publicly available information, and on some occasions, communication with the manufacturers. This reflects the best available knowledge at the time of this writing. Future iterations of these algorithms may incorporate substantial advancements, necessitating ongoing review, and potential updates.

3.1 *Introduction of Deep Learning Architectures*

Before delving deeper into the discussion of AI/ML/DL algorithms utilizing physiological signals for OSA diagnosis, it is essential to provide a concise review of the DL architectures commonly employed. While Sect. 2.1 addressed key ML models using clinical features, this section focuses specifically on DL approaches leveraging physiological signals measured by various wearable sensors.

Overall, DL models are considered more advanced and advantageous for sleep physiological data analysis than ML models. This stems from their ability to autonomously extract pertinent features from intricate datasets and learn hierarchical representations. Sleep physiology data exhibits multidimensionality and is characterized by nuanced patterns, making it well-suited for DL approaches. In contrast, manual feature extraction in ML models presents several drawbacks [18]. First, ML can introduce bias originating from the reliance on domain expertise for feature selection. Second, this approach is a labor-intensive and time-consuming process. Lastly, it may be poorly adaptable to changes in data distributions, which limits the model's ability to generalize across diverse datasets and necessitates significant effort to update or refine features as new information becomes available.

Several DL architectures have been utilized in OSA diagnosis, and they can be broadly categorized into basic and advanced structures. Basic DL architectures serve as the foundation for more complex DL models, with the latter incorporating more sophisticated mechanisms and structures to address specific challenges in managing very deep networks, refining sequence modeling, and enhancing feature extraction and representation.

3.1.1 Basic DL Architectures

1. *Dense layers (fully connected layers)* [88]: Dense layers, or fully connected layers, are the simplest form of DL models, where each neuron in a layer is

connected to every neuron in the next layer. They are often used to combine features.

2. *Convolutional Neural Network (CNN)* [89]: CNNs are specialized DL models for processing data with a grid-like topology, such as images. They use convolutional layers to efficiently recognize spatial hierarchies in data.
3. *Recurrent Neural Network (RNN)* [88]: RNNs are designed to handle sequential data, allowing previous outputs to be used as inputs while having hidden states. They are fundamental for tasks that involve sequences, such as speech recognition.
4. *Long Short-Term Memory (LSTM)* [90]: LSTMs are a special kind of RNN capable of learning long-term dependencies. They do this through mechanisms called gates that regulate the flow of information.
5. *Bi-directional Long Short-Term Memory (Bi-LSTM)* [91]: Bi-LSTMs process data in both forward and backward directions, making them powerful for capturing context in text and sequence data more effectively than unidirectional LSTMs.

3.1.2 Advanced DL Architectures

1. *Multiscale convolutional network* [92]: Multiscale convolutional networks process data at multiple resolutions to capture features at various scales. This approach enhances the model's ability to recognize patterns of different sizes.
2. *Temporal convolutional network (TCN)* [93]: TCNs apply convolutional operations across time. They are designed for sequence modeling tasks and can capture long-term dependencies in time-series data effectively.
3. *ResNet* [94]: Short for Residual Network, is a type of CNN architecture that introduced the concept of "skip connections" to enable the training of much deeper networks. These connections allow the gradient to flow through the network directly, mitigating the vanishing gradient problem and leading to significant improvements in training deep neural networks. ResNets are widely used for various computer vision tasks due to their ability to efficiently learn from data and their scalability to hundreds or even thousands of layers.
4. *ResNeXt* [95]: ResNeXt is a variation of the ResNet model that introduces a "cardinality" dimension, which represents the number of independent paths within blocks. This design improves accuracy and efficiency.
5. *Squeeze-and-excitation network* [96]: This network architecture introduces a mechanism to explicitly model the interdependencies between channels of convolutional features, enhancing the representational power of the network.
6. *Encoder-Decoder* [97]: This architecture is used for translating between different forms of data. It works by compressing an input into a latent-space representation and then expanding it back to an output of a different form, commonly used in machine translation.

7. *U-Net* [98]: U-Net is a convolutional network architecture for fast and precise segmentation of images. It's especially useful in medical image analysis, featuring a symmetric expanding path that helps in precise localization.
8. *Transformer* [99]: Transformers are models that use self-attention mechanisms to weigh the significance of different parts of the input data differently. They are highly efficient for tasks like language understanding. This model surged in popularity following its successful application in ChatGPT.

3.2 SaMD and Algorithms Integrated into Medical-Grade Wearables for OSA Diagnosis

As indicated in Sect. 1.3.3, the US FDA has cleared ten OSA-diagnosing wearables/SaMD in recent years [100–109]. These emerging wearables and SaMD can be categorized into four groups:

- PAT-based: including NightOwl (Ectosense, Belgium; now under ResMed), ANNE sleep (Sibel Inc. Niles, Illinois), and Somfit (Compumedics Limited, Australia)
- PPG-based: encompassing SleepImage SaMD (MyCardio, Denver, Colorado), Aurora SaMD (EnsoData, Madison, Wisconsin), and Belun Sleep System BLS-100 (Belun Technology Company Limited, Hong Kong)
- Respiratory effort-base: such as Wesper Lab (Wesper, New York, New York) and Sunrise (Sunrise, Belgium)
- Acoustic-based: represented by AcuPebble OX100 (Acurable, London, UK) and BresoDx1 (BresoTEC, Toronto, Ontario, Canada)

Table 9 delineates the wearable/SaMD names, 510(k) numbers, approval dates, type of sensors used and their locations, the signal channels, the dataset used for clinical validation, and the performance for OSA detection and sleep staging. Notably, SleepImage, AcuPebble, and NightOwl are not included in Table 9 as their algorithms are rule-based (NightOwl does have published ML algorithms for central sleep apnea detection but not for OSA detection to the best of our knowledge) [110]. Wesper Lab lacks publications indicating the use of AI/ML/DL algorithms and is also not included.

3.2.1 Sensor Modalities in FDA-Cleared OSA-Detecting Wearables

Modern wearable technologies for OSA detection integrate two key components: miniaturized, high-performance electronic sensors and advanced AI/ML/DL algorithms. Unlike conventional pulse oximeters, which typically obtain PPG signals from the fingertip, the FDA-cleared OSA-detecting wearables strategically incorporate cutting-edge sensors positioned across various body parts, including

Table 9 FDA 510(k) summary of medical-grade devices for OSA diagnosis with AI/ML/DL

Device name/ (510(k) no.)/ approved date/ type	Sensor location & signal channels	Dataset of clinical trial	Performance of evaluating OSA severity	Performance of sleep stage estimation
Aurora [100] (K231355) 8-Feb-2024 SaMD	Sensors: no specific criteria. Channels: PPG and oximetry.	158 adults.	AHI3 $\geq$ 5: sen 92.6%, spec 71.6%. AHI4 $\geq$ 5: sen 89.4%, spec 76.8%.	4-class sleep stage: Wake: sen 86.7%, spec 93.5%; Light NREM: sen 80.9%, spec 85.5%; Deep NREM: sen 63.4%, spec 95.9%; REM: sen 83.6%, spec 97.5%.
Somfit [101] (K231546) 30-Nov-2023 Device	Sensors on forehead: Photodiode, oximeter front end, microphone, accelerometer, and EEG amplification. Channels: PAT, pulse rate, oximetry, EEG, snoring and motion.	91 adults.	Mean difference (95% confidence interval) of Somfit AHI vs WatchPAT AHI: 0.294 (−2.661, 2.074) events/h. Mean difference (95% confidence interval) of Somfit ODI vs PSG ODI: 0.658 (−1.012, 2.326) events/h.	5-class sleep stage: Wake: sen 80.04%, spec 92.44%; N1: sen 19.67%, spec 96.96%; N2: sen 85.43%, spec 83.20%; N3: sen 65.06%, spec 98.63%; REM: sen 88.73%, spec 95.87%.
Belun Sleep System [102] (K222579) 23-Feb-2023 Device	Sensors on proximal phalanx: Optical PPG sensor and accelerometer. Channels: PPG, pulse rate, oximetry and actigraphy.	106 adults.	AHI4 $\geq$ 15: sen 87.7%, spec 86.0%; AHI4 $\geq$ 30: sen 84.0%, spec 95.1%.	3-class sleep stage: Wake: sen 60.4%, spec 96.1%; NREM: sen 90.4%, spec 69.5%; REM: sen 71.2%, spec 94.4%.
Sunrise [104] (K222262) 22-Dec-2022 Device	Sensors at chin: Accelerometer (gyroscope), PPG (sensor 2) and thermistor (sensor 2). Channels: Mandibular movements, discrete position, SpO2 and pulse rate.	289 adults in Belgium and 31 adults in France.	Belgium group: AHI $\geq$ 5: sen 99%, spec 86%; AHI $\geq$ 15: sen 92%, spec 94%; AHI $\geq$ 30: sen 81%, spec 99%. France group: AHI $\geq$ 5: sen 100%, spec 75%; AHI $\geq$ 15: sen 94%, spec 100%; AHI $\geq$ 30: sen 87%, spec 100%.	Mean difference (95% confidence interval) of TST: Belgium group, −4.50 (−41.74, 35.67) min; France group, −10.50 (−37.42, 25.79) min.

BresoDX1 [105] (K220012) 21-Dec-2022 Device	Sensors on suprasternal notch: Microphone and accelerometer. Sensors on finger: Oximeter sensor. Channels: Airflow, respiratory effort, tracheal breath sounds, tracheosternal movement, pulse rate, SpO2 and body position.	164 adults.	REI_b-based diagnosis at AHI $\geq$ 15: sen 88.5%, spec 84.9%, PPV 84.1%, NPV 89.0%.	Not reported.
ANNE Sleep [106] (K220095) 11-Jul-2022 Device	Sensors at chest: ECG sensor and accelerometer. Sensor on finger: Oximeter. Channels: PAT, pulse rate, heart rate, oximetry, snoring, body position and chest movement.	225 adults.	AHI4 $\geq$ 15: sen 90%, spec 98%.	They have TST as analysis outputs but no validation results in 510k summary.

Abbreviation: *AHI* apnea-hypopnea index without specifying the hypopnea criteria, *AHI3* apnea-hypopnea index with hypopnea defined as a $\geq$30% drop in airflow for $\geq$10 s associated with an arousal or a $\geq$3% oxygen desaturation, *AHI4* apnea-hypopnea index with hypopnea defined as a $\geq$30% drop in airflow for $\geq$10 s associated with a $\geq$4% oxygen desaturation, *ECG* electrocardiography, *EEG* electroencephalogram, *NPV* negative predictive value, *N1* non-rapid eye movement sleep, stage 1, *N2* non-rapid eye movement sleep, stage 2, *N3* non-rapid eye movement sleep, stage 3, *NREM* non-rapid eye movement, *ODI* oxygen desaturation index, *PAT* peripheral arterial tonometry, *PPG* photoplethysmography, *PSG* polysomnography, *PPV* positive predictive value, REI_b the total number of respiratory events scored × 60 divided by monitoring time (in minutes), *REM* rapid eye movement, *SaMD* software as a medical device, *sen* sensitivity, *spec* specificity, *SpO2* oxygen saturation, *TST* total sleep time the fingertip (ANNE Sleep [106], NightOwl [108], SleepImage [109]), proximal phalanx (Belun ring [102], SleepImage ring), forehead (Somfit [101]), chin (Sunrise [104]), anterior neck over the trachea (AcuPebble [103]), suprasternal notch (BresoDX1 [105], ANNE Sleep chest sensor), and chest/abdomen (Wesper Lab [107]), as shown in Table 9. Notably, ANNE Sleep employs a dual-sensor configuration, incorporating both a fingertip and a chest sensor. Additionally, Aurora [100] and SleepImage, both received clearance from the FDA as SaMD, can offer OSA diagnostic capabilities through coupling with compatible medical-grade pulse oximeters. While SleepImage currently provides two pulse oximeter sensor options (a ring and a fingertip), there is no evidence that Aurora integrates with any specific medical devices to our knowledge.

3.2.2 AI/ML/DL Model Architectures in Medical-Grade OSA-Detecting Wearables/SaMD

Information concerning AI/ML/DL model architectures (including inputs, models, and outputs) employed by Belun Sleep Platform, NightOwl, ANNE Sleep, BresoDX1, and Sunrise was extracted from peer-reviewed publications and 510(k) premarket notifications. These findings are summarized and presented in Table 10. Notably, NightOwl, BresoDX1, and Aurora are among the OSA-detection tools utilizing ML algorithms, while Belun Ring, ANNE Sleep, BresoDX1, Somfit, and Aurora employ DL algorithms [110–116]. Aurora and Somfit are not included in Table 10 due to the absence of published information regarding their algorithms. Our understanding suggests that the Somfit sleep staging algorithm, utilizing three EEG/EOG channels (differential frontal EEG and approximations of left and right EOGs), is a DL algorithm based on a fully convolutional multi-layer neural network, while its automated respiratory events scoring algorithm is rule-based. The Aurora 510(k) notification indicated that its algorithms apply "ML algorithms including multiple deep neural network machine learning models," without providing further details [100].

An analysis of current wearable solutions reveals that only the Belun Sleep Platform and Sunrise integrate dual AI/ML/DL algorithms for both sleep staging and OSA detection. Although BresoDX1 incorporates DL algorithms for respiratory event classification [114], its current algorithms for sleep assessment have not been described in recent BresoDX1 articles (though an SVM model was used in "the Patch," likely a prior BresoDX1 prototype.) [113] Notably, Sunrise utilizes ML for both functions, while the Belun Sleep Platform leverages a sophisticated DL architecture for both respiratory event detection and sleep stage classification [111, 115].

Table 10 Artificial intelligence of medical-grade devices for OSA diagnosis

Novel device	Author/year	Design of model (Inputs/structure/outputs)	Model training and testing	Performance
Belun Sleep System	Strumpf et al. 2023 [111]	*Inputs*: SpO2, pulse rate and accelerometer signals. *Model*: 8-layer ResNeXt with squeeze-and-excitation network modules for respiratory event detection; transformer with CNN for sleep stage classification. *Outputs*: bAHI numbers per 5 min; Wake/REM/NREM classification per 30 s.	Trained on 5804 subjects (8434 PSGs) from SHHS, fine-tuned on data of 128 subjects from two independent clinical trials, and tested on 84 subjects from the third independent clinical trial. Test dataset population: Adults with suspected OSA; Race: African American 62%, Caucasian 29%, Hispanic 1%, Asian 2%, others 1%, unknown 4%; OSA severity (AHI4): Normal 26%, mild 24%, moderate 23%, severe 27%.	OSA classification: AHI4 $\geq$ 5: sen 92%, spec 64%; AHI4 $\geq$ 15: sen 91%, spec 88%; AHI4 $\geq$ 30: sen 83%, spec 93%. 3-class sleep stage: Wake: sen 58%, spec 96%; NREM: sen 90%, spec 68%; REM: sen 70%, spec 94%.
NightOwl	Massie et al. 2023 [110]	*Inputs*: Manually extracted features from PPG-derived respiratory effort. *Model*: An ensemble of trees classifier. *Outputs*: Central (including mixed)/obstructive classification for each respiratory event.	Trained on 245 subjects with leave-one-out cross validation. Dataset population: Adults with suspected OSA; Race: not specified. Percentages of skin pigmentation were reported (light 69.9% and dark 29.7%); OSA severity (AHI3): Normal 9.8%, mild 22.9%, moderate 26.1%, severe 41.2%.	CA classification: cAHI $\geq$ 5: sen 78%, spec 95%; cAHI $\geq$ 10: sen 81%, spec 99%; cAHI $\geq$ 15: sen 73%, spec 98%.
ANNE Sleep	Davies et al. 2022 [116]	*Inputs*: not specified. *Model*: A combination of RNN and CNN for sleep-wake classification; respiration events are manually scored. *Outputs*: not specified.	Training procedure was not specified. Tested on 225 subjects. Test dataset population: Adults with suspected OSA; Race: White 72.9%, African American 11.6%, Asian 8.9%, more than 1 race 4.4%, American Indian 0.4%, native Hawaiian 0.4%; OSA severity (AHI4): Normal 40.4%, mild 29.3%, moderate 16.4%, severe 13.8%.	OSA classification: AHI4 $\geq$ 5: sen 96%, spec 86%; AHI4 $\geq$ 15: sen 90%, spec 97%; AHI4 $\geq$ 30: sen 65%, spec 99%. TST: Mean absolute percentage error 17%, mean difference 12.9 min.

(contiuned)

Table 10 (contiuned)

Novel device	Author/year	Design of model (Inputs/structure/outputs)	Model training and testing	Performance
BresoDX1	Montazeri Ghahjaverestan et al. 2023 [114]	*Inputs*: Manually extracted features from *X*-axis and *Z*-axis motions from the accelerometer and sound signals from the microphone. *Model*: DNN1 (1 layer CNN with 5 dense layers) and DNN2 (paralleled LSTM and 1 layer CNN with 3 dense layers) for respiratory event classification per 61 s; logistic regression model using the 61 s classification outputs and the periods of valid sleep from sleep model to generate the final output. *Outputs*: Probability of respiration events per second.	Trained on 74 subjects with a fourfold cross validation and tested on a separate set of 159 subjects from the same trial. Dataset population: Adult and overweight with a moderate degree of sleep apnea; Race: not specified; OSA severity (AHI3): Normal 33.0%, mild 27.5%, moderate 19.7%, severe 19.7%.	OSA classification: AHI3 $\geq$ 5: sen 94%, spec 63%; AHI3 $\geq$ 15: sen 90%, spec 86%; AHI3 $\geq$ 30: sen 97%, spec 91%.
The Patch[a]	Montazeri Ghahjaverestan et al. 2020 [113]	*Inputs*: Manually extracted features from *X*-axis, *Y*-axis and *Z*-axis motions from the accelerometer and sound signals from the microphone. *Model*: SVM with Gaussian kernel. *Outputs*: Sleep/wake classification per 30 s.	Trained on 45 subjects with SE <80% with a partially fourfold cross validation on 88 subjects from the same trial. Dataset population: Adults; Race: not specified; OSA severity (AHI3): Normal 30.7%, mild 22.7%, moderate 23.9%, severe 22.7%.	Sleep/wake stage: Wake: sen 71%, spec 88%.

Sunrise	Le-Dong et al. 2021 [115]	*Inputs*: Manually extracted features from three axes mandibular movements signals. *Model*: Extreme Gradient Boosting classifier. *Outputs*: Wake/light NREM/deep NREM/REM per 30 s.	Trained on 800 subjects and tested on a separate set of 226 subjects from the same trial. Test dataset population: Adults with suspected OSA; Race: not specified; OSA severity: not specified.	TST mean difference with 95% confidence interval: −13.0 (−52.9, 19.0) min. Sleep time % difference: Wake: 3.8 (−6.8, 16.8)%, Light NREM: −14.9 (−31.1, 1.8)%, deep NREM: 6.0 (−6.0, 21.2)%, REM: 8.4 (−21.3, 2.4)%.
	Pépin et al. 2020 [112]	*Inputs*: Manually extracted features from three axes mandibular movements signals. *Model*: Machine learning, not specified. *Outputs*: Wake/micro-arousals/sleep respiratory effort/normal sleep classification per 30 s.	Trained on 100 subjects and tested on a separate set of 376 subjects which were collected from same location during same period. Test dataset population: Adults with suspected OSA; Race: not specified; OSA severity: Non-OSA 12.2%, PSG-RDI $\geq$ 5 with symptoms 28.5%, PSG-RDI $\geq$ 15 59.3%.	RDI mean difference with 95% confidence interval: Non-OSA group: 1.31 (−1.05, 3.66) events/h, RDI $\geq$ 5 with symptoms: −0.69 (−3.77, 2.38) events/h, RDI $\geq$ 15: −11.74 (−20.83, −2.67) events/h.

Abbreviations: *AHI3* apnea-hypopnea index with hypopnea defined as a ≥30% drop in airflow for ≥10 s associated with an arousal or a ≥3% oxygen desaturation, *AHI4* apnea-hypopnea index with hypopnea defined as a ≥30% drop in airflow for ≥10 s associated with a ≥4% oxygen desaturation, *bAHI* Belun reported apnea-hypopnea index, *CA* central apnea, *cAHI* central apnea-hypopnea index, *CNN* convolutional neural network, *DNN* deep neural network, *NREM* non-rapid eye movement, *OSA* obstructive sleep apnea, *PPG* photoplethysmography, *PSG* polysomnography, *RDI* respiratory disturbance index, *REM* rapid eye movement, *RNN* recurrent neural network, *SE* sleep efficiency, *sen* sensitivity, *SHHS* Sleep Heart Health Study, *spec* specificity, *SpO2* oxygen saturation, *SVM* support vector machine, *TST* total sleep time

[a]The Patch is likely a prior prototype of BresoDX1

3.3 AI/ML/DL Algorithms Incorporated in Consumer-Grade Wearables

In addition to the medical-grade AI/ML/DL-powered tools, a growing market of consumer-grade wearables is emerging for OSA detection. Similar to their medical-grade counterparts, these consumer wearables often employ PPG and accelerometry to track SpO2, movement, pulse rate, and pulse rate viability (PRV)/heart rate viability (HRV) [64]. There exists the potential for some consumer-grade wearables to transition into medical-grade devices, contingent upon successful clinical validation demonstrating satisfactory accuracy in detecting OSA. A recent example is the Samsung Smart Watch Sleep Apnea Feature mobile app, which received FDA De Novo clearance as a Class II device for risk assessment (not diagnosis) of moderate-to-severe adult OSA [117].

Table 11 delineates inputs, model structures, and outputs of consumer wearables capable of OSA detection [118–127]. It covers a wide array of wearables from smart rings (Circul [122]), smartwatches (Samsung Galaxy Watch [123, 124], and HUAWEI Smartwatch GT2 [125]) to a palm patch device (WISM [120]). While these devices share common inputs such as SpO2, PPG, PRV/HRV, and motion, their outputs vary. Some focus on determining sleep-wake states, while others attempt to detect OSA using ODI. The model structures employed in these consumer wearables also exhibit diversity, ranging from ensemble learning techniques like Random Forest to DL models utilizing CNN, LSTM, or Encoder-Decoder. A notable limitation of consumer wearables, such as Circul and WISM, is their primary reliance on ODI rather than AHI.

3.4 Standalone OSA-Detecting AI/ML/DL Algorithms

Beyond the AI/ML/DL algorithms embedded within wearables, there are standalone algorithms not explicitly integrated into any devices. The majority of research in this domain utilized PPG/SpO2 signals acquired from PSG [128–135], while some leveraged signals from wrist-worn PPG and accelerometry sensors [133, 135]. These algorithms are often developed using data from open source. Publicly available databases, such as the Multi-Ethnic Study of Atherosclerosis (MESA) [22], SHHS [136], Sleep and Obstructive Sleep Apnea Monitoring with Non-Invasive Applications project (SOMNIA) [137], Stanford Technological Analytics and Genomics in Sleep Study (STAGES) [138], and Traumatic Brain Injury Study (TBI) are often employed for AI/ML/DL model training. Table 12 offers a comprehensive overview of the database utilized, the specific data inputs, model structures, and the corresponding data outputs generated by these standalone algorithms.

This review has observed an emerging trend toward employing intricate DL model architectures in standalone algorithms. This suggests a potential shift to adopt more complex DL models for enhanced OSA detection capabilities. Furthermore,

Table 11 Algorithms of consumer-grade wearables

Author/year	Novel device	Model inputs	Model structure	Model outputs
Zou et al. 2024 [118]	Wearable bracelet with PPG	Pulse interval series from PPG	One-dimensional multiscale bi-directional TCN	SA/No-SA classification per 60 s
Wang et al. 2023 [119]	Smart ring with PPG and oximeter	SpO2 and PPG were preprocessed to remove noise and segmented.	Random Forest classifier & multiscale entropy	The diagnosis of sleep apnea syndrome
Xu et al. 2023 [120][a]	WISM: pulse oximeter on the palmar thenar major muscles	SpO2, heart rate, and body movement signals	Not explicitly detailed	ODI
Fedorin et al. 2023 [121]	Samsung Galaxy Watch with green light PPG and three-axis accelerometer	Seven features from accelerometer and interbeat intervals sequence from PPG	Encoder-decoder architecture with RNN	SA/No-SA per 30 s
Zhao et al. 2022 [122][a]	Circul ring with PPG and three-axis accelerometer	SpO2 and PR feature extraction and movement measuring	Automated feature selection; and sleep/wake analysis.	ODI from potential OD events and total analyzed time
Fedorin et al. 2021, 2020 [123, 124]	Samsung Galaxy Watch with green light PPG and three-axis accelerometer	Manually extracted features including the heart rate variability, PPG shape, respiration rate, activity, and posture	Bi-LTSM	RE/non-RE classification per 60 s; sleep/wake classification per 60 s.
Chen et al. 2021 [125]	HUAWEI smartwatch GT2, including an accelerometer, a gyroscope, a geomagnetic sensor, an optical pulse rate sensor, an ambient light sensor, an air pressure sensor, and a capacitive sensor	Relevant respiratory waveforms, acceleration signal, pulse rate variability characteristics from green light PPG, and blood oxygen saturation features derived from infrared and red light PPG	Classification models	AHI and sleep-wake states

(continued)

Table 11 (continued)

Author/year	Novel device	Model inputs	Model structure	Model outputs
Chang et al. 2020 [126]	Abdominal and thoracic three-axis accelerometers, a pulsed oximeter, and an electrocardiogram sensor	Respiratory events model: manual extracted features from six channels of the abdominal and thoracic accelerometer signals and SpO2 signal; Sleep stage model: instantaneous heart rate signal converted from ECG and SpO2 signal.	Respiratory events model: LTSM; Sleep stage model: CNN.	Obstructive sleep apnea/central sleep apnea/hypopnea/ normal classification per 20 s; sleep/wake per 30 s.
Hafezi et al. 2019 [127]	Patch recording tracheal movements	Manually feature extract from three-axis accelerometer	CNN + LSTM	Apnea-hypopnea probability per seconds

Abbreviation: *AHI* apnea-hypopnea index, *Bi-LTSM* bi-directional long short-term memory, *CNN* convolutional neural network, *ECG* electrocardiography, *LSTM* long short-term memory, *OD* oxygen desaturation, *ODI* oxygen desaturation index, *PPG* photoplethysmography, *PR* pulse rate, *RE* respiratory event, *RNN* recurrent neural network, *SA* sleep apnea class, containing all subtypes of events (i.e., central apnea, obstructive apnea, mixed apnea, and hypopnea), *SpO2* oxygen saturation, *TCN* temporal convolutional network

[a]Uncertain whether the algorithms used are rule-based or AI-driven

researchers are increasingly focused on crafting bespoke models, rather than relying on standard architectures like CNNs or RNNs [130–132, 135]. These custom-designed models are engineered to more effectively capture and analyze the complex patterns inherent in sleep physiological data. The ultimate goal is to achieve superior model generalizability and robustness across diverse datasets.

4 Developing and Validating AI/ML/DL Algorithms for OSA Screening and Diagnosis

Several key factors are paramount when developing and validating AI/ML/DL models, and these include model design, selecting model datasets, and evaluating model performance [18].

Table 12 Algorithms derived from databases

Author/year	Database	Model inputs	Model structure	Model outputs
Olsen et al. 2024 [135]	Open-source database: STAGES (35 subjects), TBI (231 subjects) and MESA (1335 subjects); and 35 subjects undergoing PSG	PPG from PSG and wrist-worn device; Accelerometer signals from wrist-worn device	A DNN architecture, inspired by U-Net, DeepSleep [132] and U-Sleep [133]	SA/No-SA classification per 30 s; 4-class sleep stage per 30 s
Jiang et al. 2023 [129]	59 subjects undergoing PSG	PPG from PSG	CNN + LTSM	SA/No-SA classification per 15 s
Wei et al. 2023 [130]	110 subjects undergoing PSG	PPG from PSG Preprocess: decreases in the amplitude fluctuation of PPG and peak-to-peak interval of PPG signal are extracted as the input of deep learning network	A model named MS-Net that combined multiscale one-dimensional convolutional block with shadow one-dimensional convolutional module	SA/No-SA classification per 60 s
Huttunen et al. 2023 [131]	877 subjects undergoing PSG	PPG and SpO2 from PSG	U-Net with squeeze-and-excitation network	Normal/hypopnea/apnea classification per 1 s; 5-class sleep stage per 30 s
Liu et al. 2022 [132]	Open-source database: SHHS (5293 subjects) and Apnea-ECG (8 subjects); and 179 subjects undergoing PSG	SpO2 from PSG Preprocess: Segmented SpO2 for Bi-LTSM model; manual feature extraction from whole night SpO2 for linear regressor	This model contains four parts: a temporal encoder with Bi-LSTM, a local feature extractor using CNN, whole night feature fusion, and a connector and linear regressor	SA/No-SA classification in SpO2
Papini et al. 2020 [133]	Open-source database: SOMNIA (469 subjects) and HealthBed (33 subjects)	Manually extracted features from wrist-worn PPG	CNN	SA/No-SA classification per 30 s
Kang et al. 2019 [134]	82 subjects undergoing PSG	PPG from PSG	LSTM	Normal/hypopnea/apnea classification per 10 s

Abbreviation: *Bi-LSTM* bi-directional long short-term memory, *CNN* convolutional neural network, *DNN* deep neural network, *ECG* electrocardiography, *LSTM* long short-term memory, *MESA* Multi-Ethnic Study of Atherosclerosis, *PPG* photoplethysmography, *PSG* polysomnography, *SA* sleep apnea class, containing all subtypes of events (i.e., central apnea, obstructive apnea, mixed apnea, and hypopnea), *SHHS* Sleep Heart Health Study, *SOMNIA* Sleep and Obstructive Sleep Apnoea Monitoring with Non-Invasive Applications project, *SpO2* oxygen saturation, *STAGES* Stanford Technological Analytics and Genomics in Sleep Study, *TBI* Traumatic Brain Injury Study

4.1 Deciding Model Design

It is crucial to first understand the clinical utility and capabilities of AI solutions of interest, especially whether they are based on ML or DL. For the OSA screening settings using clinical features, where the number of available features is relatively small and the input data primarily comes from demographic information or electronic health records, training complex, data-hungry DL models from scratch might not be the best fit. Here, constructing a more focused and tailored model utilizing smaller, efficient ML models could prove to be a smart approach. Alternatively, fine-tuning powerful LLMs like ChatGPT might be worth exploring, but this area requires further investigation [23, 24]. In contrast, OSA diagnosis at home settings often involves intricate physiological signals from various sensors, which can be prone to interference from external noise. Advanced DL techniques might be better suited for handling such intricate data. There is a noticeable trend in recent AI models using physiological signals, shifting beyond traditional ML and basic CNNs/RNNs toward more complex, customized, and powerful DL approaches.

4.2 Selecting Model Datasets

Building and validating AL/ML/DL models necessitate the utilization of comprehensive, accurately labeled, and representative datasets. These datasets serve as the cornerstone for training, tuning, and external testing, ensuring their robustness and generalizability across a wide spectrum of populations. Notably, large-scale and diverse sleep studies meticulously scored by multiple experts, such as SHHS, MESA, Massachusetts General Hospital Sleep Laboratory, and Wisconsin Sleep Cohort, offer raw data from thousands of PSGs, serving as the standard reference [18]. As mentioned in Sect. 3.4, databases like SOMNIA and STAGES that include synchronized signals of PSG and wearables can also significantly bolster model training.

However, merely possessing vast, open-source datasets is not sufficient. It is critical to acknowledge the potential for inaccuracies when employing algorithms that are not specifically designed for a particular wearable device. Systematic biases can creep in due to variations in PPG sensor design and implementation across different wearables. These variations can manifest as noticeable discrepancies in signal quality or resolution, ultimately leading to performance disparities. Therefore, during algorithm development, careful consideration must be given to the unique characteristics and inherent limitations of the target wearable device. Performance optimization can be achieved by fine-tuning the models with datasets specifically designed for those devices. Take the BSP as an example. The original model was developed on a substantial sample of 5804 subjects (8434 PSGs) sourced from SHHS. It then underwent external testing and further fine-tuning using data from 128 subjects from two separate cohorts (Table 10). The resulting Gen2 DL algorithms were then subjected to rigorous external validation using 84 subjects from a distinct dataset with diverse racial composition, demonstrating satisfactory performance and generalizability in sleep staging as well as in OSA detection, particularly at AHI cutoffs of 15 and 30 [111].

4.3 Examining Model Performance

Rigorously validating algorithmic models is paramount for ensuring their unwavering reliability and real-world effectiveness. This process encompasses two crucial steps: internal validation and external validation. Internal validation, using techniques like k-fold cross-validation, scrutinizes a model's consistency within the training data. External testing, acting as the ultimate test, confirms the effectiveness of the model on completely independent datasets. It is crucial that external testing datasets come from unrelated sources, ensuring the model's diagnostic accuracy in diverse clinical contexts [41, 79]. For instance, in an attempt to distinguish central from obstructive events, NightOwl researchers recently trained an ensemble of tree classifiers on 245 subjects using leave-one-out cross-validation. While the performance was impressive, it is critical to recognize that this is an internal validation study. Without external testing from a separate dataset, the results cannot be considered conclusive [110]. Moreover, external testing datasets should ideally encompass diverse racial and ethnic groups to ensure the robustness of the model across diverse populations.

Moreover, to accurately evaluate the performance, it is vital to compare an emerging device against PSG, the gold standard for OSA diagnosis. One should also avoid uncritically accepting reported performance or making direct comparisons between the devices/algorithms as such comparisons are fraught with challenges due to frequent and subtle shortcomings in study designs, methodologies, and variability in how statistical analyses are reported [18]. These challenges may include, among others, small sample sizes, failure to compare with in-lab PSG, biased OSA severity distribution, deviation from the standard AASM 3% and 4% rules, "borrowing" PSG data for AHI calculation, reliance on "optimal device-AHI cutoffs" instead of standard cutoffs of 5, 15, and 30, incomplete or selective reporting of statistical analyses, and not leveraging a separate external testing dataset as previously discussed [18, 64].

5 Future Trends and Summary

From automated PSG scoring to OSA screening and diagnosis, AI/ML/DL algorithms have rapidly surged in recent times and transformed the landscape of sleep medicine. In this chapter, we presented the implementation of AI/ML/DL algorithms in two distinct clinical scenarios: in-clinic OSA screening leveraging clinical features and at-home OSA diagnosis utilizing PPG and accelerometry-based wearable devices.

The first scenario exemplifies how AI models can be adept at risk stratification and OSA prediction by using clinical features. These models are poised for continuous improvement and eventual integration into EMR systems, empowering clinicians to seamlessly incorporate AI-powered insights into their daily clinical workflow. They possess the potential to flag high-risk patients, prompting healthcare providers (particularly busy non-sleep providers such as family physicians) to recognize the high probability of OSA and the necessity for further sleep testing and earlier interventions. This offers significant assistance to busy clinicians, who may have limited expertise in sleep medicine or who face constraints due to time limitations, competing demands, or a reluctance to delve into lengthy sleep histories or treatment challenges [17, 43]. In essence, such AI-powered tools not only offer the potential to liberate valuable physician time but also hold promise for driving improved patient outcomes, particularly for those at high risk for cardiovascular complications.

The second scenario ventures into at-home diagnosis utilizing medical-grade OSA-detecting wearables. Among the diverse array of devices employing various mechanisms, PPG-based wearables stand out as particularly noteworthy, as they not only offer the capability for OSA diagnosis but also hold immense potential for predicting cardiovascular outcomes by harnessing physiological biomarkers like HRV, hypoxic burden [139], delta HR [140], and pulse wave amplitude drop index [141]. A significant portion of these devices are now partially or fully powered by AI/ML/DL algorithms for sleep staging and OSA detection. However, ongoing refinement of these AI models remains paramount. The current trend demonstrably gravitates toward more advanced, customized, and powerful DL approaches, surpassing the traditional ML and basic DL models.

We posit that the synergy between these two AI approaches has the potential to emerge as the primary tool for future OSA screening and diagnosis. Nevertheless, significant work remains before this vision materializes. Paramount among these challenges is the continual, rigorous performance evaluation of the latest iterations of AI models. Only through unwavering validation efforts can we ensure the accuracy and generalizability of these models for the real world.

To cultivate the development of safe, effective, and high-quality medical devices powered by AI/ML/DL models, the FDA, Health Canada, and the United Kingdom's Medicines and Healthcare Products Regulatory Agency collaborated and established ten guiding principles in 2021 [142]. These principles, also known as Good Machine Learning Practice (GMLP) in the development of trustworthy AI/ML/DL algorithms for medical purposes. In addition to GMLP, clinical validation researchers must also remain cognizant of recent initiatives to standardize sleep technology research [62, 143, 144]. These endeavors aim to facilitate clear and unambiguous comparisons across diverse devices and algorithms, ultimately preventing the misinterpretation of study outcomes.

In conclusion, innovative sleep technologies will undoubtedly continue to experience exponential growth, fundamentally redefining the landscape of clinical sleep medicine. The role of AI/ML/DL will demonstrably expand, significantly augmenting personalized care, operational efficiency, access to care, patient satisfaction, and overall population health for the foreseeable future.

References

1. Senaratna CV, Perret JL, Lodge CJ, Lowe AJ, Campbell BE, Matheson MC, et al. Prevalence of obstructive sleep apnea in the general population: A systematic review. Sleep Med Rev. 2017;34:70–81.
2. Heinzer R, Vat S, Marques-Vidal P, Marti-Soler H, Andries D, Tobback N, et al. Prevalence of sleep-disordered breathing in the general population: the HypnoLaus study. Lancet Respir Med. 2015;3(4):310–8.
3. Faulx MD, Mehra R, Reis Geovanini G, Ando SI, Arzt M, Drager L, et al. Obstructive sleep apnea and its management in patients with atrial fibrillation: An International Collaboration of Sleep Apnea Cardiovascular Trialists (INCOSACT) global survey of practicing cardiologists. Int J Cardiol Heart Vasc. 2022;42:101085.
4. Altaf QA, Dodson P, Ali A, Raymond NT, Wharton H, Fellows H, et al. Obstructive Sleep Apnea and Retinopathy in Patients with Type 2 Diabetes. A Longitudinal Study. Am J Respir Crit Care Med. 2017;196(7):892–900.
5. Young T, Peppard PE, Gottlieb DJ. Epidemiology of obstructive sleep apnea: a population health perspective. Am J Respir Crit Care Med. 2002;165(9):1217–39.
6. Iftikhar IH, Hoyos CM, Phillips CL, Magalang UJ. Meta-analyses of the Association of Sleep Apnea with Insulin Resistance, and the Effects of CPAP on HOMA-IR, Adiponectin, and Visceral Adipose Fat. J Clin Sleep Med. 2015;11(4):475–85.
7. Chien MY, Lee PL, Yu CW, Wei SY, Shih TT. Intramyocellular Lipids, Insulin Resistance, and Functional Performance in Patients with Severe Obstructive Sleep Apnea. Nat Sci Sleep. 2020;12:69–78.
8. Lee PL, Wu YW, Cheng HM, Wang CY, Chuang LP, Lin CH, et al. Recommended assessment and management of sleep disordered breathing in patients with atrial fibrillation, hypertension and heart failure: Taiwan Society of Cardiology/Taiwan Society of sleep Medicine/Taiwan Society of pulmonary and Critical Care Medicine joint consensus statement. J Formos Med Assoc. 2024;123(2):159–78.
9. Lin MT, Lai CL, Lee PL, Shen MH, Yu CJ, Fang CT, Chen CL. Timely diagnosis and treatment of sleep apnea reduce cardiovascular sequelae in patients with myocardial infarction. PLoS One. 2018;13(7):e0201493.
10. Yeboah J, Redline S, Johnson C, Tracy R, Ouyang P, Blumenthal RS, et al. Association between sleep apnea, snoring, incident cardiovascular events and all-cause mortality in an adult population: MESA. Atherosclerosis. 2011;219(2):963–8.
11. Marin JM, Carrizo SJ, Vicente E, Agusti AG. Long-term cardiovascular outcomes in men with obstructive sleep apnoea-hypopnoea with or without treatment with continuous positive airway pressure: an observational study. Lancet. 2005;365(9464):1046–53.
12. Punjabi NM, Caffo BS, Goodwin JL, Gottlieb DJ, Newman AB, O'Connor GT, et al. Sleep-disordered breathing and mortality: a prospective cohort study. PLoS Med. 2009;6(8):e1000132.
13. Perez-Pozuelo I, Zhai B, Palotti J, Mall R, Aupetit M, Garcia-Gomez JM, et al. The future of sleep health: a data-driven revolution in sleep science and medicine. NPJ Digit Med. 2020;3:42.
14. Schutte-Rodin S, Deak MC, Khosla S, Goldstein CA, Yurcheshen M, Chiang A, et al. Evaluating consumer and clinical sleep technologies: an American Academy of Sleep Medicine update. J Clin Sleep Med. 2021;17(11):2275–82.

15. Goldstein C. Current and Future Roles of Consumer Sleep Technologies in Sleep Medicine. Sleep Med Clin. 2020;15(3):391–408.
16. Chiang AA, Khosla S. Consumer Wearable Sleep Trackers: Are They Ready for Clinical Use? Sleep Med Clin. 2023;18(3):311–30.
17. Watson NF, Fernandez CR. Artificial intelligence and sleep: Advancing sleep medicine. Sleep medicine reviews. 2021;59:101512.
18. Bandyopadhyay A, Bae C, Cheng H, Chiang A, Deak M, Seixas A, Singh J. Smart sleep: what to consider when adopting AI-enabled solutions in clinical practice of sleep medicine. J Clin Sleep Med. 2023;19(10):1823–33.
19. Goldstein CA, Berry RB, Kent DT, Kristo DA, Seixas AA, Redline S, et al. Artificial intelligence in sleep medicine: an American Academy of Sleep Medicine position statement. J Clin Sleep Med. 2020;16(4):605–7.
20. Gottlieb DJ, Punjabi NM. Diagnosis and Management of Obstructive Sleep Apnea: A Review. JAMA. 2020;323(14):1389–400.
21. Jordan AS, McSharry DG, Malhotra A. Adult obstructive sleep apnoea. Lancet. 2014;383(9918):736–47.
22. Chen X, Wang R, Zee P, Lutsey PL, Javaheri S, Alcantara C, et al. Racial/Ethnic Differences in Sleep Disturbances: The Multi-Ethnic Study of Atherosclerosis (MESA). Sleep. 2015;38(6):877–88.
23. Mira FA, Favier V, Dos Santos Sobreira Nunes H, de Castro JV, Carsuzaa F, Meccariello G, et al. Chat GPT for the management of obstructive sleep apnea: do we have a polar star? Eur Arch Otorhinolaryngol. 2024;281(4):2087–93.
24. Campbell DJ, Estephan LE, Mastrolonardo EV, Amin DR, Huntley CT, Boon MS. Evaluating ChatGPT responses on obstructive sleep apnea for patient education. J Clin Sleep Med. 2023;19(12):1989–95.
25. Chung F, Yang Y, Brown R, Liao P. Alternative scoring models of STOP-bang questionnaire improve specificity to detect undiagnosed obstructive sleep apnea. J Clin Sleep Med. 2014;10(9):951–8.
26. Chung F, Abdullah HR, Liao P. STOP-Bang Questionnaire: A Practical Approach to Screen for Obstructive Sleep Apnea. Chest. 2016;149(3):631–8.
27. Marti-Soler H, Hirotsu C, Marques-Vidal P, Vollenweider P, Waeber G, Preisig M, et al. The NoSAS score for screening of sleep-disordered breathing: a derivation and validation study. Lancet Respir Med. 2016;4(9):742–8.
28. Chen H, Zheng Z, Chen R, Zeng Y, Li N, Zhu J, et al. A meta-analysis of the diagnostic value of NoSAS in patients with sleep apnea syndrome. Sleep Breath. 2022;26(2):519–31.
29. Luo J, Huang R, Zhong X, Xiao Y, Zhou J. STOP-Bang questionnaire is superior to Epworth sleepiness scales, Berlin questionnaire, and STOP questionnaire in screening obstructive sleep apnea hypopnea syndrome patients. Chin Med J (Engl). 2014;127(17):3065–70.
30. Chen NH, Johns MW, Li HY, Chu CC, Liang SC, Shu YH, et al. Validation of a Chinese version of the Epworth sleepiness scale. Qual Life Res. 2002;11(8):817–21.
31. Chiu HY, Chen PY, Chuang LP, Chen NH, Tu YK, Hsieh YJ, et al. Diagnostic accuracy of the Berlin questionnaire, STOP-BANG, STOP, and Epworth sleepiness scale in detecting obstructive sleep apnea: A bivariate meta-analysis. Sleep Med Rev. 2017;36:57–70.
32. Pivetta B, Chen L, Nagappa M, Saripella A, Waseem R, Englesakis M, Chung F. Use and Performance of the STOP-Bang Questionnaire for Obstructive Sleep Apnea Screening Across Geographic Regions: A Systematic Review and Meta-Analysis. JAMA Netw Open. 2021;4(3):e211009.
33. Albuquerque FN, Calvin AD, Sert Kuniyoshi FH, Konecny T, Lopez-Jimenez F, Pressman GS, et al. Sleep-disordered breathing and excessive daytime sleepiness in patients with atrial fibrillation. Chest. 2012;141(4):967–73.
34. Starkey SY, Jonasson DR, Alexis S, Su S, Johal R, Sweeney P, et al. Screening for Obstructive Sleep Apnea in an Atrial Fibrillation Population: What's the Best Test? CJC Open. 2021;3(4):442–9.

35. Reuter H, Herkenrath S, Treml M, Halbach M, Steven D, Frank K, et al. Sleep-disordered breathing in patients with cardiovascular diseases cannot be detected by ESS, STOP-BANG, and Berlin questionnaires. Clin Res Cardiol. 2018;107(11):1071–8.
36. Genta PR, Drager LF, Lorenzi Filho G. Screening for Obstructive Sleep Apnea in Patients with Atrial Fibrillation. Sleep Med Clin. 2017;12(1):99–105.
37. Huang WC, Lee PL, Liu YT, Chiang AA, Lai F. Support vector machine prediction of obstructive sleep apnea in a large-scale Chinese clinical sample. Sleep. 2020;43(7).
38. Duarte RLM, Rabahi MF, Magalhães-da-Silveira FJ, de Oliveira-E-Sá TS, Mello FCQ, Gozal D. Simplifying the Screening of Obstructive Sleep Apnea With a 2-Item Model, No-Apnea: A Cross-Sectional Study. Journal of clinical sleep medicine: JCSM: official publication of the American Academy of Sleep Medicine. 2018;14(7):1097–107.
39. Liu WT, Wu HT, Juang JN, Wisniewski A, Lee HC, Wu D, Lo YL. Prediction of the severity of obstructive sleep apnea by anthropometric features via support vector machine. PLoS One. 2017;12(5):e0176991.
40. Ustun B, Westover MB, Rudin C, Bianchi MT. Clinical Prediction Models for Sleep Apnea: The Importance of Medical History over Symptoms. J Clin Sleep Med. 2016;12(2):161–8.
41. Holfinger SJ, Lyons MM, Keenan BT, Mazzotti DR, Mindel J, Maislin G, et al. Diagnostic Performance of Machine Learning-Derived OSA Prediction Tools in Large Clinical and Community-Based Samples. Chest. 2022;161(3):807–17.
42. Caffo B, Diener-West M, Punjabi NM, Samet J. A novel approach to prediction of mild obstructive sleep disordered breathing in a population-based sample: the Sleep Heart Health Study. Sleep. 2010;33(12):1641–8.
43. Bazoukis G, Bollepalli SC, Chung CT, Li X, Tse G, Bartley BL, et al. Application of artificial intelligence in the diagnosis of sleep apnea. J Clin Sleep Med. 2023;19(7):1337–63.
44. U.S. Food & Drug Administration. K173974. Published July 14, 2019. Accessed January 19, 2024. https://www.accessdata.fda.gov/cdrh_docs/pdf17/K173974.pdf.
45. U.S. Food & Drug Administration. K213360. Published July 5, 2022. Accessed January 19, 2024. https://www.accessdata.fda.gov/cdrh_docs/pdf21/K213360.pdf.
46. U.S. Food & Drug Administration. K210480. Published July 6, 2021. Accessed January 19, 2024. https://www.accessdata.fda.gov/cdrh_docs/pdf21/K210480.pdf.
47. Kapur VK, Auckley DH, Chowdhuri S, Kuhlmann DC, Mehra R, Ramar K, Harrod CG. Clinical Practice Guideline for Diagnostic Testing for Adult Obstructive Sleep Apnea: An American Academy of Sleep Medicine Clinical Practice Guideline. J Clin Sleep Med. 2017;13(3):479–504.
48. Jonas DE, Amick HR, Feltner C, Weber RP, Arvanitis M, Stine A, et al. Screening for Obstructive Sleep Apnea in Adults: Evidence Report and Systematic Review for the US Preventive Services Task Force. JAMA. 2017;317(4):415–33.
49. Lee PL, Huang YH, Lin PC, Chiao YA, Hou JW, Liu HW, et al. Automatic Sleep Staging in Patients With Obstructive Sleep Apnea Using Single-Channel Frontal EEG. J Clin Sleep Med. 2019;15(10):1411–20.
50. Medicine. AAoS. The International Classification of Sleep Disorders, Third Edition (ICSD-3). 2014.
51. Malhotra A, Ayappa I, Ayas N, Collop N, Kirsch D, McArdle N, et al. Metrics of sleep apnea severity: beyond the apnea-hypopnea index. Sleep. 2021;44(7):zsab030.
52. Liu PK, Ting N, Chiu HC, Lin YC, Liu YT, Ku BW, Lee PL. Validation of photoplethysmography- and acceleration-based sleep staging in a community sample: comparison with polysomnography and Actiwatch. J Clin Sleep Med. 2023;19(10):1797–810.
53. Collop NA, Tracy SL, Kapur V, Mehra R, Kuhlmann D, Fleishman SA, Ojile JM. Obstructive sleep apnea devices for out-of-center (OOC) testing: technology evaluation. J Clin Sleep Med. 2011;7(5):531–48.
54. Ferber R, Millman R, Coppola M, Fleetham J, Murray CF, Iber C, et al. Portable recording in the assessment of obstructive sleep apnea. ASDA standards of practice. Sleep. 1994;17(4):378–92.

55. Collop NA, Anderson WM, Boehlecke B, Claman D, Goldberg R, Gottlieb DJ, et al. Clinical guidelines for the use of unattended portable monitors in the diagnosis of obstructive sleep apnea in adult patients. Portable Monitoring Task Force of the American Academy of Sleep Medicine. J Clin Sleep Med. 2007;3(7):737–47.
56. Light MP, Casimire TN, Chua C, Koushyk V, Burschtin OE, Ayappa I, Rapoport DM. Addition of frontal EEG to adult home sleep apnea testing: does a more accurate determination of sleep time make a difference? Sleep Breath. 2018;22(4):1179–88.
57. Levendowski DJ, Popovic D, Berka C, Westbrook PR. Retrospective cross-validation of automated sleep staging using electroocular recording in patients with and without sleep disordered breathing. Int Arch Med. 2012;5(1):21.
58. Lucey BP, McLeland JS, Toedebusch CD, Boyd J, Morris JC, Landsness EC, et al. Comparison of a single-channel EEG sleep study to polysomnography. J Sleep Res. 2016;25(6):625–35.
59. Stepnowsky C, Levendowski D, Popovic D, Ayappa I, Rapoport DM. Scoring accuracy of automated sleep staging from a bipolar electroocular recording compared to manual scoring by multiple raters. Sleep Med. 2013;14(11):1199–207.
60. Younes M, Younes M, Giannouli E. Accuracy of Automatic Polysomnography Scoring Using Frontal Electrodes. J Clin Sleep Med. 2016;12(5):735–46.
61. Chang S-Y, Wu B-C, Liou Y-L, Zheng R-X, Lee P-L, Chiueh T-D, Liu T-T. An Ultra-Low-Power Dual-Mode Automatic Sleep Staging Processor Using Neural-Network-Based Decision Tree. IEEE Transactions on Circuits and Systems I: Regular Papers. 2019;66(9):3504–16.
62. de Zambotti M, Goldstein C, Cook J, Menghini L, Altini M, Cheng P, Robillard R. State of the science and recommendations for using wearable technology in sleep and circadian research. Sleep. 2024;47(4).
63. Pires GN, Arnardottir ES, Islind AS, Leppanen T, McNicholas WT. Consumer sleep technology for the screening of obstructive sleep apnea and snoring: current status and a protocol for a systematic review and meta-analysis of diagnostic test accuracy. J Sleep Res. 2023;32(4):e13819.
64. Chiang AA, Jerkins E, Holfinger S, etc. OSA Diagnosis Goes Wearable: Are the Latest Devices Ready to Shine? . Manuscript submitted to JCSM. March 2024.
65. Kirby SD, Eng P, Danter W, George CF, Francovic T, Ruby RR, Ferguson KA. Neural network prediction of obstructive sleep apnea from clinical criteria. Chest. 1999;116(2):409–15.
66. Bouloukaki I, Kapsimalis F, Mermigkis C, Kryger M, Tzanakis N, Panagou P, et al. Prediction of obstructive sleep apnea syndrome in a large Greek population. Sleep Breath. 2011;15(4):657–64.
67. Zou J, Guan J, Yi H, Meng L, Xiong Y, Tang X, et al. An effective model for screening obstructive sleep apnea: a large-scale diagnostic study. PLoS One. 2013;8(12):e80704.
68. Shah N, Hanna DB, Teng Y, Sotres-Alvarez D, Hall M, Loredo JS, et al. Sex-Specific Prediction Models for Sleep Apnea From the Hispanic Community Health Study/Study of Latinos. Chest. 2016;149(6):1409–18.
69. Wang KJ, Chen KH, Huang SH, Teng NC. A Prognosis Tool Based on Fuzzy Anthropometric and Questionnaire Data for Obstructive Sleep Apnea Severity. J Med Syst. 2016;40(4):110.
70. Shin CH, Grabitz SD, Timm FP, Mueller N, Chhangani K, Ladha K, et al. Development and validation of a Score for Preoperative Prediction of Obstructive Sleep Apnea (SPOSA) and its perioperative outcomes. BMC Anesthesiol. 2017;17(1):71.
71. Traxdorf M, Tziridis K, Scherl C, Iro H, Haferkamp J. The Erlangen Questionnaire: a new 5-item screening tool for obstructive sleep apnea in a sleep clinic population – A prospective, double blinded study. Eur Rev Med Pharmacol Sci. 2017;21(16):3690–8.
72. Duarte RLM, Rabahi MF, Magalhaes-da-Silveira FJ, de Oliveira ESTS, Mello FCQ, Gozal D. Simplifying the Screening of Obstructive Sleep Apnea With a 2-Item Model, No-Apnea: A Cross-Sectional Study. J Clin Sleep Med. 2018;14(7):1097–107.
73. Kim YJ, Jeon JS, Cho SE, Kim KG, Kang SG. Prediction Models for Obstructive Sleep Apnea in Korean Adults Using Machine Learning Techniques. Diagnostics (Basel). 2021;11(4).

74. Keshavarz Z, Rezaee R, Nasiri M, Pournik O. Obstructive Sleep Apnea: A Prediction Model Using Supervised Machine Learning Method. Stud Health Technol Inform. 2020;272:387–90.
75. Zhang L, Yan YR, Li SQ, Li HP, Lin YN, Li N, et al. Moderate to severe OSA screening based on support vector machine of the Chinese population faciocervical measurements dataset: a cross-sectional study. BMJ Open. 2021;11(9):e048482.
76. Casal-Guisande M, Torres-Durán M, Mosteiro-Añón M, Cerqueiro-Pequeño J, Bouza-Rodríguez JB, Fernández-Villar A, Comesaña-Campos A. Design and Conceptual Proposal of an Intelligent Clinical Decision Support System for the Diagnosis of Suspicious Obstructive Sleep Apnea Patients from Health Profile. Int J Environ Res Public Health. 2023;20(4).
77. Aiyer I, Shaik L, Sheta A, Surani S. Review of Application of Machine Learning as a Screening Tool for Diagnosis of Obstructive Sleep Apnea. Medicina (Kaunas). 2022;58(11).
78. Huo J, Quan SF, Roveda J, Li A. Coupling analysis of heart rate variability and cortical arousal using a deep learning algorithm. PLoS One. 2023;18(4):e0284167.
79. Han H, Oh J. Application of various machine learning techniques to predict obstructive sleep apnea syndrome severity. Sci Rep. 2023;13(1):6379.
80. Zeng G, Tao S. A Generalized Linear Transformation and Its Effects on Logistic Regression. 2023;11(2):467.
81. Jurczuk K, Czajkowski M, Kretowski M. From Random Forest to an interpretable decision tree – An evolutionary approach. Proceedings of the Companion Conference on Genetic and Evolutionary Computation; Lisbon, Portugal: Association for Computing Machinery; 2023. p. 291–4.
82. Shi Y, Ma L, Chen X, Li W, Feng Y, Zhang Y, et al. Prediction model of obstructive sleep apnea-related hypertension: Machine learning-based development and interpretation study. Front Cardiovasc Med. 2022;9:1042996.
83. Zhang C, Zhou Y, Guo J, Wang G, Wang X. Research on classification method of high-dimensional class-imbalanced datasets based on SVM. International Journal of Machine Learning and Cybernetics. 2019;10(7):1765–78.
84. Hussain SF. A novel robust kernel for classifying high-dimensional data using Support Vector Machines. Expert Systems with Applications. 2019;131:116–31.
85. Li K, Pan W, Li Y, Jiang Q, Liu G. A method to detect sleep apnea based on deep neural network and hidden Markov model using single-lead ECG signal. Neurocomputing. 2018;294:94–101.
86. Chang HY, Yeh CY, Lee CT, Lin CC. A Sleep Apnea Detection System Based on a One-Dimensional Deep Convolution Neural Network Model Using Single-Lead Electrocardiogram. Sensors (Basel). 2020;20(15).
87. Ferreira-Santos D, Amorim P, Silva Martins T, Monteiro-Soares M, Pereira Rodrigues P. Enabling Early Obstructive Sleep Apnea Diagnosis With Machine Learning: Systematic Review. J Med Internet Res. 2022;24(9):e39452.
88. Goodfellow I, Bengio Y, Courville A. Deep Learning: MIT Press; 2016.
89. LeCun Y, Bengio Y, Hinton G. Deep learning. Nature. 2015;521(7553):436–44.
90. Hochreiter S, Schmidhuber J. Long short-term memory. Neural Comput. 1997;9(8):1735–80.
91. Graves A, Schmidhuber J. Framewise phoneme classification with bidirectional LSTM and other neural network architectures. Neural Netw. 2005;18(5–6):602–10.
92. Ciresan D, Meier U, Schmidhuber J. Multi-column deep neural networks for image classification. 2012 IEEE Conference on Computer Vision and Pattern Recognition; 16–21 June 20122012. p. 3642–9.
93. Bai S, Kolter JZ, Koltun V. An empirical evaluation of generic convolutional and recurrent networks for sequence modeling. arXiv preprint arXiv:180301271. 2018.
94. He K, Zhang X, Ren S, Sun J. Deep Residual Learning for Image Recognition. Proceedings of the IEEE conference on computer vision and pattern recognition (CVPR)2016. p. 770–8.
95. Xie S, Girshick R, Dollar P, Tu Z, He K. Aggregated Residual Transformations for Deep Neural Networks. Proceedings of the IEEE Conference on Computer Vision and Pattern Recognition (CVPR)2017. p. 1492–500.

96. Hu J, Shen L, Sun G, editors. Squeeze-and-excitation networks. Proceedings of the IEEE conference on computer vision and pattern recognition; 2018.
97. Cho K, Van Merriënboer B, Gulcehre C, Bahdanau D, Bougares F, Schwenk H, Bengio Y. Learning phrase representations using RNN encoder-decoder for statistical machine translation. arXiv preprint arXiv:14061078. 2014.
98. Ronneberger O, Fischer P, Brox T, editors. U-net: Convolutional networks for biomedical image segmentation. Medical image computing and computer-assisted intervention–MICCAI 2015: 18th international conference, Munich, Germany, October 5–9, 2015, proceedings, part III 18; 2015: Springer.
99. Vaswani A, Shazeer N, Parmar N, Uszkoreit J, Jones L, Gomez AN, et al. Attention is all you need. Advances in neural information processing systems. 2017;30.
100. U.S. Food & Drug Administration. K231355. Aurora 510(k) premarket notification. Published February 8, 2024. Accessed March 28, 2024. https://www.accessdata.fda.gov/cdrh_docs/pdf23/K231355.pdf.
101. U.S. Food & Drug Administration. K231546. Somfit 510(k) premarket notification. Published November 30, 2023. Accessed March 28, 2024. https://www.accessdata.fda.gov/cdrh_docs/pdf23/K231546.pdf.
102. U.S. Food & Drug Administration. K222579. Belun Sleep System BLS-100 510(k) premarket notification. Published February 23, 2023. Accessed March 28, 2024. https://www.accessdata.fda.gov/cdrh_docs/pdf22/K222579.pdf.
103. U.S. Food & Drug Administration. AcuPebble Ox100 K222950. 510(k) premarket notification. Published February 3, 2023. Accessed March 28, 2024. https://www.accessdata.fda.gov/cdrh_docs/pdf22/K222950.pdf.
104. U.S. Food & Drug Administration. K222262. Sunrise 510(k) premarket notification. Published December 22, 2022. Accessed March 28, 2024. https://www.accessdata.fda.gov/cdrh_docs/pdf22/K222262.pdf.
105. U.S. Food & Drug Administration. K220012. BresoDX1 510(k) premarket notification. Published December 21, 2022. Accessed March 28, 2024. https://www.accessdata.fda.gov/cdrh_docs/pdf22/K220012.pdf.
106. U.S. Food & Drug Administration. K220095. ANNE Sleep 510(k) premarket notification. Published July 11, 2022. Accessed March 28, 2024. https://www.accessdata.fda.gov/cdrh_docs/pdf22/K220095.pdf.
107. U.S. Food & Drug Administration. K203343. Wesper Lab 510(k) premarket notification. Published December 21, 2021. Accessed March 28, 2024. https://www.accessdata.fda.gov/cdrh_docs/pdf20/K203343.pdf.
108. U.S. Food & Drug Administration. K191031. NightOwl 510(k) premarket notification. Published March 6, 2020. March 28, 2024. https://www.accessdata.fda.gov/cdrh_docs/pdf19/K191031.pdf.
109. U.S. Food & Drug Administration. K182618. SleepImage System 510(k) premarket notification. Published August 14, 2019. Accessed March 28, 2024. https://www.accessdata.fda.gov/cdrh_docs/pdf18/K182618.pdf.
110. Massie F, Vits S, Khachatryan A, Van Pee B, Verbraecken J, Bergmann J. Central Sleep Apnea Detection by Means of Finger Photoplethysmography. IEEE J Transl Eng Health Med. 2023;11:126–36.
111. Strumpf Z, Gu W, Tsai CW, Chen PL, Yeh E, Leung L, et al. Belun Ring (Belun Sleep System BLS-100): Deep learning-facilitated wearable enables obstructive sleep apnea detection, apnea severity categorization, and sleep stage classification in patients suspected of obstructive sleep apnea. Sleep Health. 2023;9(4):430–40.
112. Pepin JL, Letesson C, Le-Dong NN, Dedave A, Denison S, Cuthbert V, et al. Assessment of Mandibular Movement Monitoring With Machine Learning Analysis for the Diagnosis of Obstructive Sleep Apnea. JAMA Netw Open. 2020;3(1):e1919657.
113. Montazeri Ghahjaverestan N, Akbarian S, Hafezi M, Saha S, Zhu K, Gavrilovic B, et al. Sleep/Wakefulness Detection Using Tracheal Sounds and Movements. Nat Sci Sleep. 2020;12:1009–21.

114. Montazeri Ghahjaverestan N, Aguiar C, Hummel R, Cao X, Yu J, Bradley TD. Sleep Apnea Detection by Tracheal Motion and Sound, and Oximetry via Application of Deep Neural Networks. Nat Sci Sleep. 2023;15:423–32.
115. Le-Dong NN, Martinot JB, Coumans N, Cuthbert V, Tamisier R, Bailly S, Pepin JL. Machine Learning-based Sleep Staging in Patients with Sleep Apnea Using a Single Mandibular Movement Signal. American journal of respiratory and critical care medicine. 2021;204(10):1227–31.
116. Davies C, Lee JY, Walter J, Kim D, Yu L, Park J, et al. A single-arm, open-label, multicenter, and comparative study of the ANNE sleep system vs polysomnography to diagnose obstructive sleep apnea. J Clin Sleep Med. 2022;18(12):2703–12.
117. U.S. Food & Drug Administration. DEN230041. Sleep Apnea Feature De Novo classification notification. Published February 6, 2024. Accessed March 28, 2024. https://www.accessdata.fda.gov/cdrh_docs/pdf23/DEN230041.pdf.
118. Zou L, Liu G. Multiscale Bidirectional Temporal Convolutional Network for Sleep Apnea Detection Based on Wearable Photoplethysmography Bracelet. IEEE J Biomed Health Inform. 2024;28(3):1331–40.
119. Wang S, Xuan W, Chen D, Gu Y, Liu F, Chen J, et al. Machine Learning Assisted Wearable Wireless Device for Sleep Apnea Syndrome Diagnosis. Biosensors (Basel). 2023;13(4).
120. Xu Y, Ou Q, Cheng Y, Lao M, Pei G. Comparative study of a wearable intelligent sleep monitor and polysomnography monitor for the diagnosis of obstructive sleep apnea. Sleep Breath. 2023;27(1):205–12.
121. Fedorin I, Smielova A, Nastenko M, Krasnoshchok I. Forecasting of breathing events during nocturnal sleep using encoder-decoder recurrent neural network based on a sensors data of consumer smartwatches. Annu Int Conf IEEE Eng Med Biol Soc. 2023;2023:1–4.
122. Zhao R, Xue J, Zhang X, Peng M, Li J, Zhou B, et al. Comparison of Ring Pulse Oximetry Using Reflective Photoplethysmography and PSG in the Detection of OSA in Chinese Adults: A Pilot Study. Nat Sci Sleep. 2022;14:1427–36.
123. Fedorin I, Slyusarenko K. Consumer Smartwatches As a Portable PSG: LSTM Based Neural Networks for a Sleep-Related Physiological Parameters Estimation. Annu Int Conf IEEE Eng Med Biol Soc. 2021;2021:849–452.
124. Fedorin I, Slyusarenko K, Nastenko M. Respiratory events screening using consumer smartwatches. Adjunct Proceedings of the 2020 ACM International Joint Conference on Pervasive and Ubiquitous Computing and Proceedings of the 2020 ACM International Symposium on Wearable Computers 2020. p. 25–8.
125. Chen Y, Wang W, Guo Y, Zhang H, Chen Y, Xie L. A Single-Center Validation of the Accuracy of a Photoplethysmography-Based Smartwatch for Screening Obstructive Sleep Apnea. Nat Sci Sleep. 2021;13:1533–44.
126. Chang HC, Wu HT, Huang PC, Ma HP, Lo YL, Huang YH. Portable Sleep Apnea Syndrome Screening and Event Detection Using Long Short-Term Memory Recurrent Neural Network. Sensors (Basel). 2020;20(21).
127. Hafezi M, Montazeri N, Zhu K, Alshaer H, Yadollahi A, Taati B, editors. Sleep Apnea Severity Estimation from Respiratory Related Movements Using Deep Learning. 2019 41st Annual International Conference of the IEEE Engineering in Medicine and Biology Society (EMBC); 2019 23–27 July 2019.
128. Olsen M, Zeitzer JM, Richardson RN, Musgrave VH, Sorensen HBD, Mignot E, Jennum PJ. A deep transfer learning approach for sleep stage classification and sleep apnea detection using wrist-worn consumer sleep technologies. IEEE Trans Biomed Eng. 2024;PP.
129. Jiang X, Ren Y, Wu H, Li Y, Liu F. Convolutional neural network based on photoplethysmography signals for sleep apnea syndrome detection. Front Neurosci. 2023;17:1222715.
130. Wei K, Zou L, Liu G, Wang C. MS-Net: Sleep apnea detection in PPG using multi-scale block and shadow module one-dimensional convolutional neural network. Comput Biol Med. 2023;155:106469.
131. Huttunen R, Leppanen T, Duce B, Arnardottir ES, Nikkonen S, Myllymaa S, et al. A Comparison of Signal Combinations for Deep Learning-Based Simultaneous Sleep Staging and Respiratory Event Detection. IEEE Trans Biomed Eng. 2023;70(5):1704–14.

132. Liu R, Li C, Xu H, Wu K, Li X, Liu Y, et al. Fusion of Whole Night Features and Desaturation Segments Combined with Feature Extraction for Event-Level Screening of Sleep-Disordered Breathing. Nat Sci Sleep. 2022;14:927–40.
133. Papini GB, Fonseca P, van Gilst MM, Bergmans JWM, Vullings R, Overeem S. Wearable monitoring of sleep-disordered breathing: estimation of the apnea-hypopnea index using wrist-worn reflective photoplethysmography. Sci Rep. 2020;10(1):13512.
134. Kang CH, Erdenebayar U, Park JU, Lee KJ. Multi-Class Classification of Sleep Apnea/Hypopnea Events Based on Long Short-Term Memory Using a Photoplethysmography Signal. J Med Syst. 2019;44(1):14.
135. Olsen M, Zeitzer JM, Nakase-Richardson R, Musgrave VH, Sorensen HBD, Mignot E, Jennum PJ. A deep transfer learning approach for sleep stage classification and sleep apnea detection using wrist-worn consumer sleep technologies. IEEE Trans Biomed Eng. 2024;PP.
136. Quan SF, Howard BV, Iber C, Kiley JP, Nieto FJ, O'Connor GT, et al. The Sleep Heart Health Study: design, rationale, and methods. Sleep. 1997;20(12):1077–85.
137. van Gilst MM, van Dijk JP, Krijn R, Hoondert B, Fonseca P, van Sloun RJG, et al. Protocol of the SOMNIA project: an observational study to create a neurophysiological database for advanced clinical sleep monitoring. BMJ Open. 2019;9(11):e030996.
138. Zhang GQ, Cui L, Mueller R, Tao S, Kim M, Rueschman M, et al. The National Sleep Research Resource: towards a sleep data commons. J Am Med Inform Assoc. 2018;25(10):1351–8.
139. Azarbarzin A, Sands SA, Taranto-Montemurro L, Redline S, Wellman A. Hypoxic burden captures sleep apnoea-specific nocturnal hypoxaemia. European heart journal. 2019;40(35):2989–90.
140. Azarbarzin A, Sands SA, Younes M, Taranto-Montemurro L, Sofer T, Vena D, et al. The sleep apnea–specific pulse-rate response predicts cardiovascular morbidity and mortality. American journal of respiratory and critical care medicine. 2021;203(12):1546–55.
141. Hirotsu C, Betta M, Bernardi G, Marques-Vidal P, Vollenweider P, Waeber G, et al. Pulse wave amplitude drops during sleep: clinical significance and characteristics in a general population sample. Sleep. 2020;43(7):zsz322.
142. U.S. Food & Drug Administration, Health Canada, and the United Kingdom's Medicines and Healthcare products Regulatory Agency. Good Machine Learning Practice for Medical Device Development: Guiding Principles. Published October 2021. Accessed March 28, 2024. https://www.fda.gov/media/153486/download.
143. de Zambotti M, Menghini L, Grandner MA, Redline S, Zhang Y, Wallace ML, Buxton OM. Rigorous performance evaluation (previously, "validation") for informed use of new technologies for sleep health measurement. Sleep Health. 2022;8(3):263–9.
144. Depner CM, Cheng PC, Devine JK, Khosla S, de Zambotti M, Robillard R, et al. Wearable technologies for developing sleep and circadian biomarkers: a summary of workshop discussions. Sleep. 2020;43(2):zsz254.

Modeling and Analysis of Mechanical Work of Breathing

Victoria Ribeiro Rodrigues, Szilard L. Beres, Paul W. Davenport, and Nicholas J. Napoli

1 Introduction

Sleep disorders, characterized by disturbances in the normal sleep pattern, are often caused by some type of respiratory disease. These can be sleep-related breathing disorders, such as Obstructive Sleep Apnea (OSA), Central Sleep Apnea (CSA), sleep-related hypoventilation, and sleep-related hypoxemia disorder. Alternatively, they may be breathing disorders that affect sleep, such as asthma, chronic obstructive lung disease, chronic upper airway obstruction, and restrictive lung disorders, all of which can impact sleep quality and continuity [5, 10, 15, 16]. One shared characteristic among these diseases is an increase in work of breathing (WoB). Thus, it is vital to properly assess WoB in individuals with sleep disorders. In this chapter, we will provide an overview of the basics of mechanical WoB measurement.

The concept of WoB refers to the mechanical energy expended by an individual to move gas into and out of the lungs during spontaneous breathing [11]. The respiratory muscles work against five primary types of forces:

1. Elastic forces, located in the lung and chest tissues when a volume change occurs
2. Flow-resistive forces, developed in the airways due to nonelastic tissue deformation

V. R. Rodrigues · S. L. Beres · N. J. Napoli (✉)
Department of Electrical and Computer Engineering, Human Informatics and Predictive Performance Optimization (HIPPO) Lab, University of Florida, Gainesville, FL, USA
e-mail: victoria.ribeiro@ufl.edu; szilard.beres@ufl.edu; n.napoli@ufl.edu

P. W. Davenport
Department of Physiological Sciences, University of Florida, Gainesville, FL, USA
e-mail: pdavenpo@ufl.edu

R. B. Berry et al. (eds.), *Handbook of AI and Data Sciences for Sleep Disorders*, Springer Optimization and Its Applications 216,
https://doi.org/10.1007/978-3-031-68263-6_5

3. Inertial forces dependent on the mass of tissues and gases
4. Gravitational forces, often considered as part of inertial forces, typically included in the measurement of elastic forces
5. Distorting forces of the chest wall, observed during high ventilations or when the subject breathes through resistances

Inertial work is typically disregarded for two reasons: First, it is generally considered negligible under most physiological conditions [17]. Second, most of the inertial work performed during the accelerative phase is recovered during the deceleration phase [24]. Gravitational forces, as mentioned before, are considered to be included in the elastic forces and therefore are not separately quantified here. For these reasons, this chapter only focuses on analyzing the elastic forces, the flow-resistive forces, and the distorting forces of the chest wall.

2 Analysis of Work of Breathing Using Pressure and Volume

The physical definition of work in a fluid system is expressed by the equation:

$$W = \int P \, dV. \tag{1}$$

Here, W represents work, P represents pressure, and V represents volume. Therefore, the work done by the respiratory system during a breathing cycle can be quantified by analyzing a pressure–volume (PV) curve, with work calculated by the area under the curve.

Alternatively, the respiratory system can be thought of as an electrical circuit, as many of the principles in the former also hold in the latter. The analogy between electrical circuits and respiratory terms is illustrated in Table 1:

Table 1 A comparison between respiratory and electrical systems highlighting analogous components and their corresponding units

Respiratory system	Electrical equivalent
Pressure (cmH_2O)	Voltage (volts)
Gas flow (l/s)	Current flow (amps)
Airway and tissue resistance ($cmH_2O \cdot s/1$)	Electrical resistance (ohms)
Volume (1)	Quantity (coulombs)
Compliance (l/cmH_2O)	Capacitance (farads)

This analogy allows us to define work using the electrical definition:

$$W = \int V dQ. \tag{2}$$

Here, W represents the wattage of the system, also known as the work, V is the voltage, and Q is the quantity of charge. In this context, work represents the energy transferred or consumed in the electrical system.

It is important to emphasize that voltage represents the electric potential difference between two points in a circuit. Consequently, the measured work depends on the specific points where electrical potentials are recorded. This principle is also applicable when quantifying respiratory work within the respiratory system. The choice of points in the respiratory system for the pressure differential determines the type of work measured.

For instance, the gold standard for measuring respiratory work involves using esophageal pressure (P_{es}) with reference to atmospheric pressure (P_{atm}). This approach allows us to assess both intrinsic and extrinsic work performed by the human respiratory system. If the goal is to exclusively quantify intrinsic work, it is sufficient to reference P_{es} to airway pressure (P_{ao}), also known as transpulmonary pressure (P_{ptp}). Similarly, if the focus is solely on extrinsic work, the pressure differential employed in Eq. 1 should be P_{ao} with reference to P_{atm}.

2.1 *Elastic and Flow Resistive Work*

An assumption typically made in the analysis of work is that a consistent configuration of the relaxed state at a specific lung volume is maintained. This assumption is facilitated for an understanding of the effort required for breathing by examining the relationship between pleural pressure and lung volume. A mirrored representation of the static pressure–volume curve for the lung, depicted in Fig. 1 (left) as $-P_{st,l}$ (static pressure of the lung), is obtained by keeping lung volume constant and airways open at various inflation levels. The curve $P_{st,w}$ (static pressure of the chest wall) is obtained when the airways are closed, and the muscles are in a relaxed state.

Assuming open airways and no distortion of the chest wall, the minimum pressure required to be generated by the respiratory muscles in order to maintain the respiratory system at a specific volume can be determined by measuring the horizontal distance between $-P_{st,l}$ and $P_{st,w}$. This pressure corresponds to the value indicated by the static pressure–volume curve of the respiratory system (P_{rs}) during relaxation, as shown in Fig. 1 (right). The work performed by the muscles in stretching the system during inspiration from functional residual capacity (FRC), represented by point A, is equal to the area enclosed by points ABCA.

To further analyze the elastic work of breathing, separate pressure–volume relationships for the lungs and thorax are illustrated in two panels in Fig. 2. The elastic work required exclusively to increase lung volume is indicated by the area

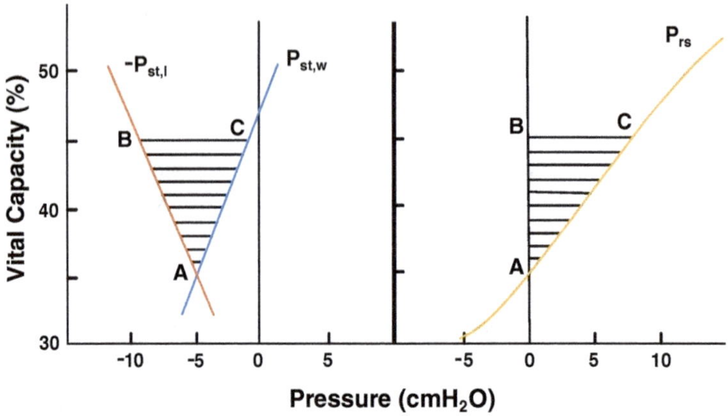

Fig. 1 Diagram displays pressure–volume relationships, with pleural pressure on the left and mouth pressure on the right. The horizontal hatching signifies the elastic work performed by the inspiratory muscles during the process of inspiration. Recreated from [24]

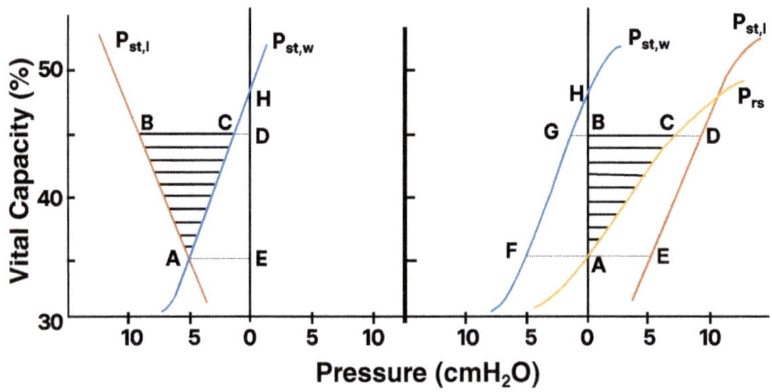

Fig. 2 Diagram displays pressure–volume relationships, with pleural pressure on the left and mouth pressure on the right. The horizontal hatching denotes the elastic work performed by the inspiratory muscles during the process of inspiration. Recreated from [24]

ABDEA. In comparison, the total elastic work needed for inspiration is the area ABCA, as shown in Fig. 1. Therefore, the elastic work required to inflate the entire system (lungs and thorax) is less than the work needed to inflate the lungs alone by the amount represented by ACDEA. This additional work is released from the energy stored in the thorax during inspiration and represented by the area AFGBA in Fig. 2 (right). This energy is equivalent to the area ACDEA; the energy is transferred back from the lungs to the thorax without any loss during expiration. As lung volumes exceed those indicated by point H in Fig. 2, the counterspringing effect disappears since both the lungs and the thorax exert elastic forces in the same direction.

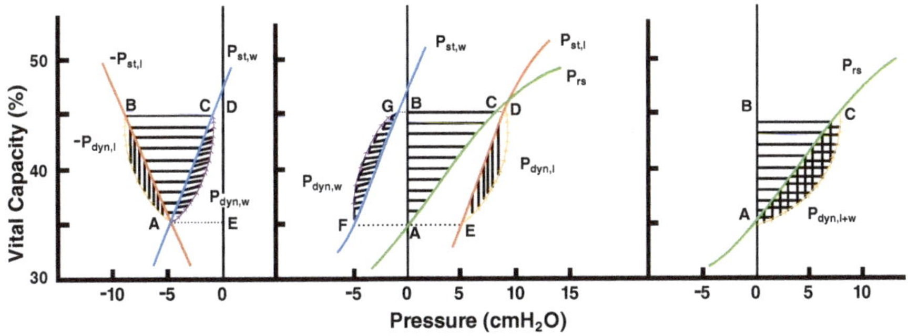

Fig. 3 Diagram illustrates different pressure–volume loops in terms of various pressures: on the left, pleural pressure; in the middle, both pleural and mouth pressure; and on the right, mouth pressure. The horizontal hatching represents inspiratory elastic work, while the vertical hatching represents the work required to overcome the flow resistance in the lung, including the airways and tissue. The oblique hatching denotes the work needed to overcome the flow resistance of the chest wall, and the cross-hatching represents the combined inspiratory work required to overcome the flow resistance of both the lung and chest wall. Recreated from [24]

To overcome flow resistance during inspiration, additional pressure must be applied to counteract the elastic forces. In Fig. 3 (left), curve $-P_{dyn,l}$ illustrates the pleural pressure relative to atmospheric pressure under dynamic conditions. The horizontal distance between $-P_{dyn,l}$ and $-P_{st,l}$ (Fig. 3, left) or $P_{st,l}$ (Fig. 3, middle) indicates the pressure required to overcome the flow resistance of the lungs, including the airways and tissues. The vertical hatching in the figure represents the work performed by the inspiratory muscles to overcome the flow resistance of the lungs.

The broken lines in Fig. 3 (left and middle) trace the pathway of the pressure required to overcome the flow resistance of the chest wall. Therefore, the horizontal distance between the broken line and $P_{st,w}$ represents the pressure needed during inspiration to counteract the flow resistance of the chest wall, known as $P_{dyn,w}$ (dynamic pressure of the chest wall). The area enclosed between $P_{st,w}$ and the broken line, represented by oblique hatching, symbolizes the work performed by the inspiratory muscles to overcome the flow resistance of the chest wall.

However, it is not possible to directly measure the area between $P_{st,w}$ and the broken line to determine the flow-resistive work of the chest wall in a spontaneously breathing subject. Attempts have been made by Otis [21] to calculate this work in a paralyzed subject during artificial respiration by subtracting the work of flow resistance of the lung and airways from the total flow-resistive work, as shown in Fig. 3 (right) with cross-hatching.

During expiration, if all the respiratory muscles were completely relaxed and the resistances of the pulmonary and chest wall were equal, the process would follow a line midway between the two static curves shown in Fig. 4 (left) or along the line B–A in Fig. 4 (right). In such a scenario, all the elastic energy stored in the lung would be utilized to overcome the flow resistances of both the lung and chest wall.

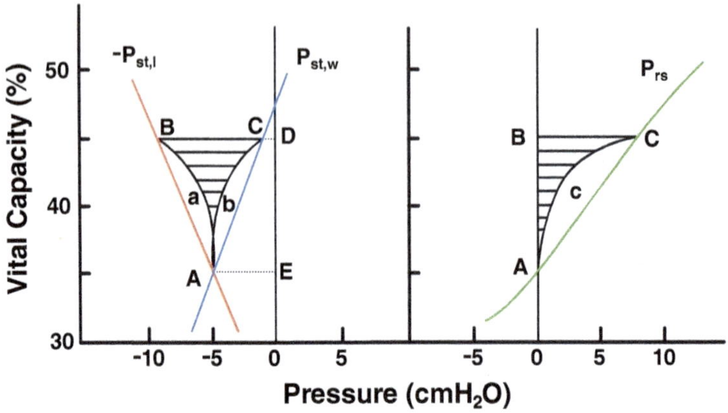

Fig. 4 Diagram represents pressure–volume relationships, with pleural pressure on the left and mouth pressure on the right. The horizontal hatching on the left side of the diagram represents the negative work performed by the inspiratory muscles during expiration. In areas a and b, we can observe the energy stored in the lung during inspiration and then expended during expiration to overcome the flow resistances of the lung and chest wall, respectively. The combined areas of a and b equal area c. Recreated from [24]

However, only a portion of this energy is used for this purpose, as indicated by areas a and b for the lung and chest wall shown in Fig. 4 (left). This can also be observed in their combined area c in Fig. 4 (right). The remaining work is employed to counteract the persistent activity of the inspiratory muscles. This is represented by the horizontal hatching, symbolizing the negative work performed by the inspiratory muscles that lengthen during expiration.

Consider the different components of mechanical work and the energy exchange among different parts of the respiratory system during the breathing cycle, as depicted in Fig. 5 [7]. It is important to note the distinction that the pressure is contributed by the inspiratory muscles when $-P_{st,l}$ is positioned to the left of $P_{st,w}$ and by the expiratory muscles when it is to the right. Figure 5 illustrates a breathing cycle starting at FRC with increased ventilation, showing the contraction of expiratory muscles.

Figure 5 analyzes the work done during a breathing cycle with increased ventilation, starting from the resting volume of the respiratory system. In Fig. 5a, the vertical hatching represents the work performed by the inspiratory muscles to overcome the flow resistance of the lung. The horizontal hatching represents the work done by the inspiratory muscles to overcome the elastic resistance of the lung. Cross-hatching indicates the work done by the inspiratory muscles to overcome the elastic resistance of the chest wall. The oblique hatching represents the work done by the inspiratory muscles to overcome the flow resistance of the chest wall. Coarse stippling represents the transfer of elastic energy from the chest wall to the lung.

In Fig. 5b, the horizontal and cross-hatching represent the work done by the elastic energy of the lung and chest wall, respectively, against the persistent activity

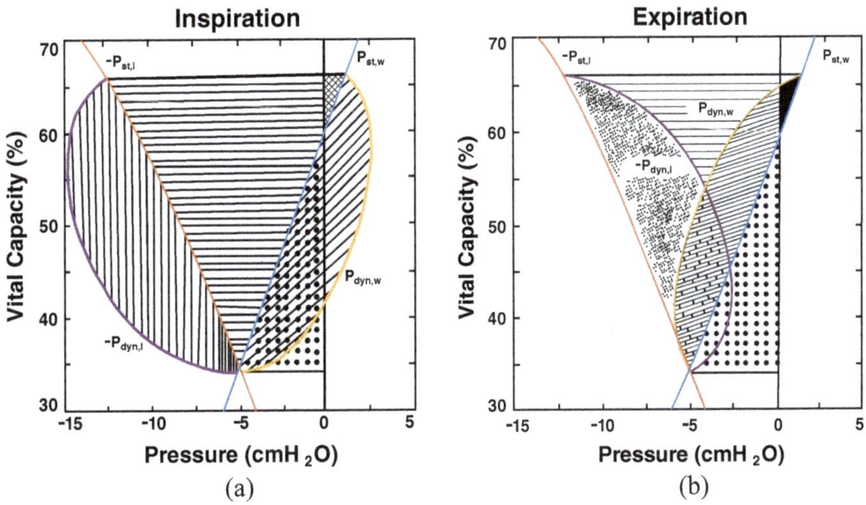

Fig. 5 Graphical analysis of work done during a breathing cycle at increased ventilation. The cycle starts at FRC. Recreated from [24]. (**a**) Inspiration. (**b**) Expiration

of the inspiratory muscles. Fine stippling indicates the work done by the elastic energy of the lung to overcome a portion of the flow resistance of the lung. Broken hatching represents the work done by the expiratory muscles to overcome the remaining flow resistance of the lung (according to the given representation, but this energy could also be utilized to overcome a portion of the flow resistance of the chest wall). The oblique hatching and solid area represent the work done by the elastic energy of the lung and chest wall, respectively, to overcome the flow resistance of the chest wall. Coarse stippling represents the transfer of elastic energy from the lung to the chest wall.

2.2 *Work Due to Chest Wall Distortion*

There are two primary forms of chest wall distortions. One form of chest wall distortion is volume shifts between the abdomen and rib cage, occurring in various conditions such as exercise or CO_2 breathing [1, 3, 12–14]. Consequently, the same lung volume (V_L) will not produce identical configurations of the respiratory system as the one observed during relaxation. When there is no blood volume shift between the periphery and chest wall, then any changes in lung volume must correspond to changes in chest wall volume (V_w) since the lung and chest wall are in series, thus

$$V_L = V_w. \tag{3}$$

Additionally, the rib cage and abdomen act as volume displacing elements in parallel, leading to

$$V_{rc} + V_{ab} = V_w. \tag{4}$$

This leads to

$$V_L = V_{rc} + V_{ab}, \tag{5}$$

where V_{rc} represents rib cage volume and V_{ab} represents abdominal volume. It is significant to note volume displacement of the rib cage and abdomen can occur independently of each other; displacement of either component can be in the opposite direction to the overall change in lung volume. Consequently, not all inspiratory muscles need to shorten during inspiration, and not all expiratory muscles need to shorten during expiration.

The second type of chest wall distortion involves the deformation of the rib cage itself, which can occur during resistive breathing or in cases of disease. During the breathing cycle, changes in the shape of the rib cage exhibit a time delay between modifications in the anteroposterior diameter and alterations in the transverse diameter [1, 4]. In healthy individuals without added external respiratory loads, this type of distortion is not significant, even during intense exercise ventilation [2].

Goldman et al. [12] conducted estimations on the mechanical work involved in altering the distribution of volume changes between the rib cage and abdomen. This estimation was based on measurements of rib cage and abdominal volume displacements, changes in lung volume, and estimates of transthoracic pressure, as seen in Fig. 6.

Figure 6a shows the conventional relaxation pressure–volume curves ($-P_{st,l}$ and $P_{st,w}$). The left ordinate represented lung volume, while the Campbell diagram

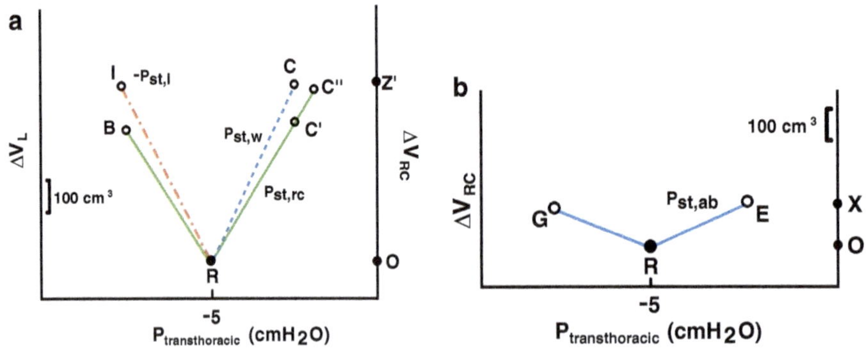

Fig. 6 Pressure–volume diagram (Campbell diagram). Recreated from [24]. (**a**) Lung volume (left y-axis) and rib cage volume (right y-axis) vs. transthoracic pressure. (**b**) Abdominal volume vs. transthoracic pressure

plotted transthoracic pressure. The analysis done in [12] involved distributing the overall change in lung volume between the rib cage and abdomen. Schematic representations of volume and transthoracic pressure changes are shown separately for the rib cage (Fig. 6a, right y-axis) and the abdomen (Fig. 6b). The total volume change was the same in both analyses, with an arbitrary distribution of 80% (Fig. 6a OZ') and 20% (Fig. 6a O'X) between the rib cage and abdomen, respectively.

It was assumed that the distribution of volume change shown was the same as that observed during relaxation at the same volumes. Segment RB represented the path followed by transthoracic pressure as the lung volume increased, where the V_{rc} equaled 80% of the total lung volume V_L. The transthoracic pressure at point C' was identical to that at point C because both points represented the overall relaxation of the chest wall and the rib cage, respectively, at the same lung volume.

In Fig. 6b, segment RG represents the trajectory of transthoracic pressure during the analyzed volume change. The transthoracic pressures at points G and E were identical to those at points I and C, respectively. The work done by the inspiratory muscles, without considering resistive work, can be calculated as the sum of the areas of triangles RBC' and RGE. This summation must be equal to the area of triangle RIC, as all these triangles share the same base (the distance between points C–I, C'–B, or E–G). Moreover, the combined heights of triangles RBC' and RGE ($V_{rc} + V_{ab}$) are equal to the height of the triangle RIC (V_L). Similarly, the combined areas of trapezoids RC'Z'OR and REXO'R should equal the area of trapezoid RCZ'OR.

Therefore, there was no difference in the amount of work calculated using the Goldman approach compared to the Campbell approach. Both estimates were based on the assumption that the distribution of volume change during breathing was the same as that during relaxation. With this understanding, let us now consider an inspiration where rib cage volume displacement accounted for 100% of the change in lung volume instead of 80% of the total.

The Campbell diagram provided the same estimate of inspiratory work as before (Fig. 6a triangle RIC). Still, the rib cage pressure–volume diagram yielded a larger estimate, namely, the area of triangle RIC". Point C" was obtained by a schematic linear extension of the rib cage's relaxation pressure–volume curve. It should be noted that the compliance of the rib cage (shown in Fig. 6a) was lower than that of the overall chest wall because the compliance of each element in a system of volume-elastic elements, arranged in parallel, had to be summed to give the overall compliance of the system.

This analysis implies that any distribution of volume change between the two chest wall pathways resulted in a distortion of the chest wall from its relaxation characteristics. The only exemption to this is observations during relaxation. As a result, additional work was required to overcome the elastic cost of this distortion [14]. Therefore, the elastic work done by the muscles of the chest wall was greater when only one of the two parallel pathways was utilized for a given change in lung volume.

3 Analysis of Work of Breathing Using Airflow

As mentioned in Sect. 2, the mechanical work to be measured is dependent on the pressure differential chosen. The gold standard measurement of work uses P_{es}, which requires a pressure catheter to be inserted through the nose to the esophagus. This makes P_{es} quite invasive and not feasible in many situations, especially when measuring work of breathing during sleep as that would require the patient to sleep with an esophageal pressure catheter. In 1950, Otis, Fenn, and Rahn proposed a mathematical equation that modeled the three main breathing resistances, namely elastic, viscous, and turbulent, using airflow [21].

3.1 Elastic Forces

When an individual fully relaxes their respiratory muscles, the lungs assume a volume similar to the end of a normal exhale. This is known as the midcapacity or relaxation volume. At this volume, the chest's elastic forces must balance out the lung's elastic forces in an equal and opposite manner. When the chest–lung system is displaced to any other volume, it generates elastic forces that counteract the displacing force. In previous research, Rahn et al. [22] introduced a method to measure these elastic forces as relaxation pressures and presented a curve illustrating the relationship between relaxation pressure and lung volume. The reciprocal slope, $\Delta P/\Delta V$, of the relaxation pressure curve represents the elastic resistance or "elastance," which refers to the pressure required to induce a unit change in volume [6, 9]. Although the relaxation pressure curve is not perfectly linear, it approximates linearity over a significant portion of its range. As an initial approximation, elastance is defined as

$$P_{el} = KV, \tag{6}$$

where K is the elastance and P_{el} is the pressure developed when the displacement from the relaxation volume is V.

3.2 Viscous and Turbulent Forces

According to [23], there are three causes of the pressure drop along the respiratory tract:

1. Viscous resistance, with the pressure drop varying linearly with the rate of flow
2. Local turbulence, resistance due to changes in the direction of flow (as in branching) and changes in the cross-sectional area of the airway, with the

pressure drop proportional to the square of the rate of flow. This type of resistance is almost entirely confined to the upper airways (larynx and distal structures).
3. Resistance due to turbulent flow, with the pressure drop varying with approximately the square of the rate of flow

From measurements made in cadavers by [23] and later validated experimentally by [20], it was determined that turbulent flow would not occur until the flow rate exceeded 5 L/s. This level of flow is rarely achieved unless during coughing episodes. Consequently, during regular breathing, only the first two factors mentioned above would affect the pressure drop. Therefore, the relationship between these forces and the flow rate of airflow may be approximated as

$$P_{alv} = k_1 \left(\frac{\mathrm{d}V}{\mathrm{d}t}\right) + k_2 \left(\frac{\mathrm{d}V}{\mathrm{d}t}\right)^2, \tag{7}$$

where P_{alv} is the pressure gradient between alveoli and the mouth that is required to move the air with a flow rate dV/dt. The constants k_1 and k_2 are the air viscance and the turbulent resistance, respectively.

3.3 *Resistance Associated with Tissue Deformation*

Estimation of the nonelastic resistance associated with tissue deformation (or flow-resistive work of the chest wall) was done in the following way. A trained subject was placed in a negative pressure ventilator, also known as an iron lung or Drinker respirator, and instructed to relax as much as possible and let the ventilator breathe for them. The pressure gradient between the inside of the respirator and the subject's mouth, along with the subject's airflow, was recorded. Assuming that the pressure recorded at any given moment represents the amount required to overcome the combined resistance and considering elastance, viscance, and turbulent resistance, the nonelastic tissue resistance can be estimated by subtracting these factors.

Consider Fig. 7, where pressure is plotted against volume for one breathing cycle. Assuming a linear correlation between elastic pressure and lung volume, the diagonal line in Fig. 7 represents the elastance. During inspiration, as the lung volume increases, the total pressure gradient between the mouth and the inside of the respirator is indicated by the distance from the y-axis to the inspiratory loop. Within this total inspiratory pressure (P_{in}) at a specific lung volume, a portion (P_{el}) represented by the distance from the y-axis to the diagonal line is required to overcome elastance. The remaining portion ($P_{in} - P_{el}$) represents the pressure needed to overcome air and tissue viscosity and turbulent resistance. The distance between the diagonal line and the loop indicated by the broken line is the pressure required to overcome the nonelastic resistance of the tissue.

During expiration, the elastic forces developed in the chest and lungs during inspiration generate the airflow. However, the total elastic force is not fully utilized

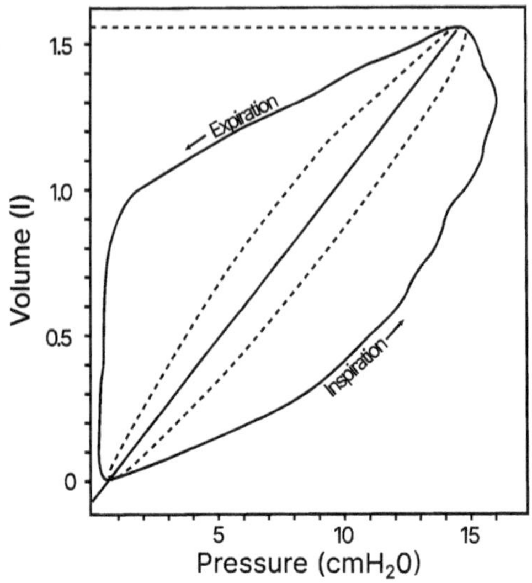

Fig. 7 Diagram of volume and pressure gradient between the respirator and the mouth during one respiratory cycle. Different regions in this figure explore different dimensions of work. The triangular area formed by the diagonal, the broken horizontal line, and the y-axis indicate the work performed during inspiration to overcome elastic resistance. The enclosed area bounded by the diagonal and the inspiration curve represents the additional work required to overcome the total viscous and turbulent resistance during inspiration. This region can be further subdivided into the work performed against nonelastic tissue resistance (the area between the diagonal and the broken line) and the work carried out to overcome air viscosity and turbulent resistance. The elastic energy accumulated during inspiration, represented by the triangle, is used for expiration. However, only the portion enclosed by the diagonal and the expiration-labeled curve is effectively utilized during this phase to counter the forces of viscosity and turbulence. The remaining energy is spent counteracting the ongoing action of the negative pressure ventilator, which opposes expiration in the initial part of this stage within the breathing cycle. Recreated from [21]

to overcome the viscous and turbulent resistances of expiration. This is because the pressure within the respirator continues to be negative, particularly during the initial phase of expiration. The pressure employed to counteract viscosity and turbulence during expiration, at any given moment, is denoted as ($P_{el} - P_{ex}$), where P_{ex} is the distance from the y-axis to the expiratory loop (or the pressure gradient between the mouth and the inside of the respirator during expiration).

By subtracting the curve from Fig. 8a from the curve from Fig. 8b, the following equation is found:

$$P_t = k_3\left(\frac{dV}{dt}\right) + k_4\left(\frac{dV}{dt}\right)^2, \tag{8}$$

where the slope represents the resistance associated with the nonelastic tissue deformation. Therefore, the summation of Eqs. 7 and 8 is defined by

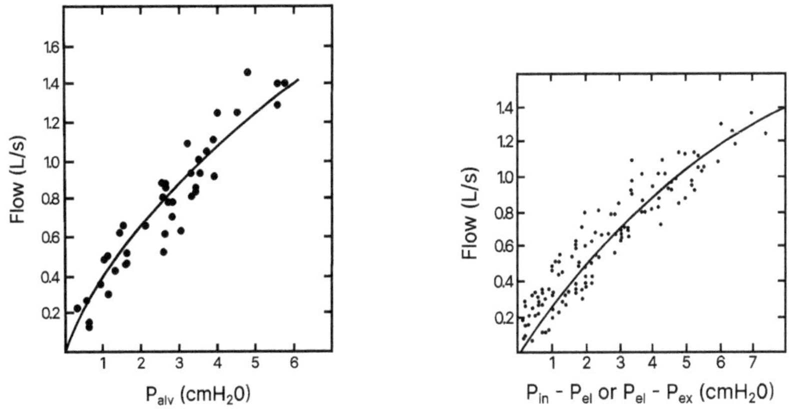

Fig. 8 Relationship between airflow and various pressure differentials. Recreated from [21]. (**a**) Relationship between airflow and the pressure gradient between alveoli and the mouth for a single subject. This curve represents Eq. 7 where $k_1 = 1.7$ and $k_2 = 1.9$. (**b**) Relationship between airflow and pressure required to overcome nonelastic resistance to breathing. This curve represents Eq. 9 where $K' = 2.7$ and $K'' = 2.1$

$$P_n = K'\left(\frac{dV}{dt}\right) + K''\left(\frac{dV}{dt}\right)^2, \tag{9}$$

where K' represents the total viscous resistance and K'' represents the total turbulent resistance. Finally, the total pressure required during breathing is given by the sum of Eqs. 6 and 9:

$$P_\Sigma = KV + K'\left(\frac{dV}{dt}\right) + K''\left(\frac{dV}{dt}\right)^2. \tag{10}$$

In this experiment, the values of the constant K were estimated for three male subjects. The estimated constants are presented in Table 2.

3.4 Sinusoidal Approach

Equation 10 can be used to estimate the work of breathing for any breathing cycle in which the airflow rate pattern is known. It can be even further generalized by describing the flow rate pattern using a mathematical expression. It is assumed that the airflow rate pattern could be approximated by a sine wave, as follows:

$$\frac{dV}{dt} = a\,sin(bt), \tag{11}$$

Table 2 Values of resistance constants estimated in [21]

Subject number	Elastic resistance	Additional resistance of air		Additional resistance of tissue		Total additional resistance	
	K	k_1	k_2	k_3	k_4	K'	K''
	cmH_2O/l	$cmH_2O/(l/s)$	$cmH_2O/(l/s)^2$	$cmH_2O/(l/s)$	$cmH_2O/(l/s)^2$	$cmH_2O/(l/s)$	$cmH_2O/(l/s)^2$
1	8.0	1.7	1.9	1.0	0.2	2.7	2.1
2	9.4	3.2	0.8	1.0	0	4.2	0.8
3	8.2	2.9	1.4	0.6	0.1	3.5	1.5
Mean	8.5	2.6	1.4	0.9	0.1	3.5	1.5

where $\frac{dV}{dt}$ is the flow rate of airflow, a is the maximal flow rate, and the frequency of breathing is given by the expression $b/2\pi = f$.

The differential expression for work is $dW = PdV$, which in substitution from Eqs. 10 and 11 becomes

$$dW = KV\,dV + K'a^2 sin^2(bt)\,dt + K''a^3 sin^3(bt)\,dt. \tag{12}$$

Integration of Eq. 12 will lead to the total work done in a single inspiration.

$$W = \int_0^{V_T} KV\,dV + \int_0^{\pi/b} (K'a^2 sin^2(bt)\,dt + K''a^3 sin^3(bt)\,dt). \tag{13}$$

After simplifying Eq. 13, observe

$$W = \underbrace{\frac{1}{2}KV_T^2}_{\text{elastic}} + \underbrace{\frac{1}{4}K'\pi^2 f V_T^2}_{\text{viscous}} + \underbrace{\frac{2}{3}K''\pi^2 f^2 V_T^3}_{\text{turbulent}}, \tag{14}$$

where each term corresponds to the mechanical work done to overcome elastic resistance, viscous resistance, and turbulent resistance, respectively.

The mean rate of doing work, denoted as $\dot{W}$, is the work per breath multiplied by the frequency of breathing. It can be calculated as

$$\dot{W} = \frac{1}{2}KfV_T^2 + \frac{1}{4}K'\pi^2(fV_T)^2 + \frac{2}{3}K''\pi^2(fV_T)^3. \tag{15}$$

Further expansion of this equation can be done by dividing the tidal volume (V_T) into alveolar volume (V_A) and dead space (V_D) such as $V_T = V_A + V_D$. The updated equation can be written as

$$\dot{W} = \frac{1}{2}Kf\left(\frac{\dot{V}_A}{f} + V_D\right)^2 + \frac{1}{4}K'\pi^2(\dot{V}_A + fV_D)^2 + \frac{2}{3}K''\pi^2(\dot{V}_A + fV_D)^3, \tag{16}$$

where alveolar ventilation $\dot{V}_A = V_A f$. This new equation allows us to examine the work changes as a factor of frequency. Figure 9 depicts this relationship when alveolar ventilation is 6 L/min and dead space is 0.2 L.

3.5 Non-sinusoidal Work of Breathing

Equation 14 effectively fulfills its purpose when estimating the work of an "ideal" breath, characterized by a single frequency, and is applicable only to a single breath. However, this assumption has been challenged in the past [18] and has more recently been investigated [19].

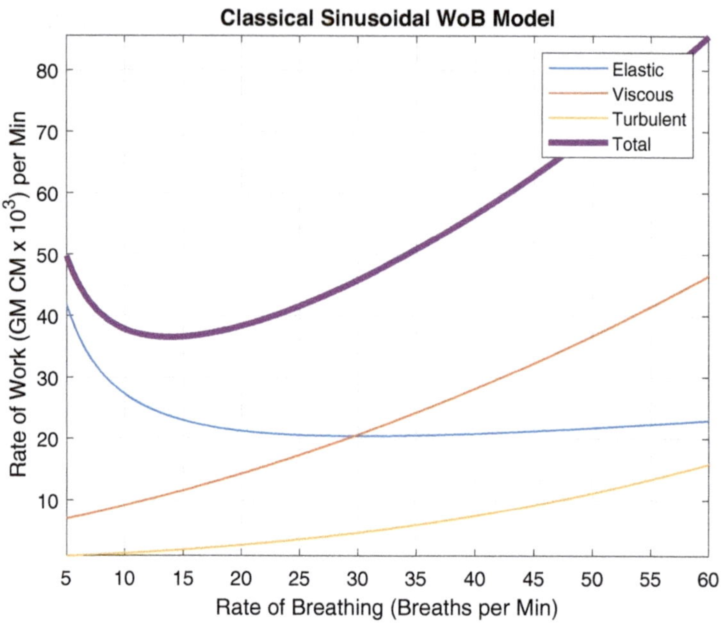

Fig. 9 The inspiratory work of breathing over a minute is modeled using sinusoidal waves, as described by [21]. This model illustrates the relationship between elastic, viscous, turbulent, and total work of breathing per minute when alveolar ventilation is 6 L/min and dead space is 0.2 L. Reprint from [19]

The sinusoidal breathing model relies on the assumption that the breathing rate is the same as the breathing frequency. Breathing rate (B_{Rate}) is typically defined as the number of breaths in a minute (breaths per minute, BPM), as shown in Eq. 17:

$$B_{Rate}(\text{BPM}) = \frac{1}{T} \cdot 60 = f \cdot 60, \tag{17}$$

where f is the frequency in hertz and T is the period of the breath in seconds. However, the work [19] argues that B_{Rate} should not be considered the frequency of breathing for realistic breathing signals, as these two characteristics of breathing are distinct and equivalent only in a special case.

Assuming the definition of the airflow pattern in Eq. 11, a sinusoidal breath is segmented into stages (inspiratory and expiratory) and frequency is now defined as

$$f = \frac{1}{T_{Tot}} = \frac{1}{T_I + T_E} = \frac{1}{2 \cdot T_E} = \frac{1}{2 \cdot T_I}, \tag{18}$$

where T_I represents the time for the inspired breath, T_E represents the time for expired breathing, and T_{Tot} represents the full period of the inspired and expired time of one cycle of a breath. In this ideal sinusoidal example, where $\frac{1}{2 \cdot T_I} = \frac{1}{2 \cdot T_E}$

(or simplistically, $T_I = T_E$), the terms "frequency" and "breathing rate" are equivalent and can be used interchangeably. However, in real breathing dynamics, the time of inspiration is rarely equivalent to the time of expiration. Therefore, when the overwhelming majority of breathing occurs with non-sinusoidal continuous waveforms, the previously mentioned equation does not hold, and

$$f \neq \frac{1}{T_{Tot}} = \frac{1}{T_I + T_E} \neq \frac{1}{2 \cdot T_E} \neq \frac{1}{2 \cdot T_I}, \tag{19}$$

when $T_I \neq T_E$. Therefore, breathing rate cannot refer to the frequency content of the breath, making Eq. 17 simply false.

To further illustrate the difference between breathing rate and frequency, two idealized flow patterns are shown in Fig. 10a. While both of them have the same T_{TOT} of 5 seconds, one has a T_I of 2.5 seconds (blue), and the other has a T_I of 1.25 seconds (orange). Therefore, even with two completely different inspiratory frequencies, the breathing rate is the same—12 BPM. Figure 10b shows the opposite

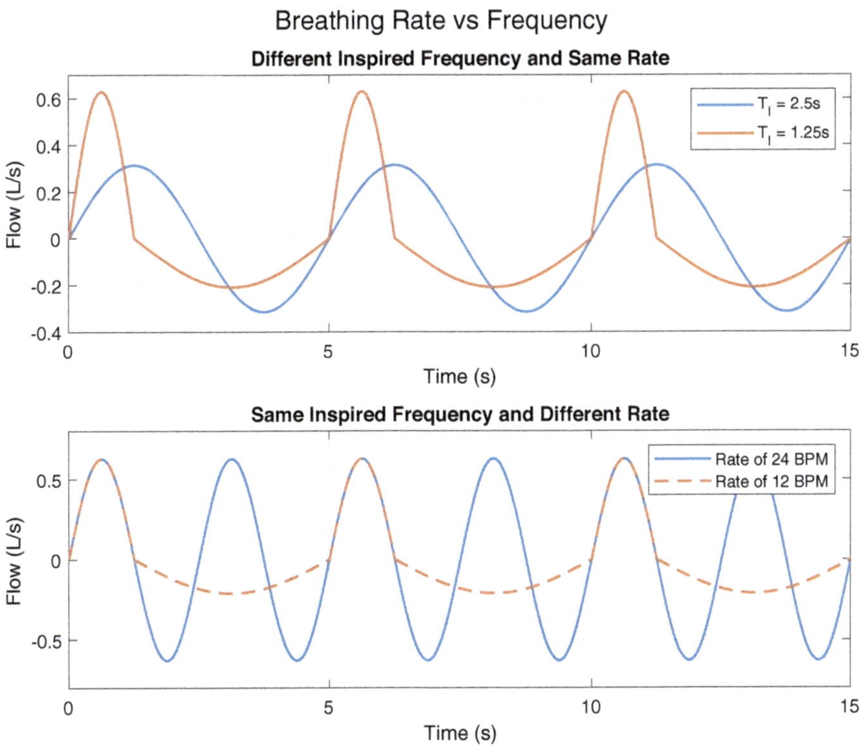

Fig. 10 Breathing Rate vs. Frequency: (**a**) The inspiratory frequencies are different, but the breathing rates are the same. (**b**) The breathing rates are different, but the inspiratory frequencies are the same. Reprint from [19]

case. Here, the inspiratory frequencies are the same, but one has a T_{Tot} of 2.5 seconds (blue), and the other one has a T_{Tot} of 5 seconds (orange). Assuming that both breathing patterns stay continuous for over a minute, the breathing rates are different even though the inspiratory frequency is the same.

Moreover, even if $T_I = T_E$, the respiratory airflow pattern cannot be characterized by a single frequency but instead consists of multiple frequencies. The branching structure of the airways introduces different sizes and lengths, each with its resonant frequencies, resulting in a range of frequencies in the airflow pattern. Turbulence, caused by irregularities and changes in airway diameter, generates fluctuations in the airflow, contributing to a broad spectrum of frequencies. Additionally, pathological conditions such as mucus, inflammation, or airway narrowing can introduce additional resonant frequencies or disrupt the normal airflow pattern, further contributing to the multifrequency nature of respiratory airflow.

3.6 Frequency and Breathing Rate as Function of Work

For simplicity, assume that an inspiratory breath is composed of a single frequency and that expiration is passive. The same conditions as originally presented in the classical sinusoidal model (seen in Fig. 9) are maintained: the same dead space ($V_D = 200cc$), alveolar ventilation ($V_A = 6$ L/min), and mean coefficients of resistance ($K = 8.52\,\text{cmH}_2\text{O/L}$, $K' = 3.5\,\text{cmH}_2\text{O/(L/s)}$, and $K'' = 1.5\,\text{cmH}_2\text{O/(L/s)}^2$). The differentiation between breathing rate and breathing frequency shown in Eq. 17 is applied to Eq. 15. B_{Rate} is distributed across Eq. 16 to evaluate how the frequency of the inspiratory breath impacts WoB across the elastic, viscous, and turbulent components, as shown, respectively, by

$$\dot{W}_{Elastic} = \frac{1}{2} B_{Rate} K \left(\frac{V_A}{B_{Rate}} + V_D \right)^2 \tag{20}$$

$$\dot{W}_{Viscous} = \frac{1}{4} K' \pi^2 B_{Rate} f \left(\frac{V_A}{B_{Rate}} + V_D \right)^2 \tag{21}$$

$$\dot{W}_{Turbulent} = \frac{2}{3} K'' \pi^2 B_{Rate} f^2 \left(\frac{V_A}{B_{Rate}} + V_D \right)^3 . \tag{22}$$

Figure 11 depicts these equations across different breathing rates and inspiratory frequencies along with a comparison to the classical model. The inclusion of the classical sinusoidal work model serves to illustrate the extent of error introduced when more realistic breathing patterns are incorporated into the modeling framework. The classical sinusoidal model also provides valuable insights into state transitions within breathing patterns. To the left of the intersection, $T_I < T_E$; to the right, $T_I > T_E$; and at the intersection, $T_I = T_E$ creating a genuine sinusoidal waveform. An instantaneous inspiration flow limit is imposed in Fig. 11b, c and

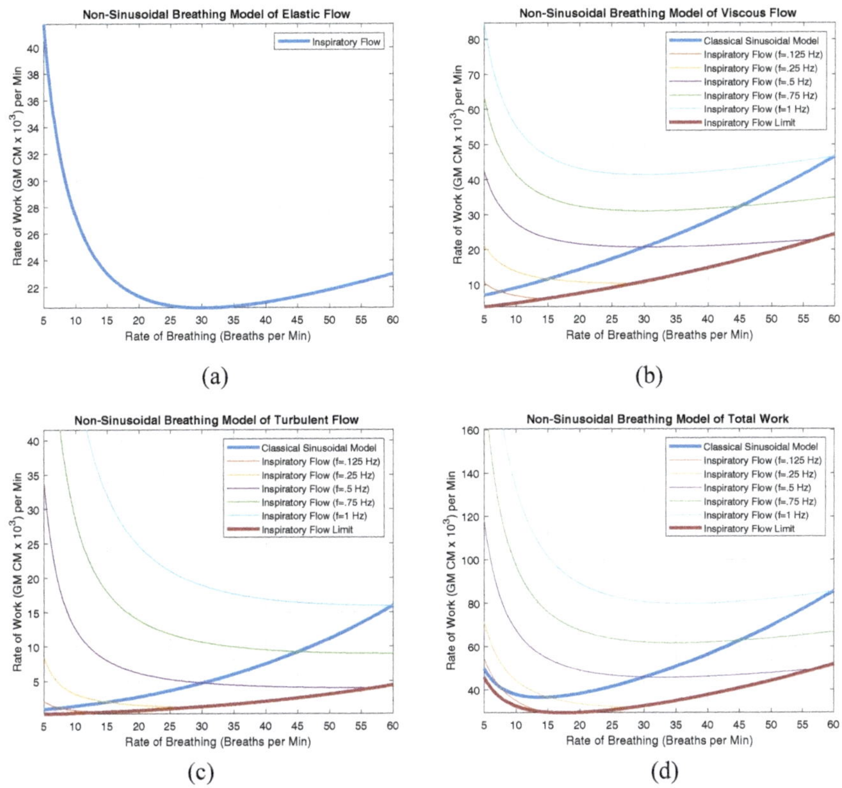

Fig. 11 Work of breathing at various inspiratory frequencies and rates of breathing. Reprint from [19]. (**a**) Model of elastic component of WoB. (**b**) Model of viscous component of WoB. (**c**) Model of turbulent component of WoB. (**d**) Model of total WoB

d, restricting the range of the model since the T_I is bound by the breathing rates T_{Tot}. This limit is further constrained to emulate a minimum expiratory time of 10% of T_{Tot}, equivalent to a 90% duty cycle. The exponential decline in total work is evident across all the instantaneous flow frequencies as the breathing rate increases. The decrease in work can be attributed to the need to maintain alveolar ventilation at a rate of 6 liters per minute, which requires larger and deeper breaths at lower breathing rates. As the respiratory rate increases, the tidal volume, V_T, of each breath may decrease, leading to shallower breaths.

4 Conclusion

Since Campbell's groundbreaking work on pressure–volume curves in 1958 [8], there has been a continuous effort within the scientific community for accurate and precise models of respiratory work. Yet, the past three decades have seen limited progress, leaving the invasive esophageal pressure catheter as the gold standard for measuring WoB and its components. This lack of progress highlights the critical need for reliable noninvasive methods, especially in the context of sleep disorders caused by respiratory diseases.

Numerous gaps persist within the field concerning noninvasive methods that can precisely estimate both intrinsic and extrinsic work. Most current methods assume a sinusoidal pattern for breathing rates, even though humans do not breathe sinusoidally [19]. This discrepancy can introduce potential errors in the accuracy of these models and the actual measurements obtained using gold standard techniques. Non-sinusoidal models have demonstrated superior precision in aligning with the gold standard and further development of these models holds promise for enhancing our understanding of lung-related diseases, optimizing human breathing in challenging environments, like high altitude or during exercise, and designing life support systems that better cater to the unique needs of individuals with sleep disorders.

Acknowledgments The authors would like to acknowledge the Office of Naval Research for supporting this research (Contract Number N000142212653).

Competing Interests The authors have no conflicts of interest to declare that are relevant to the content of this chapter.

References

1. E. Agostoni and P. Mognoni. Deformation of the chest wall during breathing efforts. *Journal of Applied Physiology*, 21(6):1827–1832, November 1966.
2. E. Agostoni, P. Mognoni, G. Torri, and G. Miserocchi. Forces deforming the rib cage. *Respiration Physiology*, 2(1):105–117, January 1966.
3. E. Agostoni and G. Torri. An analysis of the chest wall motions at high values of ventilation. *Respiration Physiology*, 3(3):318–332, December 1967.
4. Emilio Agostoni. A graphical analysis of thoracoabdominal mechanics during the breathing cycle. *Journal of Applied Physiology*, 16(6):1055–1059, November 1961.
5. Raanan Arens and Hiren Muzumdar. Sleep, sleep disordered breathing, and nocturnal hypoventilation in children with neuromuscular diseases. *Paediatric Respiratory Reviews*, 11(1):24–30, March 2010.
6. L. E. Bayliss and G. W. Robertson. THE VISCO-ELASTIC PROPERTIES OF THE LUNGS. *Quarterly Journal of Experimental Physiology and Cognate Medical Sciences*, 29(1):27–47, March 1939.
7. E. J. Moran (Edward James Moran) Campbell, E. Agostoni, and J. Newsom Davis. *The respiratory muscles: mechanics and neural control*. Saunders, Philadelphia, 2d ed. edition, 1970.
8. Edward James Moran Campbell. *The respiratory muscles and the mechanics of breathing*. Lloyd-Luke, 1958.
9. Robert B. Dean and Maurice B. Visscher. THE KINETICS OF LUNG VENTILATION: An Evaluation of the Viscous and Elastic Resistance to Lung Ventilation with Particular Reference to the Effects of Turbulence and the Therapeutic Use of Helium. *American Journal of Physiology-Legacy Content*, 134(3):450–468, September 1941.

10. Kevin Gipson, Mengdi Lu, and T. Bernard Kinane. Sleep-Disordered Breathing in Children. *Pediatrics In Review*, 40(1):3–13, January 2019.
11. Christine A. Gleason and Sherin U. Devaskar. *Avery's Diseases of the Newborn*. Elsevier, September 2011. Publication Title: Avery's Diseases of the Newborn.
12. M. D. Goldman, G. Grimby, and J. Mead. Mechanical work of breathing derived from rib cage and abdominal V-P partitioning. *Journal of Applied Physiology*, 41(5):752–763, November 1976.
13. G. Grimby, M. Goldman, and J. Mead. Respiratory muscle action inferred from rib cage and abdominal V-P partitioning. *Journal of Applied Physiology*, 41(5):739–751, November 1976.
14. K Konno and J Mead. Static volume-pressure characteristics of the rib cage and abdomen. *Journal of Applied Physiology*, 24(4):544–548, April 1968.
15. Mei-Yu Lee, Ching-Chi Lin, Sheng-Yeh Shen, Chung-Hsin Chiu, and Shwu-Fang Liaw. Work of Breathing in Eucapnic and Hypercapnic Sleep Apnea Syndrome. *Respiration*, 77(2):146–153, 2009.
16. Walter T. McNicholas, Daniel Hansson, Sofia Schiza, and Ludger Grote. Sleep in chronic respiratory disease: COPD and hypoventilation disorders. *European Respiratory Review*, 28(153):190064, September 2019.
17. Jere Mead. *Measurement of Inertia of the Lungs at Increased Ambient Pressure. Journal of Applied Physiology*, 9(2):208–212, September 1956.
18. Joseph Millic-Emilli. Work of Breathing. In Ronald G. Crystal and John B West, editors, *The lung: scientific foundations*. Lippincott-Raven, Philadelphia, 2nd ed edition, 1997.
19. Nicholas J. Napoli, Victoria R. Rodrigues, and Paul W. Davenport. Characterizing and Modeling Breathing Dynamics: Flow Rate, Rhythm, Period, and Frequency. *Frontiers in Physiology*, 12, 2022.
20. A. B. Otis and D. F. Proctor. Measurement of alveolar pressure in human subjects. *American Journal of Physiology-Legacy Content*, 152(1):106–112, December 1947.
21. Arthur B. Otis, Wallace O. Fenn, and Hermann Rahn. Mechanics of Breathing in Man. *Journal of Applied Physiology*, 2(11):592–607, May 1950.
22. Hermann Rahn, Arthur B. Otis, Leigh E. Chadwick, and Wallace O. Fenn. THE PRESSURE-VOLUME DIAGRAM OF THE THORAX AND LUNG. *American Journal of Physiology-Legacy Content*, 146(2):161–178, May 1946.
23. Fritz Rohrer. Der Strömungswiderstand in den menschlichen Atemwegen und der Einfluss der unregelmässigen Verzweigung des Bronchialsystems auf den Atmungsverlauf in verschiedenen Lungenbezirken. *Pflüger's Archiv für die Gesamte Physiologie des Menschen und der Thiere*, 162(5-6):225–299, October 1915.
24. Charis Roussos, editor. *The thorax - Part 1*. Number v. 85 in Lung biology in health and disease. M. Dekker, New York, 2nd ed., rev. and expanded edition, 1995.

A Probabilistic Perspective: Bayesian Neural Network for Sleep Apnea Detection

Minhee Kim, Xin Zan, and Xiaochen Xian

1 Introduction

Sleep apnea, a common respiratory disorder, affects approximately 15% of men and 5% of women in the adult population and 1%–5% of infants and children in the juvenile population. This sleep disorder not only disrupts sleep by causing breathing difficulties but also leads to daytime sleepiness, fatigue, and inattention. It poses a significant risk for severe health issues, including heart disease, stroke, and cardiovascular dysfunction. Beyond health, sleep apnea affects society through increased medical and psychiatric morbidity, motor vehicle accidents, reduced work productivity, and heightened mortality rates. Consequently, there is a critical need for accessible and accurate diagnosis methods.

Polysomnography (PSG) is the established method for diagnosing sleep apnea, but its high labor cost and manual inspection requirements limit its accessibility, leaving many cases undiagnosed. Machine learning (ML) methods, especially those analyzing physiological signals such as electrocardiogram (ECG), airflow, blood oxygen saturation, and snoring signals, have emerged as promising alternatives [1, 2].

M. Kim (✉)
University of Florida, Gainesville, FL, USA
e-mail: mkim3@ufl.edu

X. Zan
Department of Industrial and Systems Engineering, University of Iowa, Iowa City, IA, USA
e-mail: xin-zan@uiowa.edu

X. Xian
H. Milton Stewart School of Industrial and Systems Engineering, Georgia Institute of Technology, Atlanta, GA, USA
e-mail: xxian@gatech.edu

R. B. Berry et al. (eds.), *Handbook of AI and Data Sciences for Sleep Disorders*,
Springer Optimization and Its Applications 216,
https://doi.org/10.1007/978-3-031-68263-6_6

However, the application of existing ML models, designed for tasks like image processing or speech recognition, to sleep apnea detection presents challenges due to the unique characteristics of the sleep apnea disorder and the diagnostic process. A prominent challenge is the uncertainty throughout the entire pipeline of sleep apnea diagnosis, from biological processes of sleep to PSG measurement and diagnostic decisions [3, 4]. The pervasive uncertainty significantly comprises the reliability and clinical implementation of most existing ML models [4]. It can be categorized into two types: aleatoric (data) and epistemic (model) uncertainties [5]. In particular, aleatoric uncertainty is inherent to the heterogeneity in biological process of sleep across patients and the variability in PSG measurement system [3, 6]. This type of uncertainty is related to inherent randomness or ambiguity in data and is therefore irreducible. On the other hand, epistemic uncertainty arises from a lack of knowledge about the training data or the optimal model to establish a predictive relationship between PSG signals and apnea diagnosis. For example, this form of uncertainty may arise when annotating particularly difficult epochs of PSG signals or when a model fails to generalize [4, 6]. Unlike aleatoric, epistemic uncertainty can be mitigated by applying higher quality training data or by employing a higher capacity ML model. Moreover, the limited labeled data often found in sleep apnea detection, resulting from high manual labeling costs, can lead to inaccurate modeling and increased uncertainty in diagnosis results when applying ML models. Therefore, it is crucial to provide uncertainty estimates alongside detection results to guide clinical decisions, such as timely interventions and appropriate treatments.

This necessity further leads to the concept of active learning in ML, where models actively select the most informative data points for learning [7]. In the context of sleep apnea, where data labeling is laborious and expensive, active learning can be particularly useful as it targets gaps in existing datasets to collect new, valuable data, thereby improving model accuracy. The hypothesis is that a model guided by its "curiosity" will be more effective given a limited amount of labeled data. If the model provides systematic uncertainty quantification, it can highlight areas of high uncertainty, directing physicians to focus on these regions for future labeling and analysis.

Motivated by these facts, this chapter introduces Bayesian neural networks (BNNs), which combine the flexibility and accuracy of typical ML models with systematic uncertainty quantification. This approach addresses the challenges in sleep apnea detection, making BNNs a suitable tool for advancing diagnosis and treatment strategies in this field.

2 What Is Bayesian Neural Network?

Unlike conventional neural networks (NNs) that are treated as deterministic functions, BNN views the NN as a probabilistic model and quantifies the uncertainties with Bayesian inference. A BNN places a prior distribution over the network's

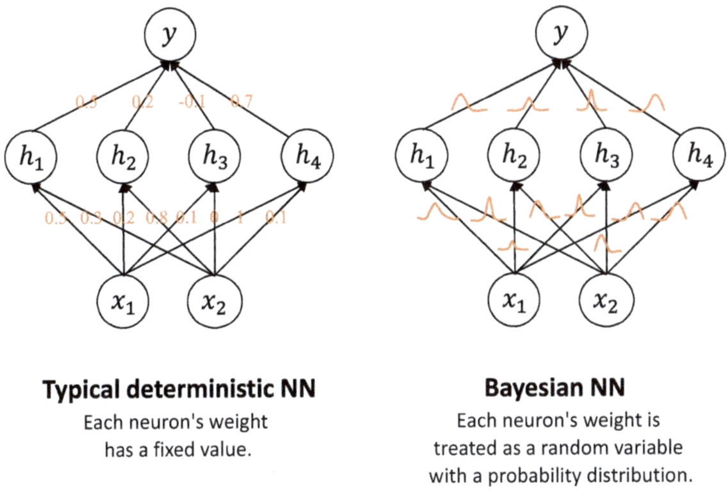

Fig. 1 Comparison between conventional deterministic neural network and BNN

weights and yields posterior distributions over the weights given the observed data. Figure 1 illustrates the comparison between a conventional deterministic NN and BNN. Several works have employed BNN models for classifying and diagnosing sleep apnea based on features extracted and selected from different physiological signals, including thoracic effort signals [8], oximetry signals [9, 10], and nasal pressure and airflow signals [11]. BNN has been reported to provide high accuracy and enhanced generalization capabilities in apnea classification as it controls the distribution of the weights and the network complexity. In addition, BNN is expected to be advantageous with a limited size of training dataset, which is a common problem present in apnea diagnosis [9, 12].

Although BNNs offer high accuracy, robustness to overfitting, and uncertainty quantification, one major challenge is that exact Bayesian inference is computationally intractable for most of the (deep) NN structures. To overcome this challenge, various approximations have been proposed including Laplace approximation [13], variational inference [14, 15], expectation propagation [16], and Hamiltonian methods [17]. For example, Graves [14] applied data sampling-based variational inference and improved the scalability to a large amount of data [14]. Unfortunately, the method showed unsatisfactory performance in practice, due to noises from Monte Carlo approximations within the stochastic gradient computations. Alternatively, Soudry et al. [16] used expectation propagation for modeling networks with binary weights [16]; however, the method did not provide posterior variance estimations for continuous weights. In addition, one common drawback is that these approaches still come with a significant computational cost. To reduce the computational cost, bootstrapping has been applied by separately training many randomly initialized models on the different subsets of training data [18]. Although this approach is more computationally efficient than the conventional

BNN approaches, it can easily lead to unreliable uncertainty estimations. For instance, it has been shown that the prediction on the test data very far from the training data can be still associated with unjustified high confidence [15].

Recently, Gal and Ghahramani [15] developed Monte Carlo dropout (MC dropout), which combines approximate BNN inference with dropout [15]. Dropout is a stochastic regularization technique widely used to prevent coadaptation and overfitting in NNs [19]. The key idea of dropout is to randomly remove (drop) some neurons and their connections from the NN during each iteration of stochastic gradient descent. At the test time, all neurons are present, and the trained weights are multiplied by the probability of keeping (not dropped) neurons. In contrast with conventional dropouts, which drop neurons only at training time, MC dropout trains a model with dropout and also performs a dropout at the test time. In this way, dropout can be interpreted as a variational inference approximation under certain conditions [15]. MC dropout has drawn considerable attention recently, due to its simplicity, scalability, and computational efficiency compared with the conventional BNN approaches. In the following sections, we will employ MC dropout to model the uncertainty stemming from unknown model parameters.

3 How Can Bayesian Neural Network Be Used for Sleep Apnea Detection?

In this section, we will explore the application of BNNs for automated detection of sleep apnea, specifically focusing on obstructive sleep apnea (OSA), a common type of sleep apnea characterized by increased airway resistance often linked to airflow limitation, chest-abdominal paradox, or snoring.

3.1 Problem Formulation

The task of automatic sleep apnea detection is framed as a regression problem. The objective is to predict the latent severity of apnea, measured as the drive-over-flow ratio, using data from fixed 3-second breath cycles. Four key physiological signals are used as model inputs: nasal airflow, ventilatory drive, snoring, and blood oxygen saturation. We implement two versions of NNs for this task: a deterministic convolutional NN (CNN) and a Bayesian CNN (BCNN). Both models share the same architecture, except that the BCNN includes additional dropout layers, enabling MC dropout for uncertainty quantification. During training, the deterministic CNN is trained with mean squared error (MSE) loss, while the BCNN utilizes negative log-likelihood (NLL) loss to effectively incorporate Bayesian principles.

3.2 Data and Preprocessing

The performance of the BCNN is evaluated using a dataset from a sleep study conducted at a local Florida sleep center. This dataset includes a selected PSG recording featuring 15 different physiological signals, including the four signals mentioned in Sect. 3.1. The subject of this study has been diagnosed with OSA, a common type of sleep apnea characterized by an increase in airway resistance that is often associated with airflow limitation, chest–abdominal paradox, or snoring [20]. Following the literature, we employ the respiratory resistance surrogate, defined as the ratio of drive to flow, as the ground-truth label for assessing breath-by-breath OSA severity.

For preprocessing, each signal is downsampled to 100 Hz (i.e., 300 data points for the fixed 3-second breath cycles) and normalized based on the mean and standard deviation during periods free of apnea events for each subject. The signals are segmented using overlapping sliding windows, each corresponding to a 3-second moving breath cycle. The training dataset comprises 1000 instances from one recording. The test dataset consists of 250 instances. The ground-truth label for each instance, referred to as the resistance surrogate, is calculated by the total absolute value of the drive signal over the total absolute value of the flow signal within each moving breath cycle. Figure 2 provides an illustration of the four selected signals across ten breath cycles in 30 seconds.

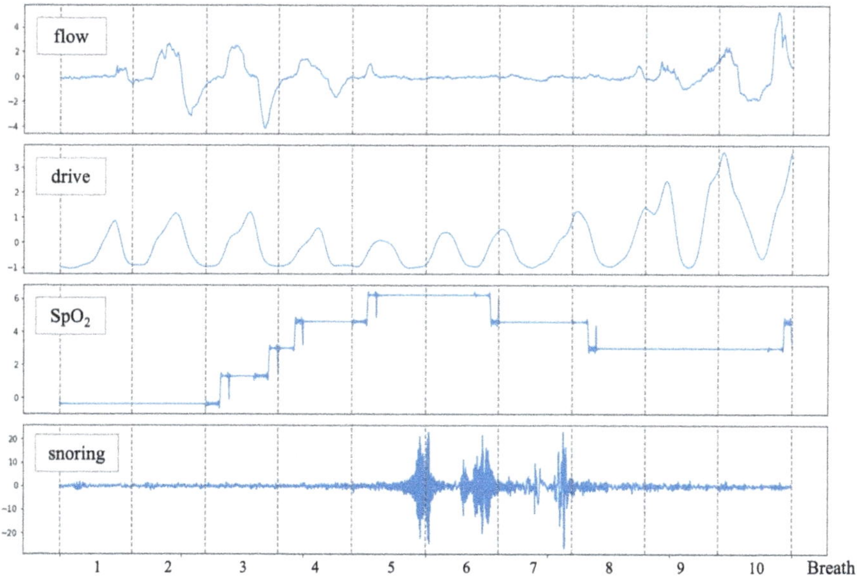

Fig. 2 Visualization of four key signals used as inputs of NNs

3.3 *Results*

3.3.1 Comparison of CNN and BCNN

To evaluate the performance of our models, we employed four metrics: MSE, mean absolute errors (MAEs), Pearson correlation coefficient, and Spearman rank correlation coefficient. The results, summarized in Table 1, show that the BCNN outperforms the CNN across all metrics. Specifically, the BCNN achieves lower MSE, lower MAE, and higher values for both Pearson and Spearman correlation coefficients.

A detailed comparison of the true labels and the predictions from CNN and BCNN over various instances is presented in Fig. 3. This comparison illustrates that the BCNN's predictions align more closely with the true labels than those of the CNN. Notably, the CNN struggles with predicting small label values indicating low apnea likelihood or severity (e.g., instances 100-150).

3.3.2 Decomposition of Uncertainty Quantification

We further investigate the uncertainty quantified by the BNN by categorizing it into two types: aleatoric and epistemic uncertainties [5]. Aleatoric uncertainty

Table 1 Prediction performance comparison of CNN and BCNN

	MSE	MAE	Pearson corr	Spearman corr
CNN	0.0074	0.0654	0.7756	0.3831
BCNN	0.0056	0.0549	0.8372	0.5172

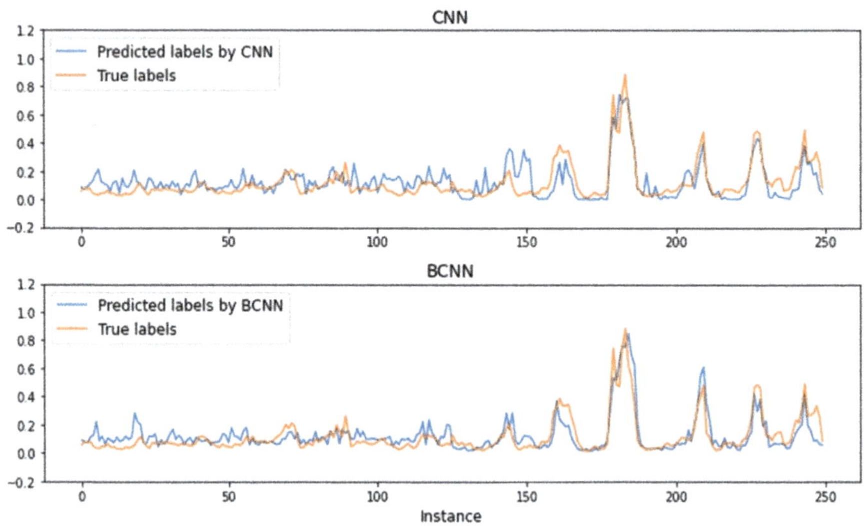

Fig. 3 Comparison of the prediction results of CNN (top) and BCNN (bottom) versus true labels

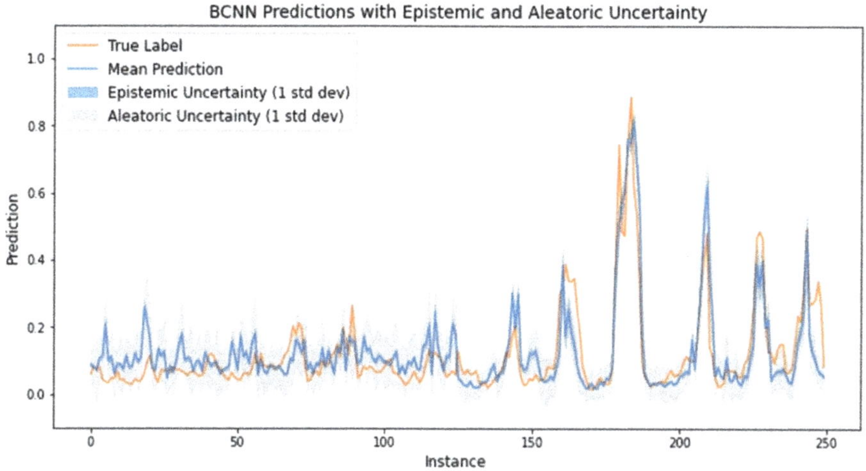

Fig. 4 Overview of BCNN predictions with epistemic and aleatoric uncertainty

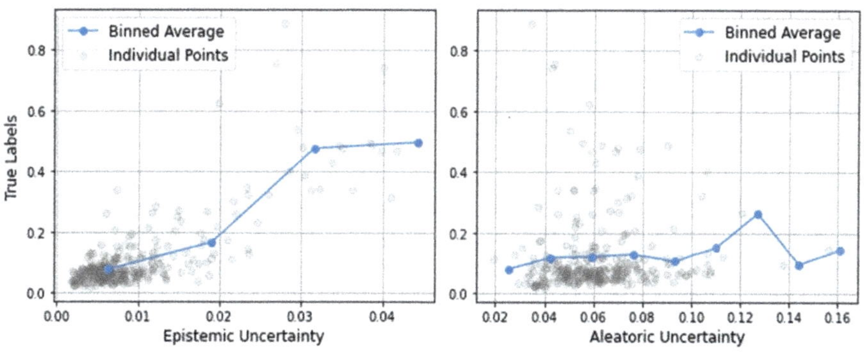

Fig. 5 Epistemic (left) and aleatoric (right) uncertainty versus true labels

stems from inherent randomness in observations (data noise), while epistemic uncertainty arises from limitations in our model knowledge. It is known that aleatoric uncertainty cannot be reduced by collecting more data, while the epistemic uncertainty can. In order to better understand the prediction uncertainty and allocate further resources (e.g., should we collect more data to improve our prediction results?), it is crucial to decompose the quantified uncertainty into these two types.

Here, we follow the procedure based on the previous work [15, 21] for uncertainty decomposition. Figure 4 illustrates the decomposition of epistemic and aleatoric uncertainties. The constancy of aleatoric uncertainty across various instances suggests that a homoscedastic noise model is appropriate for our dataset. This will be elaborated in detail later.

Figure 5 displays the relationship between the uncertainties and the true label values. Figures 4 and 5 indicate a positive correlation between epistemic uncertainty and label values. High epistemic uncertainty in instances with greater label values suggests that the BCNN model is less effective in learning features of instances with higher apnea likelihood and severity. This is an expected outcome, given the relative scarcity of high-severity apnea instances in the dataset. This insight into the model's uncertainty can guide future data collection and model improvement efforts, particularly for instances with high apnea severity.

3.3.3 Comparison of Homoscedastic and Heteroscedastic Uncertainties

Inspired by the results in Fig. 5, we conducted a comparative analysis of model performance under homoscedastic and heteroscedastic uncertainty assumptions. Homoscedastic uncertainty presumes that aleatoric uncertainty, referring to the inherent randomness in data, has a uniform variance across different instances. This assumption simplifies the ML model by treating all data points as equally uncertain but may not always reflect the true nature of complex healthcare data characterized by variability in physiological states, subjects, measurement techniques, etc. By contrast, heteroscedastic uncertainty allows for the variance of aleatoric uncertainty to vary among different instances, which may align more closely with the realities of healthcare data. In the study of sleep apnea, heteroscedasticity may be particularly relevant as it accommodates differences in signal stability and noise across various sleep stages and patient conditions. By acknowledging and modeling this variability, heteroscedastic models can adapt to diverse data sources and conditions, potentially yielding more precise and reliable predictions. Our comparison of the two assumptions aims to examine how effectively each uncertainty model captures the complex and dynamic nature of physiological signal data and handles the intrinsic uncertainty and ambiguity inherent in diagnosing sleep apnea.

The comparative results are summarized in Table 2. The results indicate that the model assuming homoscedastic uncertainty outperforms the one based on heteroscedastic uncertainty in terms of predictive accuracy. Similar to Figs. 3, 6 further shows the prediction results assuming homoscedastic and heteroscedastic uncertainties. The figure shows that homoscedastic assumption leads to slightly more accurate fitting results than heteroscedastic one. Specifically, the homoscedastic model outperforms the heteroscedastic one for instances with low label values (i.e., low apnea likelihood and low apnea severity). In addition, the homoscedastic model can better estimate the peaks with sharp changes that cannot be well estimated by the heteroscedastic one or deterministic CNN model as observed in Fig. 3.

Table 2 Prediction performance comparison of homoscedastic and heteroscedastic BCNNs

	MSE	MAE	Pearson corr	Spearman corr
Homoscedastic	0.0041	0.0469	0.8827	0.5820
Heteroscedastic	0.0056	0.0549	0.8372	0.5172

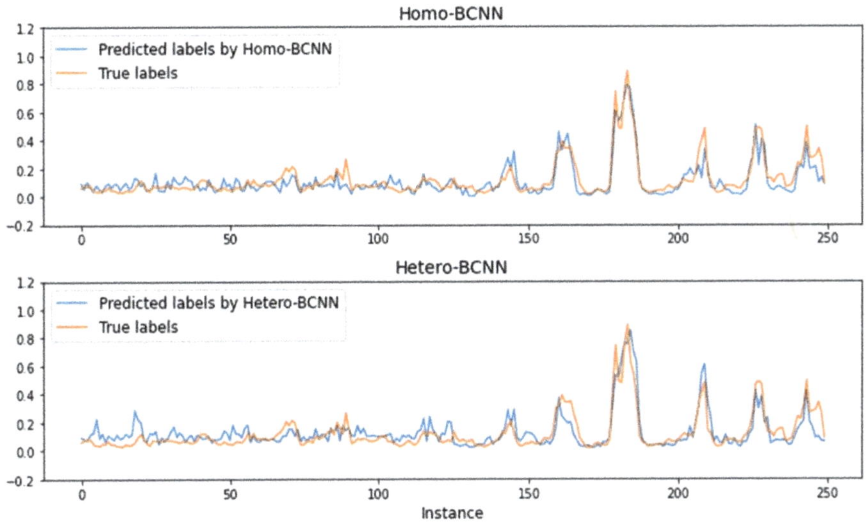

Fig. 6 Comparison of the prediction results of BCNN assuming homoscedastic uncertainty (top), heteroscedastic uncertainty (middle), and true labels (bottom)

These findings appear counterintuitive regarding the superior performance of the homoscedastic model, especially given the inherently heterogeneous nature of sleep processes, a characteristic that would seemingly favor a heteroscedastic approach to accommodate variable uncertainty across data [3, 6]. Under a close examination, we find that this is attributed to the applied dataset. Since the dataset in our study is derived from consistent measurement equipment and processing methods and predominantly encompasses data from the same rapid eye movement (REM) sleep stage, it is logical that the noise characteristics (aleatoric uncertainty) would be relatively uniform across all instances. This aligns with expectations considering the nature of aleatoric uncertainty, which is linked to observation noise.

This uniformity in aleatoric uncertainty suggests that the variation in the applied dataset is more likely attributable to the underlying phenomena being measured (i.e., sleep apnea severity) rather than inconsistencies or errors in the measurement process itself. Therefore, a homoscedastic uncertainty model, which assumes a consistent level of observational noise across all instances, is more appropriate and effective for this particular dataset for the task of sleep apnea detection. It should be noted that heteroscedastic uncertainty models have a broader applicability and are more appropriate in a general case when the acquired dataset encompasses a wide range of data sources, measurement techniques, conditions, sleep stages, or subjects.

3.3.4 Effect of Training Dataset Size

Lastly, we investigate how the size of the training dataset affects the performance of BCNN. It is widely known that NN models generally require substantial amounts of data to deliver satisfactory results. However, BCNNs have been recognized for their ability to perform well with relatively smaller datasets [22]. Bayesian methods, by their nature, integrate over all possible models (in a probabilistic sense) rather than committing to a single model, as is the case with deterministic approaches. This integration effectively compensates for the lack of data by considering a wider range of hypotheses about the underlying data generation process.

To explore this aspect, we conducted experiments to measure the accuracy of both the deterministic CNN and the BCNN with varying sizes of training data. The results of these experiments are depicted in Fig. 7. As anticipated, there is a general trend of improving performance with the increase in the number of training data samples for both CNN and BCNN models. This improvement is consistent with the understanding that more data provide a richer learning environment, allowing models to capture and generalize patterns more effectively. Another thing to note is that BCNN performs relatively well even with a limited amount of data.

These findings highlight the robustness of BCNNs against limited training data size, elaborating their suitability for applications like sleep apnea detection where acquiring large datasets can be challenging. The ability of BCNNs to deliver reliable performance even with limited data highlights their potential as a powerful tool in medical diagnostics and other fields where data scarcity is a common issue.

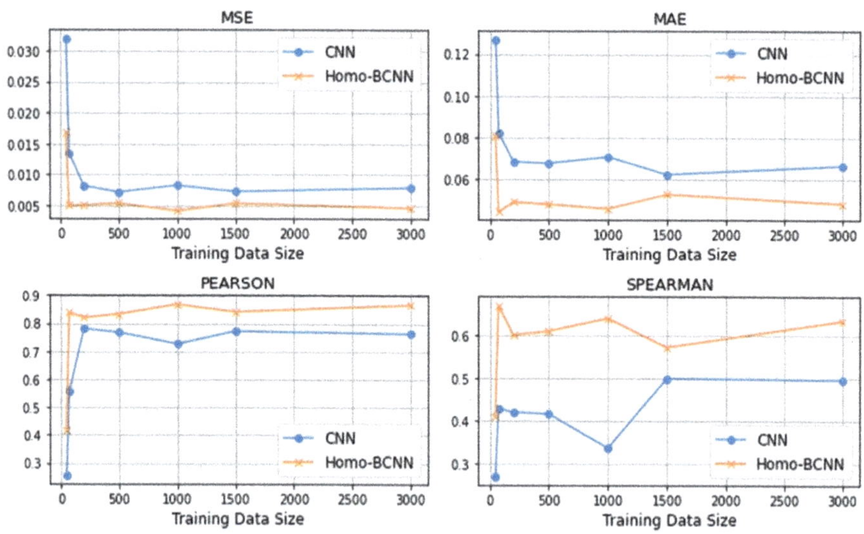

Fig. 7 Prediction accuracy with varying training size for CNN and homoscedastic BCNN

4 Concluding Remarks

This chapter has provided a comprehensive exploration of the application of BNNs, specifically BCNNs, for the detection of sleep apnea. Through various analyses and comparisons, we have demonstrated the effectiveness and potential of BCNNs in this problem, highlighting their advantages over traditional deterministic NNs. Key findings of our chapter include:

1. **Superior Numerical Performance of BNNs**: Across various metrics such as mean squared errors, mean absolute errors, and correlation coefficients, the BNN consistently outperformed its deterministic counterpart in accurately predicting the latent severity of apnea. This means that BNNs provide more precise and reliable predictions of latent severity of apnea. The superior performance of BNN implies that the PSG data used for diagnosing sleep apnea commonly contain inherent variability and noise that deterministic models struggle to handle. This is expected and consistent with clinical practice, as PSG data involve a range of physiological signals collected from various sensors and are therefore subject to various forms of noise and variability. Additionally, manual labeling and diagnosis of sleep apnea in PSG data can introduce subjective errors, which BNNs are better equipped to manage due to their probabilistic nature. Such accurate predictions of apnea severity are expected to help clinicians in timely and appropriate interventions, thus improving the overall management of sleep apnea. For example, efficient and precise prediction of severe sleep apnea can prompt immediate initiation of Continuous Positive Airway Pressure (CPAP) therapy and supports enhanced patient self-management [23]. Furthermore, precise predictions can assist in customizing treatment plans to fit individual patient needs, ensuring that each patient receives the most effective therapy based on their specific condition.
2. **Uncertainty Quantification**: The decomposition of uncertainty into aleatoric (inherent noise in data) and epistemic (uncertainty in the model) components using BNNs can offer insightful perspectives to guide further data collection and clinical decision-making. Not all uncertainties can be addressed by refining ML models, but understanding these different uncertainties enables clinicians to make more informed decisions for diagnosing and managing sleep apnea more effectively. For example, high epistemic uncertainty may indicate the need for more data to make a confident diagnosis. This can guide clinicians to prioritize further data collection where it matters most and tailor treatments more effectively. On the other hand, unexpectedly high aleatoric uncertainty suggests variability that may be linked to sensor issues or patient movement during sleep studies. Recognizing this can lead clinicians to consider necessary improvements in PSG technology or adjustments in data collection protocols, thereby enhancing the quality and reliability of the data. Moreover, analyzing different levels of uncertainty in predictions across various instances through heteroscedastic models can deepen the understanding of how symptoms and diagnostic capabilities vary under different conditions. When selecting models

with uncertainty quantification in practice, it is crucial for clinicians to choose a model that aligns well with their specific data and clinical requirements. The balance between model simplicity and complexity is essential to ensure that the model is both effective in its predictions and manageable for practical use. Being aware of the dataset's characteristics and the specific diagnosis challenges aids clinicians in selecting the most suitable model, maximizing the benefits of uncertainty quantification in improving patient outcomes.

3. **Robustness to Training Data Size**: BNNs maintained good performance even with smaller datasets. The robustness to limited data availability makes BNNs particularly attractive for medical applications like sleep apnea detection, where large labeled datasets may not always be feasible. This ensures that even with limited patient data, more reliable diagnostics can still be made, making BNNs a valuable tool in resource-constrained diagnostic settings. This capability is vital for enabling the early diagnosis and treatment of sleep apnea on a broad scale, potentially mitigating serious complications such as heart disease and stroke that can arise from delayed or inaccurate diagnoses. In clinical practice, BNNs' ability to perform well with few labeled training data also significantly reduces the manual effort required for annotating PSG data. This reduction is highly desirable for practitioners, saving labor-intensive and costly labeling efforts and leveraging the advantages of AI technology to improve diagnostic processes.
4. **Future Directions**: While this study underscores the potential of BNNs in sleep apnea detection, further research is needed to refine these models for clinical application. This includes enhancing model interpretability (the ability to understand and explain how a computational model makes its predictions) and decision-making (using model outputs to make final clinical decisions). The model interpretability enables clinicians to understand and explain the rationale behind a model's outputs for integrating this technology seamlessly into apnea diagnostic processes in clinical practice. In addition, understanding and interpretation of various uncertainties by BNNs are also valuable to provide intelligent and informed insights, guiding clinicians in making more precise and targeted interventions. Another promising research venue is integrating other ML techniques to further enhance manual labeling efficiency, thereby streamlining diagnosis processes and improving operational efficiencies. For example, active learning is a powerful tool to enhance the model's training efficiency, where the model actively queries for the most informative data points to improve itself. This strategic learning technique focuses annotation efforts specifically on data points that the model identifies as ambiguous or uncertain, which significantly reduces the time-consuming and labor-intensive burden of data annotation for model training. This technique not only optimizes the use of existing data but also helps in quickly adapting the model to new or evolving clinical scenarios.

In conclusion, the application of BNNs in sleep apnea detection represents a significant advancement in the field of medical diagnostics. Currently, the emphasis on applying NNs for sleep apnea largely revolves around developing new NN designs or selecting suitable existing designs. However, this chapter aims to extend this trend by underscoring the importance of a probabilistic approach and the promising capabilities of BNNs in this field. The unique capabilities of BNNs to handle uncertainties and work effectively with limited data can improve the accuracy and accessibility of sleep apnea diagnostics. Moving forward, continued research and development in this area will be crucial to fully realize the potential of BNNs in enhancing patient care and outcomes in sleep medicine and beyond.

References

1. Sheikh Shanawaz Mostafa, Fábio Mendonça, Antonio G. Ravelo-García, and Fernando Morgado-Dias. A systematic review of detecting sleep apnea using deep learning. *Sensors*, 19(22):4934, 2019.
2. Maziar Hafezi, Nasim Montazeri, Shumit Saha, Kaiyin Zhu, Bojan Gavrilovic, Azadeh Yadollahi, and Babak Taati. Sleep apnea severity estimation from tracheal movements using a deep learning model. *IEEE Access*, 8:22641–22649, 2020.
3. Dae Y Kang, Pamela N DeYoung, Justin Tantiongloc, Todd P Coleman, and Robert L Owens. Statistical uncertainty quantification to augment clinical decision support: a first implementation in sleep medicine. *NPJ digital medicine*, 4(1):142, 2021.
4. Ivo Pascal de Jong, Andreea Ioana Sburlea, and Matias Valdenegro-Toro. Uncertainty quantification in machine learning for biosignal applications–a review. *arXiv preprint arXiv:2312.09454*, 2023.
5. Eyke Hüllermeier and Willem Waegeman. Aleatoric and epistemic uncertainty in machine learning: An introduction to concepts and methods. *Machine Learning*, 110:457–506, 2021.
6. Hans van Gorp, Iris AM Huijben, Pedro Fonseca, Ruud JG van Sloun, Sebastiaan Overeem, and Merel M van Gilst. Certainty about uncertainty in sleep staging: a theoretical framework. *Sleep*, 45(8):zsac134, 2022.
7. Wei-Ning Hsu and Hsuan-Tien Lin. Active learning by learning. In *Proceedings of the AAAI Conference on Artificial Intelligence*, volume 29, 2015.
8. Oscar Fontenla-Romero, Bertha Guijarro-Berdinas, Amparo Alonso-Betanzos, and Vicente Moret-Bonillo. A new method for sleep apnea classification using wavelets and feedforward neural networks. *Artificial Intelligence in Medicine*, 34(1):65–76, 2005.
9. JV Marcos, R Hornero, D Alvarez, Ian T Nabney, F Del Campo, and C Zamarrón. The classification of oximetry signals using Bayesian neural networks to assist in the detection of obstructive sleep apnoea syndrome. *Physiological measurement*, 31(3):375, 2010.
10. Daniel Álvarez, Gonzalo César Gutiérrez-Tobal, Fernando Vaquerizo-Villar, Verónica Barroso-García, A Crespo, CA Arroyo, F Del Campo, and R Hornero. Automated analysis of unattended portable oximetry by means of Bayesian neural networks to assist in the diagnosis of sleep apnea. In *2016 global medical engineering physics exchanges/pan American health care exchanges (GMEPE/PAHCE)*, pages 1–4. IEEE, 2016.
11. Gonzalo C Gutiérrez-Tobal, Julio de Frutos, Daniel Álvarez, Fernando Vaquerizo-Villar, Verónica Barroso-García, Andrea Crespo, Felix Del Campo, and Roberto Hornero. A Bayesian neural network approach to compare the spectral information from nasal pressure and thermistor airflow in the automatic sleep apnea severity estimation. In *2017 39th Annual International Conference of the IEEE Engineering in Medicine and Biology Society (EMBC)*, pages 3741–3744. IEEE, 2017.
12. Nuno Pombo, Nuno Garcia, and Kouamana Bousson. Classification techniques on computerized systems to predict and/or to detect apnea: A systematic review. *Computer methods and programs in biomedicine*, 140:265–274, 2017.
13. D.J.C. MacKay. *Bayesian methods for adaptive models*. PhD thesis, California Institute of Technology, 1992.

14. A. Graves. Practical variational inference for neural networks. In *Advances in Neural Information Processing Systems 24*, pages 2348–2356, 2011.
15. Y. Gal and Z. Ghahramani. Dropout as a Bayesian approximation: Representing model uncertainty in deep learning. In *Proceedings of the 33rd International Conference on International Conference on Machine Learning - Volume 48*, pages 1050–1059, 2016.
16. D Soudry, I Hubara, and R Meir. Expectation backpropagation: Parameter-free training of multilayer neural networks with continuous or discrete weights. In *Advances in Neural Information Processing Systems 27*, pages 963–971, 2014.
17. J.T. Springenberg, A. Klein, S. Falkner, and F. Hutter. Bayesian optimization with robust Bayesian neural networks. In *Advances in Neural Information Processing Systems 29*, pages 4134–4142, 2016.
18. I. Osband, C. Blundell, A. Pritzel, B. Van Roy, and B. Van Roy. Deep exploration via bootstrapped DQN. In *Advances in Neural Information Processing Systems 29*, pages 4026–4034, 2016.
19. G.E. Hinton, N. Srivastava, A. Krizhevsky, I. Sutskever, and R.R. Salakhutdinov. Improving neural networks by preventing co-adaptation of feature detectors. *arXiv preprint arXiv:1207.0580*, 2012.
20. Richard B Berry, Scott Ryals, and Mary H Wagner. Use of chest wall EMG to classify hypopneas as obstructive or central. *Journal of Clinical Sleep Medicine*, 14(5):725–733, 2018.
21. Minhee Kim and Kaibo Liu. A Bayesian deep learning framework for interval estimation of remaining useful life in complex systems by incorporating general degradation characteristics. *IISE Transactions*, 53(3):326–340, 2020.
22. Hao Wang and Dit-Yan Yeung. A survey on Bayesian deep learning. *ACM computing surveys (CSUR)*, 53(5):1–37, 2020.
23. Cathy A Goldstein, Richard B Berry, David T Kent, David A Kristo, Azizi A Seixas, Susan Redline, M Brandon Westover, Fariha Abbasi-Feinberg, R Nisha Aurora, Kelly A Carden, et al. Artificial intelligence in sleep medicine: an American academy of sleep medicine position statement. *Journal of Clinical Sleep Medicine*, 16(4):605–607, 2020.

Automatic and Machine Learning Methods for Detection and Characterization of REM Sleep Behavior Disorder

Matteo Cesari and Irene Rechichi

1 Rapid Eye Movement Sleep Behavior Disorder

Rapid eye movement (REM) sleep behavior disorder (RBD) is a sleep disorder characterized by dream enactment during REM sleep (presented in form of vocalizations, jerks, and motor behaviors) and by abnormal muscular activity in REM sleep. The polysomnography (PSG) electrophysiological hallmark of RBD is therefore the presence of muscular tone in REM sleep, a phenomenon known as REM sleep without atonia (RWA). Patients with RBD might experience a wide range of conditions, from unnoticed sleep disruption to severe injuries to themselves or the bed partners [1].

Diagnostic criteria for RBD are described by the International Classification of Sleep Disorder (ICSD) [2], and modifications to these criteria have been recently proposed by the International RBD Study Group (IRBDSG) [3]. Both criteria require demonstration of RWA for RBD diagnosis. The two criteria differ for the documentation of dream enacting behaviors. While for the ICSD a clinical history of dream enactment is sufficient, the IRBDSG guidelines recommend that for a definite RBD diagnosis dream enactment is recorded during video-PSG (v-PSG).

RBD can manifest as isolated (formally known as idiopathic), as well as associated with other conditions. Isolated RBD (iRBD) is a condition when RBD occurs in the absence of associated comorbidities or known provoking factors. Several studies have shown that patients with iRBD, when followed up over years,

M. Cesari (✉)
Department of Neurology, Medical University of Innsbruck, Innsbruck, Austria
e-mail: matteo.cesari@i-med.ac.at

I. Rechichi
Department of Control and Computer Engineering, Politecnico di Torino, Torino, Italy
e-mail: irene.rechichi@polito.it

R. B. Berry et al. (eds.), *Handbook of AI and Data Sciences for Sleep Disorders*,
Springer Optimization and Its Applications 216,
https://doi.org/10.1007/978-3-031-68263-6_7

convert to an overt alpha-synucleinopathy (i.e., Parkinson's disease (PD), dementia with Lewy bodies (DLB), and multiple system atrophy (MSA)) [1]. The conversion rate has been shown to be up to 73.5% after 12 years of follow-up [4]. Thus, iRBD is by now recognized as an early stage of alpha-synucleinopathies [1]. When not isolated, RBD can be associated with intake of medications, overt neurodegenerative disorders, narcolepsy, autoimmune diseases, and brainstem lesions [1].

Rule-based and artificial intelligence (AI) algorithms have been developed and applied also in the field of RBD. This chapter summarizes them and is structured in this way. Section 2 describes rule-based algorithms for automatic RWA quantification, as demonstration of RWA is required for RBD diagnosis. Section 3 introduces machine learning (ML) and deep learning (DL) algorithms which have been developed for the purpose of identifying patients with RBD. Section 4 describes the ML and DL algorithm which have been developed for predicting the conversion to overt alpha-synucleinopathies in iRBD patients. Finally, Sect. 5 concludes the chapter presenting future perspectives.

To provide a comprehensive literature review in this area, the authors searched for eligible papers in PubMed.[1]

2 Rule-Based Methods for RWA Quantification

As introduced in Sect. 1, RWA is the polysomnographic hallmark of RBD. Both the ICSD [2] and the IRBDSG diagnostic guidelines [3] require the PSG and the electromyographic (EMG) activity to be visually inspected by a sleep expert and manually scored by a neurologist, in order to properly quantify RWA. Therefore, the implementation of the scoring rules entails a time-consuming process, often prone to inter- and intra-rater variability [5]. This vulnerability led to the need and the subsequent development of rule-based methods for the scoring of RWA.

Different rule-based approaches have been proposed in the literature to pursue quantification of motor activity during sleep and express it in the form of indices. The proposed algorithms exploit the surface EMG activity of the submentalis, mentalis, and flexor digitorum superficialis (FDS), by applying various signal processing techniques. These methods rely mostly on the variations in amplitude observed during the REM stage, by using observation windows of different lengths. Some of the most popular metrics, summarized in Table 1, were first developed with the aim of differentiating between healthy subjects and RBD patients and were thoroughly investigated and cross-compared in a previous study on a cohort

[1] Search terms: ((machine learning) OR (deep learning) OR classifier OR (artificial intelligence) OR algorithm OR (data driven)) AND ((rapid eye movement sleep behavior disorder) OR (REM sleep behavior disorder)). Date of the search: July 18, 2023.

Table 1 Summary of the rule-based methods presented in this section along with proper reference. For each method, the following are included: EMG source, preprocessing specifications, window length, population under study, and performance metric (in terms of area under the curve). The acronym *ND* refers to subjects with neurodegenerative diseases. The acronym OSAS refers to subjects with obstructive sleep apnea syndrome

Index	EMG source	Filter	Epoch length	Population	Type	Performance	Reference
RAI	Chin	Bandpass 10–100 Hz	1 s	35 controls (10 age-matched)	Semi-automatic	0.83 (AUC)	[13, 14]
				31 RBD			
				10 MSA			
				5 OSAS			
STREAM	Chin	Bandpass 10–70 Hz	3 s	6 controls	Semi-automatic	0.84 (AUC)	[7]
				23 ND (9 RBD)			
FRI	Chin	Bandpass 10–70 Hz	3 s	29 controls	Semi-automatic	0.81 (AUC)	[8]
		Notch 50 Hz		21 RBD			
				43 PD			
Automated	Chin	Bandpass 50–300 Hz	3 s	60 controls	Semi-Automatic	0.93 (AUC)	[9, 14]
SINBAR	Bilateral FDS			20 RBD			

of healthy controls, patients with iRBD, PD patients with RBD, and PD patients without RBD [6].

As previously stated, these methods analyze the EMG signal and define, in most cases, abnormal motor activity by using as a baseline the amplitude values observed during quiet REM sleep or NREM sleep. This is the case in the Supra-Threshold REM Activity Metric (STREAM), which accounts for the variations in motor activity described as variance across windows of 3-second length, i.e., *mini-epochs* [7]. In more detail, the index is expressed as the percentage of 3-s mini-epochs in REM sleep with variance above the baseline threshold, which is defined as the variance computed during NREM sleep in a low-activity condition. Other indices, namely the Frandsen Index (FRI) and the computerized Sleep Innsbruck Barcelona (SINBAR) method, employ an analogous window length.

The FRI [8] defines an *activity curve*, based on the filtered EMG signal, and performs event detection whenever the activity curve is found above a defined detection threshold. Such threshold was heuristically explored by multiplying the baseline level, i.e., a measure of the lowest activity curve throughout the night, with an even factor in the range of 2–16, with steps of 2. Other parameters, including the duration of the events, the inter-event interval, and the amount of REM sleep, were also taken into account to define the best detection combination.

In 2014, a computerized version of the SINBAR RWA quantification method was proposed [9]. This method provided an automatic computation of the SINBAR metrics for the quantification of RWA by computing the phasic, tonic, *any* activity, and the SINBAR index in the mentalis and FDS muscles, following the guidelines published by the group in [10]. The combination of automatic quantification and manual artifact correction led to a significant decrease in the number of false positives, making it a reliable tool for the scoring of RWA. For this reason, the computerized version of the SINBAR index [9] was also the first algorithm to be implemented and fully integrated in a PSG system; it is also the only one currently employed in the clinical and diagnostic routine. An open-access version of the automatic SINBAR method has been recently proposed [11].

Lastly, the REM Atonia Index (RAI) was proposed with the aim of quantifying the amplitude of the rectified submentalis EMG on a cohort of patients with iRBD and healthy controls [12]. An improved version, allowing for noise reduction and limiting the effect of motion artifacts, has been proposed in [13], and its validity as first-line screening item has also been demonstrated in a comparison study [14]. The RAI accounts for the percentage of atonia during REM sleep and is defined on the continuous interval [0, 1], where 0 represents complete loss of atonia; a threshold of 0.8 or 0.9 has been proposed to discriminate between healthy subjects and RBD patients and proved to be indicative of altered atonia during REM sleep.

As previously specified, these methods are rule-based, meaning that they consist of a set of rules defined by humans to score RWA. A limitation of these scoring approaches is that they simply use thresholds to identify RWA. Although some of the described methods incorporate a noise correction step, it has been shown that these metrics often require the manual correction of artifacts, caused, for instance, by sleep apneas, which are known to substantially increase the EMG amplitude in the mentalis and submentalis muscles [15], leading in most cases to false positives or wrong values of the indices. Furthermore, although RWA is the electrophysiological hallmark of RBD, it constitutes only a necessary condition for its diagnosis, and it is not therefore specific for the identification of patients with RBD. To overcome the limitations of rule-based RWA quantification methods, researchers have investigated the use of machine and deep learning algorithms for directly classifying and identifying patients with RBD. Due to the properties of the algorithms, these methods directly learn features and/or patterns characterizing patients with RBD. These algorithms could therefore be potentially employed as decision-support methods and are summarized in the next section.

3 Machine and Deep Learning Algorithms for RBD Identification

In recent years, ML has been widely employed in healthcare, finding applications in the computer-assisted diagnosis, prediction and monitoring of diseases. These models have also been employed in the study of sleep: for instance, by defining pipelines and frameworks for the automatic scoring of polysomnography. Consequently, a huge number of these models have also been employed in the study of RBD, to provide for automated screening or decision-support frameworks. These methods rely on various physiological sources (or biosignals) and may be feature driven—i.e., variables are used to extract information from data—or data driven—i.e., the algorithms work on the signal itself. These approaches will be described in the following subsections, grouped according to the signal employed.

3.1 Algorithms Using Data from Polysomnography

A first attempt to the ML-based detection of RBD was provided by exploring the biosignals collected during polysomnography, through a feature-driven approach. Traditional PSG offers a wide variety of biosignals recorded during sleep, including the electroencephalogram (EEG), EMG, electrocardiogram (ECG), and electrooculogram (EOG). These enclose a great amount of information that can be extracted by means of various features, later employed and used to differentiate RBD subjects from healthy ones, or controls with other sleep disorders.

This section describes the studies presenting with this approach; the papers are grouped according to the employed signal.

3.1.1 Algorithms Based on Multiple Polysomnographic Features

Different approaches combining multiple PSG signals were proposed in the literature.

Cooray et al. [16] proposed an automatic pipeline for the detection of RBD subjects. The analysis was performed using PSG data from 106 subjects (53 RBD, 53 age-matched controls). The method envisaged an initial automatic sleep staging, through the use of 156 features extracted from the EMG, EEG, and EOG signals, used to train a Random Forest (RF) classifier. The EEG features were extracted in the time domain (statistical metrics), frequency domain (power metrics), and nonlinear (entropy measures and energy operators). The Discrete Wavelet Transform (DWT) was employed to extract features from the EOG channel. As regards the EMG, some of the metrics described in Sect. 2 were computed and employed as features for the sleep stage classification algorithm. Subsequently, an automatic RBD detection algorithm was developed; this relied on three traditionally established RWA metrics (RAI, STREAM, and FRI, *cf.* Section 2), features extracted from the sleep architecture, and an additional feature investigating the EMG characteristics, namely the fractal exponent. This set of features was used as input to a random forest (RF) classifier (500 trees, 3 samples per split) and proved to be efficient in detecting RBD subjects, with a test accuracy of 96% (manual sleep scoring) and 92% (automated sleep scoring). The RAI proved to be the most important feature in the RF classifier, followed by the proportion of non-REM (NREM) sleep stage 3 and the atonia index ratio between REM and NREM stage 2 sleep.

In a later work [17], the same authors proposed a fully automated RBD detection pipeline through a lower number of signals; this was attained by disposing of the EEG channels. Therefore, the analysis relied solely on the EOG, EMG, and ECG sources. The population in the study, built from various available datasets, included 50 patients with RBD and 50 age-matched, healthy controls. Features from the EMG and EOG were extracted in an analogous fashion as the previous work [16]; additionally, features from the single-lead ECG recorded during PSG were extracted and included in the ML pipeline. These included regularity measures (such as the beat-to-beat interval), nonlinear (various entropy measures and Poincaré plots statistical measures), and spectral features (peak power of the ECG signal). Different source combinations were tested: specifically, (i) EMG+ECG, (ii) EMG alone, and (iii) ECG alone. The models employed to attain RBD detection were RF classifiers (500 trees, number of split: $\sqrt{M}$, where M equals the number of features employed), and a tenfold CV was adopted as validation technique. The best combination resulted to be the ECG+EMG, yielding an RBD detection accuracy of $93 \pm 10\%$; in this configuration, the EMG features were ranked as more informative, especially the EMG fractal exponent, the REM atonia index, and the atonia index ratio between NREM and REM segments. As regards the classification pursued through the EMG sensor alone, a similar performance was achieved, with accuracy of $93 \pm 9\%$, respectively. A decrease in detection performance is observed when considering the ECG sensor alone, with $62 \pm 20\%$ accuracy. These metrics remain consistent when shifting to an entirely automated pipeline, i.e., entailing automatic sleep staging as a first step. Indeed, the combination of EMG and ECG achieved an overall accuracy of 92 ± 9.8%. EMG alone attained an overall accuracy of 90 ± 11%, reasonably comparable with the one obtained after manual sleep staging. Though in the study above the ECG sensor alone proved promising but did not achieve the best results, the authors discussed its classification potential. Based on these assumptions and on the evidence that RBD subjects present with lower heart rate variability (HRV) [18], recent works undertook RBD detection based on single-lead ECG, or ECG-derived features only, attaining a higher performance. These will be discussed in the following sections (*cf.* Sect. 3.2.5).

Christensen et al. [19] tackled classification of neurological subjects (RBD and PD) against non-neurological subjects (healthy controls and patients with periodic limb movement disorder, PLMD), based on EEG and EOG. A total of five channels (3 EEG and 2 EOG) were employed in the analysis. First, unsupervised *topic models* were used to cluster different signal characteristics in the EEG and EOG overnight. Briefly, based on spectral content, *words* were derived from EEG and EOG signals. A Latent Dirichlet Allocation algorithm was then used to classify the words into several topics. EOG signals led to three topics (with good correspondence with absence of eye movement, slow, and rapid eye movements), while EEG led to six topics (which showed a good correspondence with human-defined sleep stages). Features describing stability and fragmentation of the different topics were then extracted and used in a logistic regression classifier to differentiate the neurological and non-neurological subjects. When considering a combination of EEG and EOG, the logistic regression achieved in the training dataset an area under the receiver operating characteristic curve (AUC) of 93%, with true positive rate (TPR) and true negative rate (TNR) of 93.8% and 87.5%, respectively. Validation performance was reasonably comparable, with 91.4% TPR, though it featured a slight decrease in TNR (68.8%). High performances were attained when considering EEG alone, with analogous results. The EOG topics were not as effective, reaching an AUC of 79.3%, with TPR below 70%.

3.1.2 Algorithms Based on EMG Alone

A first application of ML for identification of RBD based only on EMG was proposed by Kempfner et al. [20]. The proposed method aimed to discriminate between abnormal muscle activity during REM and physiological REM atonia, on a cohort of 48 subjects (16 patients with iRBD, 16 PLMD, and 16 age-matched, healthy controls). The work proposed an index—i.e., the Kempfner Index (KEI)—as a ML-derived measure of RWA. In addition to the chin EMG, the study considered for the analysis also the bilateral tibialis anterior (TA) channels, as well as the bilateral EOG channels—which, within the scope of this study, were considered as EMG signals. For each channel, an envelope was built by smoothing the filtered (bandpass 10–70 Hz) and rectified signal. The signals were then divided into 3-s mini-epochs. Each EMG channel of each subject was then normalized, in order to make its amplitude comparable across different subjects. A one-class support vector machine (OC-SVM) was then trained considering the amplitude of the normalized EMG channels in REM sleep of 75% healthy controls. Such a classifier divided these values into *inliers* (i.e., low-amplitude EMG) and *outliers* (i.e., high-amplitude EMG). After training, the classifier was applied to the patients and remaining control subjects, and for each subject the KEI was calculated as the percentage of 3-s mini-epochs in REM sleep classified as outliers by the OC-SVM. By using this index, iRBDs were distinguished from the remaining subjects with a validation AUC of 0.989, when combining all the channels. Great discriminative potential was provided by the bilateral tibialis muscles alone (AUC = 0.974) and their combination with the EOG channels (AUC = 0.993).

In the wave of including multiple EMG sources for better performance, Cesari et al. in [21] proposed a data-driven, probabilistic model of RWA, based on the mentalis and tibialis EMG signals, which appeared to outperform [20] in an ML-based detection of RBD. The study included a cohort of 27 healthy controls, 29 patients with RBD, and 36 patients with PLMD. The mean absolute amplitude value (MAAV) was employed as feature to describe the EMG activity during sleep; it was computed on 1-second mini-epochs, based on previous findings presented in [12] and on the fact that 3-second mini-epochs were found to be too long to capture small EMG twitches. In order to compare MAAV values across subjects, the values were normalized for each subject. On the assumption that the control group presented resting EMG during REM, the healthy subjects cohort was partitioned into three subgroups and was used to create a probabilistic model of atonia, by fitting univariate Gaussian distributions to the MAAV values in REM sleep. Based on the trained Gaussian distributions, it was possible to estimate, for each 1-s mini-epoch, the probability of muscular activity. Muscular activity was then defined when such probability was over 90%. Once the muscular activities were identified, the following muscle activity features were computed: (i) percentage of REM mini-epochs containing muscular activity, (ii) percentage of NREM mini-epochs containing muscular activity, (iii) median distance between muscular activity during REM sleep, and (iv) median distance between muscular activity during NREM sleep; these yielded a total of 12 features for each subject (i.e., four features for each EMG channel). Three different classifiers were chosen and employed as an ensemble method to distinguish the three patient groups: an RF, an SVM (linear kernel), and an SVM (with radial basis function kernel). Their outputs, interpreted as classification probability, were merged through the Dempster–Shafer fusion method; the class presenting with higher classification probability was selected as the output of the ensemble classifier. The classifiers' hyperparameters, namely the number of trees and depth for the RF and the box constraint for the two SVM models, were optimized with a Bayesian approach; fivefold cross-validation was adopted, yielding an RBD-wise validation accuracy of 81.52 ± 8.20%, when considering features from both REM and NREM movements, and an average three-class overall accuracy of 70.76 ± 7.75%.

This method was externally validated on a cohort of 240 subjects, including controls, patients with high periodic limb movement index, PD patients with and without RBD [22]. Feature normalization was also adopted, to outweigh the possible inter-clinical variability deriving from different acquisition systems; hence, each muscle activity feature extracted in the external validation cohort was multiplied by a scale factor, directly proportional to the characteristics in the control group in the previous study [21]. In detecting RBD, the model achieved comparable results with respect to [21], both in the normalization and non- normalization configuration, thus demonstrating the robustness of the detection algorithm. In more detail, in this second cohort, the externally validated model achieved an average overall three-class accuracy of 72.08% (normalized features), which rises up to 77.60% when excluding PD patients from the classification; the authors ascribe this increase to the fact that PD sleep is intrinsically fragmented and may be subjected to various movements during REM and NREM, other than RBD-typical ones. Class-wise accuracy for RBD was of 84.17% considering the whole group (non-normalized features) and of 85.60% when excluding PD patients—this latter rised up to 87.20% when employing normalized features.

Although not aiming to directly classifying patients with RBD, the algorithm presented by Fairley et al. [23] for automatic discrimination of muscular phasic activity (typically seen in patients with RBD) is also worth mentioning. The study included six participants, which were analyzed considering separate left and right recordings for TA EMG. The TA signals were inspected along 1-second length epochs; according to previous studies by the same authors [24], one epoch manually scored as *phasic* when presenting with activity of amplitude four times the background and duration in the range of 100–500 ms. In order to automatically identify 1-s mini-epochs with phasic activity, the mini-epochs were first processed by means of a Discrete Time Wavelet Transform, by employing mother wavelets in the Daubechies and Symlet families. This approach proved to be suitable for describing the complexity of EMG activity, which is known to shift across various frequency bands, especially when phasic twitches occur. In particular, low levels of wavelet decomposition (i.e., levels 1–4) were employed. Feature extraction was carried out from the coefficients, and a total of 24 features were extracted, including statistical measures (standard deviation, skewness, and kurtosis) and entropy measures (Shannon entropy). Dimensionality reduction was attained through principal component analysis and the feature/variable selection algorithm; this latter was implemented along with the forward floating search method, making use of a recursive algorithm for the minimization of the objective function, in order to find the optimal set of l features (from the initial d measurements) to be employed in the classification. The objective function employed in this work relied on the average scattering between the classes in the dataset. Binary classification between phasic and non-phasic EMG segments was performed through a linear classifier, based on the Mahalanobis distance. To countervail overfitting, two validation loops were considered. In the inner loop different classification configurations were tested, varying, at each iteration, the number of features retained for the analysis (range: 1–15)—or the number of components (range: 1–24), in the case of PCA—for a total of 8 iterations. The external loop envisaged a total of 30 iterations: first, a 80–20 hold-out cross-validation scheme was adopted; then, the training set was further subdivided following a 75 (training)–25 (test)% proportion, to ensure generalization capability of the tested model. The classification results were presented in terms of TPR and TNR, which were found to be above 90% for all tested configurations and for all subjects. In particular, the best model attained a TPR of 97% and a TNR of 99%.

This work envisaged the manual exclusion of all artifacts, whereas the results presented by Cesari et al. in [21, 22] proved to be substantially unaffected by artifacts due to snoring, sleep apnea, and ECG crosstalk, and only technical artifacts due to electrode detachment were excluded from the recordings.

An analogous window length (1 second) was adopted in the analysis by Rechichi et al. [25]. The authors proposed a method for the automatic detection of RBD subjects, based on the spectral analysis of the chin EMG recorded during REM sleep. The analysis included a total of 38 subjects (22 RBD and 16 HC) from a public repository (CAP Sleep Database [26, 27]), and external validation was carried out on an additional private repository (18 RWA-positive subjects). A Welch modified periodogram (Hamming window) was applied to the EMG epochs, in order to estimate the power spectral density (PSD), and three spectral features were extracted; namely, (*i*) the mean frequency of the PSD, which virtually represents the spectral centroid, (*ii*) the spectral edge Frequency at 50% of the total power, representing the median frequency, and (*iii*) the spectral edge frequency at 95% of the total power—this latter accounting for the frequency below which the 95% of the total power of the signal is to be found. Two supervised models were employed to pursue RBD automatic detection, on the first dataset: the K-Nearest Neighbor (KNN) an SVM, with a hold-out cross-validation, and a 70/30 proportion (train/test). The classifiers' hyperparameters were optimized by means of a Bayesian approach, and a fivefold CV was adopted in this training phase; the final optimized models were (*i*) K (number of neighbors): 10, and Spearman distance for the KNN, and (*ii*) linear kernel and C (maximum penalty) of 2.09 for the SVM. The optimized models achieved an overall accuracy of 86.96% and 82.61% for the KNN and SVM, respectively, with TPR of 93.33% and 86.67%, in a 5-fold CV. The performance on the test set (30% of the initial dataset) featured a slight decrease for the KNN model, attaining an overall accuracy of 81.82% and 85.71% TPR; this reduction seemed to be due to the fact that the model was optimized on a different data batch. Subsequently, as described above, the models underwent external validation, through a one-class assessment. Model performance, estimated in terms of average accuracy, proved to be very high, showing a 94.45% for the linear SVM and 100% for the KNN; the authors claim that this latter might reasonably undergo a decrease when introducing a larger number of subjects in the external validation. Finally, starting from the classifiers' outputs, the authors propose a distance-based model for assessing the degree of REM dissociation—i.e., the extent of RWA. In more detail, the Dissociation Index (DI) is defined in the range of 0–1, where a value of 1 represents maximum dissimilarity from the healthy reference. Within this framework, RBD subjects are compared to a data-driven *healthy model* by means of Euclidean distance. A similarity neighborhood is defined, and the obtained distance values are later mapped onto the DI through a normalization process, in order to provide an independent and reproducible metric, to be implemented in the follow-up practice, for instance, in neurological patient care.

3.1.3 Algorithms Based on EEG Alone

Based on the promising outcomes yielded by the EEG features described in Sect. 3.1.1, various studies undertook RBD detection based solely on EEG. Previously, some studies observed differences in EEG signals when comparing RBD subjects and healthy controls. In particular, the former appear to feature an increased delta power during sleep with respect to the age-matched, healthy population [28], and longer duration of slow-wave sleep.

Hensen et al. employed the EEG signal during REM sleep in order to detect RBD [29]; the population in the study included ten RBD subjects and ten healthy controls. A total of six EEG channels, recorded during PSG, were included in the analysis; given that the EEG signals are easily affected by noise, the signals were first bandpass filtered in the frequency range of 0.75–32 Hz with a finite-impulse response filter. Feature extraction envisaged the computation of the absolute power in the five clinically relevant EEG frequency bands: δ, θ, α, β—this latter further divided into β_1 (13–21 Hz) and β_2 (21–30 Hz). A total of 30 features were extracted for each subject, and feature normalization was performed by means of a subject-specific rescaling. Classification was carried out with two different classifiers: a Bayes probabilistic classifier and a KNN; the study does not report information about the model parameters. The Bayes classifier attained a TPR and TNR of 90% when employing all 30 features; when using only five features, the classifier performed quite well, achieving 80% in both metrics. The KNN classifier did not perform as well, reaching a TPR and TNR of 50% and 80%, respectively. However, from the feature analysis, the frequency band in the β_2 range proved to be one of the most discriminative for classifying the RBD group.

In a following work with a larger cohort, Bisgaard et al. investigated a similar approach [30] to pursue RBD detection. The study included 34 RBD subjects and 42 controls; the six EEG channels commonly recorded during PSG (F3, F4, C3, C4, O1, and O2) were included in the analysis. All signals were rectified and filtered and subsequently subdivided into 3-second mini-epochs, in order to proceed with feature extraction. Three features were extracted from each mini-epoch: (i) the signal-to-noise correlation, (ii) the peak amplitude of the signal, and (iii) the *iRBD feature*—i.e., a variable accounting for EMG-related content in the EEG. To compute this latter, the variance of each mini-epoch was compared to the baseline (median variance) of the surrounding mini-epochs, which constitute a *reference window*. Detection of RBD subjects was carried out in an unsupervised manner, employing first a K-means clustering, and second, a simplified K-means model, with only one cluster. Hold-out validation was employed to assess the model performance; an overall accuracy of 83% was attained in the training set, with 67% and 95% TPR and TNR, respectively. The performance on the test set featured, as expected, a slight decrease, with 78% accuracy and 63% and 90% TPR and TNR, respectively. These performances are in line with the ones presented in [29], though the cited study embraced a supervised approach to identifying RBD.

In a more recent study, Dimitriadis et al. tackled the supervised classification of different sleep disorders based on EEG [31], employing online available data from the CAP Sleep Database [26, 27]. The work encompassed the analysis of the EEG channels available in the repository, which are at least three for each subject. Artifacts were reduced through the use of independent component analysis and maximum overlap discrete wavelet transform, and the resulting, filtered signals were further downsampled to 256 Hz. The channels included in the analysis were P4-O2, F4-C4, C4-P4, and C4-A1, for a total of three bipolar sources and one monopolar; 22 RBD subjects were included in the analysis, along with 16 HC and other 69 subjects divided into six different sleep disorders classes. The signals were analyzed in a 30-second, epoch-wise fashion. The work employed the cross-frequency coupling (CFC) to pursue detection of sleep disorders. In more detail, the phase–amplitude coupling was employed to process the EEG signals; this was estimated between the phase of the slower EEG rhythm and the amplitude of the faster observed oscillation. Amplitude-to-amplitude CFC was also estimated, between the envelopes of the EEG series (computed via the Hilbert transform). Finally, an RF classifier was implemented, with 1000 trees and a number of splits $\sqrt{M}$, where M equaled the total number of features in the dataset, and a tenfold CV scheme was adopted to assess the model performance during training. The best result was achieved when using the P4-O2 channel, with a model average accuracy of 74% and RBD-related metrics of 77.3% (TPR), 81% (F1-score), and 85% (precision or PPV). The other considered channels performed worse, achieving at most a 64% F1-score, in the case of the C4-A1 sensor. These considerations lay the basis of the fact that RBD detection through a single channel-based analysis might be possible.

Indeed, in a recent work, Rechichi et al. [32] performed RBD detection using a single EEG channel. The study included 38 subjects (22 RBD) from the CAP Sleep Database [26, 27], as in [31], and an additional set of 20 subjects (10 RBD) from a private dataset. Following the assumption that RBD subjects present with altered slow-wave-sleep structure, higher power in the delta bands, and longer duration of the stage, this work focused on the analysis of both REM segments and slow-wave sleep segments. The authors selected the C4-A1 (or C3-A2) channel for the analysis, which was divided into both 2-second mini-epochs and 30-second epochs, from which different features were extracted. Time-domain features (amplitude and statistical measures) were extracted on 30-second epochs, whereas spectral and nonlinear features (power and entropy variables) were extracted on 2-second mini-epochs. Feature selection was performed through a Minimum Redundancy Maximum Relevance approach, and the top five ranked features were implemented in the classification framework. The study explored four different classifiers, namely a SVM, KNN, Naïve-Bayes Classifier, and a Decision Tree (DT). Hyperparameter optimization, with a Bayesian approach, was applied to each model, and a fivefold CV scheme (ten iterations) was employed in order to prevent overfitting of the models. When considering only the features extracted from the REM segments, the best model (KNN, with $K = 3$ and Chebyshev distance) achieved an accuracy of 83.91 ± 0.81%, with TPR 86.46 ± 2.95%. The averaged accuracy across all tested models was of 80.29 ± 0.03%. Discrimination capability of the slow-wave sleep features was also explored; the highest performance was obtained through a SVM classifier (cubic kernel, C = 2.56), attaining a model accuracy of 86.21 ± 2.11, with 91.23 ± 5.24 TPR. The averaged accuracy of all models was 81.10 ± 0.03, slightly higher than the one obtained by employing the REM features only. Finally, a combination of these two feature sets—comprising both REM and SWS features—was tested. This configuration achieved an accuracy of 90.80 ± 0.8%, with a TPR of 95.83 ± 2.95%, through a DT (cross entropy used as split criterion and maximum splits of 4), significantly higher than the other two configurations, suggesting that both stages are to be explored for the detection of RBD.

3.2 Algorithms Using Other Modalities

Although PSG is the gold-standard method to diagnose RBD, several authors have investigated whether other signals and technologies could be useful to automatically identify patients with RBD. This section presents an overview of studies that, employing other modalities than PSG, used ML and DL algorithm for this purpose. The studies are divided depending on the modality used.

3.2.1 Algorithms Using Actigraphy

Actigraphy consists in the recording of movement activity over time through accelerometers, and actigraphy devices are typically worn on the wrist. In clinical scenarios, simple algorithms estimate resting and activity periods based on the identified movements [33]. In recent years, however, more and more ML applications have been proposed in order to use actigraphy for better identification of sleep [34], and two algorithms have been proposed for RBD diagnosis.

Brink-Kjaer et al. [35] included in their study 21 patients with iRBD and 42 controls, for whom at least seven nights of high-frequency actigraphy recordings and respective sleep diary information were available. Furthermore, patients and controls filled in the Innsbruck RBD inventory and a three-item questionnaire screening for common synucleinopathy prodromes. From actigraphy, the activity count calculated in 1-, 15-, and 30-second bins was computed. Several other features from actigraphy recordings were also computed, including the number of no activity periods, an index describing twitch activity, and Hjorth parameters. Features derived from the information included in the sleep diary (e.g., sleep efficiency, total sleep time, etc.) were also obtained. The authors attempted discrimination of patients with iRBD from controls with an ensemble of 400 decision trees. Leave-one-out cross-validation scheme was used. When the classifier used only actigraphy features alone, it achieved an accuracy of 92.9%. The combination of the classifier with the Innsbruck RBD inventory and the questions lead to the accuracy of 94.0%.

In another study, Raschellà et al. [36] attempted discrimination of PD patients with and without RBD with actigraphy data. In their work, actigraphy was recorded at both wrists for two consecutive weeks. During the two weeks, patients underwent, in addition, two in-lab v-PSGs. A total of 18 PD patients without RBD and 8 with RBD were included. Actigraphy allowed calculating a total of 29 features accounting for both the characteristics of isolated, single movement episodes, and global movement patterns over the course of the nights. Movement episodes were identified based on thresholding the amplitude of acceleration magnitude and activity rates described the pattern of these movement episodes across the night. First of all, the authors built a classification algorithm using the actigraphy data recorded in-lab in a tenfold cross-validation scheme. In the training sets, the most discriminative features were selected, which were then used to build classifiers for home recordings, where 20 PD patients were used as test set. In the in-lab nights, PD with RBD was discriminated from PD without RBD with an average accuracy of 92.9% with a support vector machine. The home recordings allowed discriminating the two groups with an accuracy of 96% after seven nights of recordings and with an accuracy of 100% after 14 nights.

3.2.2 Algorithms Using Imaging Techniques

Cesari et al. investigated the combination of night 3D videos and ML to discriminate patients with iRBD from other patients with motor disorders during sleep [37]. A total of 53 patients with iRBD and 128 people without RBD were included in the study. Simultaneously, to in-lab v-PSG, a time-of-flight sensor was used to obtain depth images, which contained information on the distance between the sensor and the surface reflecting the infrared light emitted from the sensor itself. From the depth images, movements were automatically identified with a pipeline described in previous works [38]. In short, motion maps were obtained from the derivative of depth images, and movements were identified with optimized thresholds. Movements were identified in four different regions of interest (ROIs, i.e., lower body, upper body, head, and hands) and the movements divided into categories according to their duration: short (0.1 s–2 s), medium (2 s–15 s), and long (15 s–300 s). For each ROI and duration interval, two features were calculated: the 3D rate (defined as the number of identified movements in REM sleep per hour of REM sleep) and the 3D ratio (defined as the total movement duration time in REM sleep per hour of REM sleep). To compute these features, the manual annotations of REM sleep from the scored v-PSG were used. In order to discriminate patients with iRBD from the remaining ones, logistic regression classifiers with ridge regularization were trained in ten repetitions of tenfold cross-validation, by trying different combinations of features. The best test performances (accuracy: 0.866 ± 0.007 and F1-score: 0.783 ± 0.010) were obtained considering short movements in all ROIs.

In another work, Lee et al. [39] investigated whether ML algorithms applied to diffusion tensor imaging (DTI) could allow to differentiate 20 patients with iRBD from 20 sex- and age-matched controls. The authors extracted conventional DTI measures and measures of structural connectomic profiles. These features were calculated both on a global level and separately for different brain regions. Feature selection was performed with Student's t-tests, by keeping for the classification only features that were significantly different between the groups. The dataset was divided into 80% training set and 20% test set, which were used to train and test SVM classifiers. The best classification performances in the test set were achieved when considering conventional DTI measures only (accuracy = 87.5% and area under the receiver operating curve = 0.900), thus showing that DTI might be a helpful instrument to identify patients with iRBD.

3.2.3 Algorithms Using EEG

While EEG is ready available in PSG recordings, some research groups have investigated whether EEG recorded in the context of event-related potentials (ERPs) could be useful to identify patients with iRBD. In particular, one research group proposed two ML applications in this field.

Kim et al. [40] proposed an explainable DL algorithm to differentiate patients with iRBD from controls using ERPs recorded during visuospatial attention tasks. In total, 16 patients with iRBD and 19 controls were included in the study. EEG was recorded during a Posner cueing task, which was used to examine visuospatial attention. The recorded EEGs were used to derive 2D images of cortical currents. Such 2D images were then given in input to a convolutional neural network (CNN) classifier (three convolutional layers and three fully connected layers) to differentiate patients with iRBD from controls. Training was performed based on a transfer learning approach. Data from 34 subjects (all controls excluding one patient with iRBD) were used to pretrain the network. The data from the remaining patient with iRBD and data randomly chosen from controls were then used to fine-tune the network. In pretraining, 10% of data were used for validation, and in fine-tuning 20% of the data were used for test. Heatmaps were used to identify the contribution of each cortical point to the classifier output. On the test data, the classifier had an accuracy of 96.82% ± 1.78%, and it was shown that the area mostly contributing to the classification was the regions around rostral mid-frontal gyrus, superior parietal lobule, and right lateral occipital sulcus.

In another study, the same group of authors [41] further expanded their work by proposing, instead of a 2D CNN, a 3D CNN to discriminate 49 patients with iRBD from 49 controls. As in the previous work, EEG was recorded during a Posner cueing task. Preprocessed EEG was transformed into 3D images, representing cortical currents. The CNN consisted of three repetitions of a convolutional layer, batch normalization layer, and max-pooling layer, followed by two fully connected layers and one output layer, performing classification. The strategy for training and testing the classifier was the same as the one proposed in the previous work. In the test set, the algorithm achieved an accuracy of 99.81% ± 0.32%, superior to the previously proposed 2D CNN.

3.2.4 Algorithms Using Clinical Characteristics

Chong-Wen et al. [42] developed an ML model to distinguish PD patients with and without RBD based on clinical characteristics. Their population consisted of 169 PD patients (of whom 69 with RBD). For each patient, several variables were collected, which included demographic variables, motor function variables, variables describing non-motor symptoms, and information on drug use. The dataset was divided into 70% training and 30% test set in a stratified way. Three classifiers were tested: logistic regression, decision tree, and random forest. In the test set, the random forest achieved the best results (AUC = 0.807 and accuracy = 83.05%). Among all the variables investigated, an index describing sleep quality was the most important one for the classification.

In another study [43], Byeon also attempted to discriminate PD patients with and without RBD based on clinical characteristics. The cohort included 350 PD patients, of which 47.7% had RBD. The variables used for the prediction included demographic data, health behaviors, environmental factors, disease history, PD related motor signs, and neuropsychological characteristics. Also, in this case, several ML algorithms were trained and tested: random forest, discriminant analysis, classification and regression tree, neural network, and logistic regression. The best classifier (accuracy = 0.71) was also in this case the random forest model, with age being the most important variable for the classification.

3.2.5 Algorithms Using Other Modalities

In a recent study from Salsone et al. [44], the authors investigated whether an ML model could distinguish 20 patients with iRBD from 12 controls by using ECG data recorded over 24 hours. In particular, the authors divided the recordings into windows of 5 minutes (with 50% overlap), automatically identified artifacts and R-waves and finally calculated RR intervals and heart rate variability (HRV). Several features were derived from HRV, including time-domain features (e.g., average of RR intervals and standard deviation of RR intervals), frequency-domain features (e.g., spectral power in low and high frequencies), nonlinear features (e.g., sample entropy and Lyapunov exponent), and features from Poincaré plot. Features were calculated in sleep and in wake. Furthermore, the authors calculated night-to-day ratios for spectral features. Leave-one-out cross-validation scheme was employed to train a logistic regression, random forest, and XGBoost classifier. The random forest model achieved the best performances (accuracy, sensitivity, and specificity over 90%), thus showing the ability of features extracted from only ECG from wakefulness and sleep to discriminate patients with iRBD from controls.

Jeancolas et al. [45] investigated whether voice characteristics could be useful to discriminate with ML model patients with early PD, patients with iRBD, and controls, based on the fact that speech disorders are among the first symptoms to appear in PD. Speech samples were acquired from 117 patients with early PD, 41 with iRBD, and 98 healthy controls. The speech tasks were composed of sustained vowels, free speech, fast syllable repetitions, slow syllable repetitions following a given pace, short sentences repetition, and reading tasks. The authors focused on two classification tasks: early PD vs controls and iRBD vs controls. By employing ten runs of tenfold cross-validation, the authors trained three support vector machines: one employing the features extracted at the speech task level, one employing the same features calculated on small frames, and one employing the features calculated on the speech envelope. The final prediction was obtained based on majority voting of the classifiers. Patients with iRBD were distinguished from controls with a balanced accuracy of 63% $\pm$ 8%, showing that, although most patients with iRBD had no perception of speech impairment, it was possible to identify changes in speech that could discriminate them.

4 Machine and Deep Learning Algorithms for Prediction of iRBD Patient Conversion to Overt Alpha-Synucleinopathy

As introduced in Sect. 1, iRBD is recognized as an early stage of alpha-synucleinopathies. Patients with iRBD would represent therefore the ideal cohort to test neuroprotective and disease-modifying drugs to slow down or even stop the neurodegeneration. However, designing a clinical trial for iRBD patients is complicated, due to the fact that the conversion time can be longer than 10 years. Identifying iRBD patients converting in a short term (i.e., less than 5 years) and/or having biomarkers that inform on the progression of the neurodegeneration would be therefore very helpful to design such trials [46, 47].

ML and DL algorithms in this topic are scarce. Only two studies are directly related to this topic. The first one presents a DL algorithm that, using resting state EEG, can identify iRBD patients converting to overt alpha-synucleinopathies [48]. The second one presents an ML algorithm that, using FDG-PET images, reveals trajectories of neurodegeneration in iRBD [49]. The literature search revealed also another paper worth mentioning, indirectly related to the topic, but which will not be described in detail. This study presents an ML algorithm that can predict conversion from prodromal RBD (i.e., an early stage of RBD) to RBD in patients with PD. In other words, this study deals with the progression from early stage RBD to full-blown RBD in patients with PD, and it shows, via a random forest classifier, that micro-sleep instability can identify PD patients in proximity to develop RBD [50].

The study of Ruffini et al. [48] included 121 patients with iRBD and 85 healthy controls (HCs). After a follow-up of 4 $\pm$ 2 years, 14 patients with iRBD converted to PD and 13 to DLB, while the rest remained iRBD. All subjects underwent resting state EEG, recorded at sampling frequency of 256 Hz, for a variable duration. EEG was recorded at 14 scalp electrodes. The authors generated spectrograms using fast Fourier transform (FFT) after detrending blocks of 1 s with Hann window (FFT resolution was 2 Hz). Twenty-second 14 channel artifact-free epochs were collected for each subject, using a sliding window of 1 s. The analysis was restricted to the frequency content between 2 and 44 Hz. The number of spectrograms was restricted to 148 for each subject, representing a total length of 2.5 min of data. The spectrograms were centered and normalized to unit variance for each frequency and channel. The authors focused on two classification problems: (i) HC vs PD (i.e., healthy controls vs the iRBD converting to PD) and (ii) HC+RBD vs PD+DLB (i.e., healthy controls and patients remaining iRBD vs the converters). Two main architectures were implemented: a CNN and a stacked recurrent neural network (RNN). The CNN was a four hidden-layer CNN with max-pooling and dropout as only regularization. The RNN consisted of three stacked cells (long short-term memory or gated recurrent unity). Each cell used 32 hidden units and dropout as regularization. For training, subjects of the minority class were randomly replicated. For testing leave-pair-out strategy was applied, thus always having balanced classification problem. The performances were evaluated on subject basis. For the classification HC vs PD, the CNN and RNN obtained accuracy of 79% and 81% respectively, while for the classification HC+RBD vs PD+DLB 73% and 72%, respectively, thus showing that these DL architectures might be useful to identify patients with iRBD at proximity of conversion to overt alpha-synucleinopathies.

In the study of van Veen et al. [49], the authors included resting state fluorodeoxyglucose (FDG)-positron emission tomography (PET) scans of: 20 HC, 20 patients with PD, and 20 patients with Alzheimer's disease (AD) as the reference cohort; 49 HC, 21 patients with PD and 36 patients with AD, and 23 patients with DLB as the evaluation cohort; and of 20 patients with iRBD as the progression cohort. These latter underwent a second FDG-PET brain scan after 3.7 years. As a preprocessing step, all images were spatially normalized to an FDG-PET template. As the first step, a feature space was obtained. In particular, the reference cohort was employed to reduce the large number of voxels to a limited number of orthogonal dimensions explaining the major sources of variance in the data with the scaled subprofile model and principal component analysis (SSM/PCA). Each subject in the evaluation cohort and progression cohort was then mapped to this feature space, obtaining a total of 59 subject scores. Second, the subject scores were used as features in the evaluation cohort to train and test a generalized matrix learning vector quantization (GLMVQ) model aiming to distinguish the four groups in the evaluation cohort. Ten repetitions of tenfold cross-validation were used for this, and hyperparameters were optimized with grid search. Oversampling and undersampling were performed to have balanced classes during training, and features were normalized with z-transformation. During testing, such a model obtained a balanced accuracy of $66.4 \pm 14.6\%$ to distinguish the four classes. When this model was applied to the progression cohort, it was noticed that at the first scan, most of the iRBD patients (16/20) were classified as HC and 4 as PD. At the second scan only six were classified as HC, two as AD, one as DLB, and the remaining as PD. Four iRBD patients converted to PD in between the two scans: Two were classified in the PD class, one in the AD class, and one in the DLB class at follow-up. The authors state that this study is a proof of concept showing that the GLMVQ model could potentially inform on the trajectory of development of neurodegeneration in iRBD patients.

5 Outlook

This chapter provided an overview of rule-based and ML and DL algorithms and applications in the context of RBD. While the rule-based algorithms aim to automatize the quantification of RWA, mostly through the use of thresholds, the majority of the presented ML/DL algorithms deal, instead, with the problem of directly identifying/diagnosing patients with RBD. Most of them use data from PSG for this purpose. The fast development of novel consumer sleep technologies [51] will very likely bring a shift of research focus on developing new techniques using data recorded with these technologies combined with ML/DL models and algorithms. As seen in the chapter, the ML applications in order to identify patients with iRBD with higher risk of phenoconversion are so far limited. Future research should further tackle this problem, as having reliable biomarkers predicting phenoconversion and/or tracking neurodegeneration is fundamental to initiate clinical trials. ML algorithms offer the possibility to combine different modalities and signals and therefore might have an important role in this context. It should also be highlighted that none of the presented studies include a multicenter cohort, and the sample size is always relatively small. Stronger collaboration efforts and data sharing are therefore highly needed to advance further the field.

References

1. Birgit Högl, Ambra Stefani, and Aleksandar Videnovic. "Idiopathic REM sleep behaviour disorder and neurodegeneration—an update". In: *Nature Reviews Neurology* 14.1 (2018), pp. 40–55.
2. American Academy of Sleep Medicine. *International classification of sleep disorders*. 3rd. Darien, IL: American Academy of Sleep Medicine, 2014.
3. Matteo Cesari et al. "Video-polysomnography procedures for diagnosis of rapid eye movement sleep behavior disorder (RBD) and the identification of its prodromal stages: guidelines from the International RBD Study Group". In: *Sleep* 45.3 (2022), zsab257.
4. Ronald B Postuma et al. "Risk and predictors of dementia and parkinsonism in idiopathic REM sleep behaviour disorder: a multicentre study". In: *Brain* 142.3 (2019), pp. 744–759.
5. Donald L Bliwise et al. "Inter-rater agreement for visual discrimination of phasic and tonic electromyographic activity in sleep". In: *Sleep* 41.7 (2018), zsy080.
6. Matteo Cesari et al. "Comparison of computerized methods for rapid eye movement sleep without atonia detection". In: *Sleep* 41.10 (2018), zsy133.
7. Joseph W Burns et al. "EMG variance during polysomnography as an assessment for REM sleep behavior disorder". In: *Sleep* 30.12 (2007), pp. 1771–1778.
8. Rune Frandsen et al. "Analysis of automated quantification of motor activity in REM sleep behaviour disorder". In: *Journal of sleep research* 24.5 (2015), pp. 583–590.
9. Birgit Frauscher et al. "Validation of an integrated software for the detection of rapid eye movement sleep behavior disorder". In: *Sleep* 37.10 (2014), pp. 1663–1671.
10. Birgit Frauscher et al. "Normative EMG values during REM sleep for the diagnosis of REM sleep behavior disorder". In: *Sleep* 35.6 (2012), pp. 835–847.
11. Annika Röthenbacher et al. "RBDtector: an open-source software to detect REM sleep without atonia according to visual scoring criteria". In: *Scientific Reports* 12.1 (2022), p. 20886.

12. Raffaele Ferri et al. "A quantitative statistical analysis of the submentalis muscle EMG amplitude during sleep in normal controls and patients with REM sleep behavior disorder". In: *Journal of sleep research* 17.1 (2008), pp. 89–100.
13. Raffaele Ferri et al. "Improved computation of the atonia index in normal controls and patients with REM sleep behavior disorder". In: *Sleep medicine* 11.9 (2010), pp. 947–949.
14. Michela Figorilli et al. "Comparison between automatic and visual scorings of REM sleep without atonia for the diagnosis of REM sleep behavior disorder in Parkinson disease". In: *Sleep* 40.2 (2017), zsw060.
15. Matteo Cesari et al. "Flexor digitorum superficialis muscular activity is more reliable than mentalis muscular activity for rapid eye movement sleep without atonia quantification: A study of interrater reliability for artifact correction in the context of semiautomated scoring of rapid eye movement sleep without atonia". In: *Sleep* 44.9 (2021), zsab094.
16. Navin Cooray et al. "Detection of REM sleep behaviour disorder by automated polysomnography analysis". In: *Clinical Neurophysiology* 130.4 (2019), pp. 505–514.
17. Navin Cooray et al. "Proof of concept: Screening for REM sleep behaviour disorder with a minimal set of sensors". In: *Clinical Neurophysiology* 132.4 (2021), pp. 904–913.
18. Paulo Bugalho et al. "Heart rate variability in Parkinson disease and idiopathic REM sleep behavior disorder". In: *Clinical Autonomic Research* 28 (2018), pp. 557–564.
19. Julie AE Christensen et al. "Data-driven modeling of sleep EEG and EOG reveals characteristics indicative of pre-Parkinson's and Parkinson's disease". In: *Journal of neuroscience methods* 235 (2014), pp. 262–276.
20. Jacob Kempfner et al. "Rapid eye movement sleep behavior disorder as an outlier detection problem". In: *Journal of Clinical Neurophysiology* 31.1 (2014), pp. 86–93.
21. Matteo Cesari et al. "Validation of a new data-driven automated algorithm for muscular activity detection in REM sleep behavior disorder". In: *Journal of neuroscience methods* 312 (2019), pp. 53–64.
22. Matteo Cesari et al. "External validation of a data-driven algorithm for muscular activity identification during sleep". In: *Journal of Sleep Research* 28.6 (2019), e12868.
23. Jacqueline A Fairley et al. "Wavelet analysis for detection of phasic electromyographic activity in sleep: influence of mother wavelet and dimensionality reduction". In: *Computers in biology and medicine* 48 (2014), pp. 77–84.
24. Jacqueline A Fairley et al. "Computer detection approaches for the identification of phasic electromyographic (EMG) activity during human sleep". In: *Biomedical signal processing and control* 7.6 (2012), pp. 606–615.
25. Irene Rechichi et al. "Assessing rem sleep behaviour disorder: From machine learning classification to the definition of a continuous dissociation index". In: *International Journal of Environmental Research and Public Health* 19.1 (2021), p. 248.
26. Mario Giovanni Terzano et al. "Atlas, rules, and recording techniques for the scoring of cyclic alternating pattern (CAP) in human sleep". In: *Sleep medicine* 3.2 (2002), pp. 187–199.
27. Ary L Goldberger et al. "PhysioBank, PhysioToolkit, and PhysioNet: components of a new research resource for complex physiologic signals". In: *circulation* 101.23 (2000), e215–e220.
28. Jessica Massicotte-Marquez et al. "Slow-wave sleep and delta power in rapid eye movement sleep behavior disorder". In: *Annals of neurology* 57.2 (2005), pp. 277–282.
29. Ingeborg H Hansen et al. "Detection of a sleep disorder predicting Parkinson's disease". In: *2013 35th Annual International Conference of the IEEE Engineering in Medicine and Biology Society (EMBC)*. IEEE. 2013, pp. 5793–5796.
30. Sissel Bisgaard et al. "EEG recordings as a source for the detection of IRBD". In: *2015 37th Annual International Conference of the IEEE Engineering in Medicine and Biology Society (EMBC)*. IEEE. 2015, pp. 606–609.
31. Stavros I Dimitriadis, Christos I Salis, and Dimitris Liparas. "An automatic sleep disorder detection based on EEG cross-frequency coupling and random forest model". In: *Journal of Neural Engineering* 18.4 (2021), p. 046064.

32. Irene Rechichi et al. "Single-Channel EEG Detection of REM Sleep Behaviour Disorder: The Influence of REM and Slow Wave Sleep". In: *International Work-Conference on Bioinformatics and Biomedical Engineering*. Springer. 2022, pp. 381–394.
33. Michael T Smith et al. "Use of actigraphy for the evaluation of sleep disorders and circadian rhythm sleep-wake disorders: an American Academy of Sleep Medicine systematic review, meta-analysis, and GRADE assessment". In: *Journal of Clinical Sleep Medicine* 14.7 (2018), pp. 1209–1230.
34. Matthew R Patterson et al. "40 years of actigraphy in sleep medicine and current state of the art algorithms". In: *NPJ Digital Medicine* 6.1 (2023), p. 51.
35. Andreas Brink-Kjaer et al. "Ambulatory Detection of Isolated Rapid-Eye-Movement Sleep Behavior Disorder Combining Actigraphy and Questionnaire ". In: *Movement Disorders* 38.1 (2023), pp. 82–91.
36. Flavio Raschellà et al. "Actigraphy enables home screening of rapid eye movement behavior disorder in Parkinson's disease". In: *Annals of Neurology* 93.2 (2023), pp. 317–329.
37. Matteo Cesari et al. "Improved automatic identification of isolated rapid eye movement sleep behavior disorder with a 3D time-of-flight camera". In: *European Journal of Neurology* (2023).
38. Markus Waser et al. "Automated 3D video analysis of lower limb movements during REM sleep: a new diagnostic tool for isolated REM sleep behavior disorder". In: *Sleep* 43.11 (2020), zsaa100.
39. Dong Ah Lee et al. "Application of machine learning analysis based on diffusion tensor imaging to identify REM sleep behavior disorder". In: *Sleep and Breathing* 26.2 (2022), pp. 633–640.
40. Hyun Kim et al. "Characterization of attentional event-related potential from REM sleep behavior disorder patients based on explainable machine learning". In: *Computer Methods and Programs in Biomedicine* 234 (2023), p. 107496.
41. Hyun Kim et al. "Spatiotemporal characteristics of cortical activities of REM sleep behavior disorder revealed by explainable machine learning using 3D convolutional neural network". In: *Scientific Reports* 13.1 (2023), p. 8221.
42. Wu Chong-Wen, Li Sha-Sha, and E Xu. "Predictors of rapid eye movement sleep behavior disorder in patients with Parkinson's disease based on random forest and decision tree". In: *Plos one* 17.6 (2022), e0269392.
43. Haewon Byeon. "Exploring the predictors of rapid eye movement sleep behavior disorder for Parkinson's disease patients using classifier ensemble". In: *Healthcare*. Vol. 8. 2. MDPI. 2020, p. 121.
44. Maria Salsone et al. "A Machine Learning Approach for Detecting Idiopathic REM Sleep Behavior Disorder". In: *Diagnostics* 12.11 (2022), p. 2689.
45. Laetitia Jeancolas et al. "Voice characteristics from isolated rapid eye movement sleep behavior disorder to early Parkinson's disease". In: *Parkinsonism & Related Disorders* 95 (2022), pp. 86–91.
46. Aleksandar Videnovic et al. "Clinical trials in REM sleep behavioural disorder: challenges and opportunities". In: *Journal of Neurology, Neurosurgery & Psychiatry* 91.7 (2020), pp. 740–749.
47. Mitchell G Miglis et al. "Biomarkers of conversion to α-synucleinopathy in isolated rapid-eye-movement sleep behaviour disorder". In: *The Lancet Neurology* 20.8 (2021), pp. 671–684.
48. Giulio Ruffini et al. "Deep learning with EEG spectrograms in rapid eye movement behavior disorder". In: *Frontiers in neurology* 10 (2019), p. 806.
49. Rick van Veen et al. "FDG-PET combined with learning vector quantization allows classification of neurodegenerative diseases and reveals the trajectory of idiopathic REM sleep behavior disorder". In: *Computer Methods and Programs in Biomedicine* 225 (2022), p. 107042.
50. Matteo Cesari et al. "A data-driven system to identify REM sleep behavior disorder and to predict its progression from the prodromal stage in Parkinson's disease". In: *Sleep Medicine* 77 (2021), pp. 238–248.
51. Massimiliano de Zambotti et al. "Sensors capabilities, performance, and use of consumer sleep technology". In: *Sleep medicine clinics* 15.1 (2020), pp. 1–30.

Sleep Cyclic Alternating Pattern (CAP) as a Neurophysiological Marker of Brain Health

S. A. Bottari, R. Ferri, M. S. Jaffee, and John B. Williamson

1 Sleep Characteristics and Polysomnography

Normal human sleep is divided into two states: non-rapid eye movement (NREM) and rapid eye movement (REM) sleep. NREM sleep accounts for approximately 75–80% of total sleep time in adults and is further divided based on electroencephalogram (EEG) characteristics into three stages (N1, N2, and N3) through which sleep progressively deepens [1]. N1 is the lightest stage of sleep, where an individual transitions from wake to sleep. Alpha rhythms (8–13 Hz), which are the dominant waveform during wakefulness, reduce during N1 sleep and are intermixed with beta (>13 Hz) and theta oscillations (4–7 Hz). N2 sleep is progressively deeper

S. A. Bottari
Brain Rehabilitation Research Center, Malcom Randall VA Medical Center, Gainesville, FL, USA

Center for OCD, Anxiety, and Related Disorders, Department of Psychiatry, University of Florida, Gainesville, FL, USA

Department of Clinical and Health Psychology, College of Public Health and Health Professions, University of Florida, Gainesville, FL, USA
e-mail: sbottari@ufl.edu

R. Ferri
Sleep Research Center, Oasi Research Institute – IRCCS, Troina, Italy
e-mail: rferri@oasi.en.it

M. S. Jaffee
Department of Neurology, University of Florida, Gainesville, FL, USA

Center for Brain Injury, Rehabilitation, and Neuroresilience (BRAIN), University of Florida, Gainesville, FL, USA
e-mail: michael.jaffee@neurology.ufl.edu

R. B. Berry et al. (eds.), *Handbook of AI and Data Sciences for Sleep Disorders*, Springer Optimization and Its Applications 216,
https://doi.org/10.1007/978-3-031-68263-6_8

and occupies the majority of total sleep time [2]. EEG activity during N2 sleep is notable for sleep spindles (11–16 Hz) and k-complexes intermixed with theta waves and slow oscillations (0.5–2 Hz). N3 is the deepest stage of sleep and is commonly referred to as slow-wave sleep (SWS) due to a predominance of slow oscillations in EEG activity. Following N3 sleep, individuals progress to REM sleep, which accounts for approximately 20–25% of total sleep time. REM sleep is characterized by rapid eye movements, loss of muscle tone, and predominantly beta frequency waves with some theta rhythms.

Most dreams occur during REM sleep, although studies have demonstrated that nightmares in some psychiatric disorders, e.g., post-traumatic stress disorder (PTSD) can occur in either REM or NREM sleep [3]. Also, night terrors, typically a pediatric sleep disorder, occur in NREM sleep [4], though night terrors may also persist into adulthood [5]. In adults, the amount of SWS is greatest in the first third of the night and decreases in subsequent cycles, while the amount of REM sleep increases throughout the night and is greatest in the final 2–3 cycles. The stage of sleep disruption is often diagnostically critical. For example, REM sleep behavior disorder may appear similarly to night terrors by patient report, but treatment and prognosis differ dramatically with the former a strong indicator of future development of Parkinsonism [6].

Laboratory-based polysomnography (PSG) is considered the gold standard for objective measurement of sleep. PSG is an overnight sleep study that involves the continuous, simultaneous recording of many relevant physiological parameters, including brain activity (EEG), eye movements (electrooculography; EOG), muscle activity (electromyography; EMG), and heart rhythm (electrocardiography; ECG). Electrodes can also be attached to the legs to monitor periodic limb movements, and airflow can be monitored to assess for sleep-disordered breathing. Interpretation of PSG data typically involves sleep stage scoring, where the continuous recording is divided into 20- to 30-second epochs which are then classified into different sleep stages based on visual inspection by a trained technologist. This standardized assessment of PSG provides information about the temporal organization of sleep or its macrostructure. For instance, common macrostructure metrics derived from PSG include total sleep time, sleep latency, REM latency, sleep efficiency, time awake after sleep onset, and percent of the night spent in N1–N3 or REM sleep. However, this approach does not provide information regarding EEG features and phasic

J. B. Williamson
Brain Rehabilitation Research Center, Malcom Randall VA Medical Center, Gainesville, FL, USA

Center for OCD, Anxiety, and Related Disorders, Department of Psychiatry, University of Florida, Gainesville, FL, USA

Department of Clinical and Health Psychology, College of Public Health and Health Professions, University of Florida, Gainesville, FL, USA

Center for Cognitive Aging and Memory, College of Medicine, University of Florida, Gainesville, FL, USA
e-mail: John.williamson@ufl.edu

phenomena of sleep occurring outside of the 20- to 30-second scoring epoch. These phenomena constitute the microstructure of sleep and provide important additional information regarding the dynamic characteristics of sleep.

Common sleep microstructure metrics include arousals, sleep spindles, cyclic alternating pattern, and spectral EEG analysis. These dynamic characteristics of sleep are important to assess, as they can be indicative of pathological sleep processes even in the context of normal sleep macrostructure [7].

2 Cyclic Alternating Pattern and NREM Instability

The cyclic alternating pattern (CAP) may be a measure of NREM sleep instability and fragmentation [8]. Early non-systematic reports of cyclic variations in EEG and relationship to behaviors were described in the context of coma recovery and prognosis and in Creutzfeldt-Jakob disease [9]. The first formal description of CAP was articulated in 1985 [10]. CAP is a periodic EEG activity occurring during NREM sleep that is characterized by sequences of CAP cycles defined by an A phase (transient electrocortical events that are distinct from background EEG activity) and by the following B phase (return to background EEG activity). The A phase is composed of three subtypes: A1, A2, and A3. The A1 subtype promotes EEG synchronization and is thought to contribute to the process of SWS build up and maintenance. In contrast, the A2 and A3 subtypes are associated with more desynchronized EEG patterns during the transition from NREM to REM sleep [11].

Measuring CAP, initially a laborious process, has been made more accessible via automated tools, which use artificial intelligence spectra quantification approaches. For example, Hartmann and Baumert report on a highly precise automated system for CAP analysis, which has been reported in detail elsewhere [12]. In their approach, they use machine learning algorithms, specifically a recurrent neural network (RNN) approach for CAP scoring in comparison to standard classification methods. They show strong performance against standard classification methods using publicly available data. Their methods apply and compare several difference AI approaches including a long short-term memory (LSTM) network, which was more effective than other classification algorithms such as linear discriminant analysis, k-nearest neighbor or feed-forward neural network.

The detection system has been further refined by the group, achieving on average a second-by-second A phase inter-rate reliability of 0.55, quantified by the Cohen's kappa coefficient, which is within expected event-based inter-rater reliability between human scorers of 0.42 to 0.75 [13]. The detection system, similar to their prior work, implements a deep learning recurrent neural network (RNN) that was trained with manually scored recordings from children to recognize CAP A subtypes in pediatric EEG recordings. Measurements with severe clipping, which are often found in recordings with a low bit rate or physical range, and unipolar signals do not meet the requirements of the automated A phase detection system. In the first step, the raw signal of one central EEG channel is filtered and processed to remove power line interference, high-frequency noise, cardiac activity, and eye movement artifacts. Multiple features in the time and frequency domain such as Hjorth activity, Shannon entropy, Teager Energy Operator (TEO), band power descriptor, and differential EEG variance are subsequently extracted from the processed signal and passed as input to the RNN classifier.

The Fβ score may be used as cost function to deal with the biasing issues of a low number of A phase representations in overnight EEG recordings and to concentrate on the sensitivity and precision of the scoring. Further, the precision of the detection system is increased by selecting only A phases that are detected in two central EEG channels. Post-processing the output of the A subtype detection system may be accomplished by applying the rules for CAP sequences [8, 14] yielding several quantifiable parameters for statistical analysis. CAP rate is the most extensively used parameter for clinical purposes.

CAP rate is a measure of arousal instability; it may be increased when sleep is disturbed by internal or external factors, and it correlates closely with subjective ratings of sleep quality such that higher values of CAP rate are associated with poorer sleep quality [8]. In addition, CAP rate in normal sleepers shows low intraindividual variability from night to night, suggesting that it may be a representative signal of general sleep quality [15].

3 Relationship of Slow Wave Sleep to Neurobehavioral States and Outcomes

Slow-wave sleep quality is important to cognitive performance and there is increasing empirical evidence of roles in cognitive processing including memory consolidation and insight formation [16, 17]. Further, poor sleep, including poor slow-wave sleep may contribute to difficulties with attention, increased negative affect, social function, and poor behavioral inhibition [18–20]. While a good night's sleep has measurable effects on cognition the following day [21], the performance of tasks (e.g., a motor learning task) also impacts slow-wave sleep in the evening [22]. Thus, poor slow-wave sleep has a complex role in psychiatric and other cognitively relevant conditions. Slow-wave sleep disruption as measured via CAP has been shown to be disrupted in psychiatric conditions including major depressive disorder (MDD), and post-traumatic stress disorder (PTSD) [23], as well as in people with vestibular migraine headaches [24] and in neurogenerative disorders including Parkinson's disease [6] and Alzheimer's disease [25]. Further, CAP rates are sensitive to normal cognitive functioning variations in healthy people [26].

It is important to consider that what is "normal" relative to CAP rate is not well established and, further, it appears to vary across the lifespan. A meta-analysis of CAP rates across the lifespan incorporating 186 healthy individuals from 10 studies reported that A1 CAP subtypes were significantly more numerous in adolescents compared with other groups, and A2 and A3 CAP subtypes were significantly more numerous in older adults. The biggest difference in CAP rates was evident when comparing infants and older adults, with the latter having the highest rates. Overall, CAP rate increased with age and sleep depth [27]. Age is thus an important factor in the interpretation of CAP in clinical research studies.

3.1 Anxiety, Post-Traumatic Stress Disorder, and Sleep Disruption

Anxiety and trauma-related conditions such as post-traumatic stress disorder (PTSD) are associated with clinically significant sleep disruption. In fact, sleep disruption is the most common symptom complaint in PTSD, with between 50–70% of patients presenting with a diagnosable co-occurring sleep disorder [28]. Core features of PTSD contribute to sleep disruption and sleep disruption contributes to symptoms of PTSD. Common complaints include nightmares, distressed awakenings, night terrors, insomnia, and nocturnal panic attacks [29]. Further, sleep quality is also a vulnerability factor for the development of PTSD, suggesting that sleep quality and PTSD are mechanistically linked [28]. A meta-analysis of sleep quality in PTSD showed decreased slow-wave sleep, increased REM sleep, and longer sleep latencies [30].

3.2 CAP and PTSD

Only one published study has examined CAP dynamics in veterans with and without PTSD, and it found that CAP frequency was higher in those without PTSD, contrary to their original hypothesis [23]. The authors suggest that this difference may be due to increased use of psychotropic medication in the PTSD group, which is known to affect CAP rate [31–33]. Another possibility is that patients with PTSD often have other comorbidities and it has been postulated that PTSD and chronic stress more broadly may contribute to accelerated aging, which would be consistent with an elevated CAP rate [34]. There may be a healthy band range issue (sleep depth vs. other physiological processes that increase CAP rate). Although not in PTSD patients specifically, alterations in CAP, namely a reduction in the A1 subtype and increase in the A2 and A3 subtypes, have been noted in individuals suffering from frequent nightmares [35], a common symptom in PTSD. Similar alterations in CAP have been reported in REM sleep behavior disorder [36], restless leg syndrome [37], insomnia [38], and paradoxical insomnia [39], all of which are highly comorbid with PTSD. Thus, while few studies have directly assessed CAP parameters in patients with PTSD, evidence from related disorders suggests that there may be increased levels of instability during NREM sleep, especially given subjective reports of fragmented sleep and nocturnal hyperarousal. Nightmares are associated with NREM instability measured via CAP [35], higher REM [35, 40], and lower high-frequency heart rate variability [40].

CAP rates may be a relevant treatment effect marker in PTSD. In a recent pilot study investigating the effects of transcutaneous vagus nerve stimulation (tVNS) on sleep quality in veterans with PTSD, CAP rate, using an AI-driven RNN approach, appeared to be both responsive to tVNS and logically associated with other factors thought to be important in the afferent path affected by tVNS. This path includes structures critical to the function of slow-wave sleep including the nucleus of the solitary tract. Effects on the limbic system occur via activation of the nucleus of the solitary tract. Further, the locus coeruleus, the brain's primary source of norepinephrine is part of the afferent path of the vagus [41]. Noradrenergic regulation may be a causal factor in CAP rates and NREM instability. tVNS has been shown to affect critical structures in the afferent path in healthy people [42, 43]. In this study, the effect of one hour of tVNS administered in a PSG clinic on sleep and autonomic function (high-frequency heart rate variability, a well-validated indicator of beat-to-beat changes in heart rate variability caused by parasympathetic nervous system [vagal] control) was tested. Thirteen veterans with PTSD completed two nights of PSG at a University clinic during which they received 1 hour of tVNS or sham stimulation in a randomized order. A small increase in N3 sleep ($d = 0.23$) and a small-to-moderate decrease in REM sleep ($d = -0.48$) on nights of active tVNS relative to sham stimulation were reported. Further, tVNS was also associated with a moderate to large reduction in CAP rate ($d = -0.65$). Moreover, greater high-frequency heart rate variability during NREM was associated with a reduced CAP rate and NREM alpha power [44]. Replication and longitudinal assessment are necessary to establish reliability of this effect and meaning.

It is notable that decreased sleep quality is not only the most common symptom complaint in patients with PTSD, but also it is both associated with the severity of PTSD symptoms and the level of PTSD symptoms after psychotherapeutic treatment [45]. Further, often sleep symptoms persist after successful treatment for PTSD, as defined as a clinically significant reduction in symptoms of PTSD. Sleep disruption is also a vulnerability factor for suicide in these patients [46]. Thus, clarification of the nature of sleep disruptions is critical to address what appears to be both a symptom and a vulnerability factor in response to traumatic events.

3.3 CAP and Depression

More is known about the association of CAP differences and depression, though the quality of available data remains low. In a preliminary study, the sleep quality of children and adolescents of mothers with (classified as high risk for depression) and without (classified as low risk for depression) history of MDD were compared. The high-risk group children were found to have an altered distribution of CAP phase A subtypes (reduction of A1 over A2–3 ratio) compared with the low-risk group children [47]. Longitudinal follow-up is necessary to determine if this is a pathogenic prognostic marker of vulnerability to the development of depression. However, CAP rates are also altered in patients with current depression. In a relatively large study of patients with MDD, $n = 78$ with MDD and $n = 15$ healthy controls, CAP rate was higher in patients with MDD, whereas no difference in conventional PSG metrics were identified [48]. Further, changes in CAP rate appear to be important in subjective report of sleep quality. In a study of 15 patients with MDD and matched healthy controls, CAP analysis once again demonstrated greater sensitivity in patients with MDD than did conventional PSG analyses. Further, with treatment, the degree of improvement in CAP was associated with the degree of subjective symptom improvement [49].

It should be noted that there are mixed results reported in the literature which suggest we do not have a full understanding of the relationship of mood disorders to sleep architecture. For example, in patients with both insomnia and depression, it is known that persistent poor sleep is associated with higher likelihood of depressive episodes. In a single blind, 6-week drug study (nefazodone hydrochloride followed by placebo) in 15 patients with both MDD and insomnia, improvements in sleep latency and sleep efficiency and subjective sleep quality were identified but there were no differences in REM, NREM, or CAP rates [50].

3.4 Neurodegenerative Disease and Sleep Disruption

In addition to the previously mentioned relationship of REM Sleep Behavior Disorder to the eventual development of Parkinson's disease, sleep disturbance is a symptom of the most common cause of cognitive decline in older adults, Alzheimer's disease (AD) [51]. Changes in slow-wave sleep are directly associated with the degree of amyloid and tau pathology evident in patients with AD [52]. Specifically, loss of slow wave sleep activity is associated with Aβ aggregation as measured by PET [52, 53]. Further, reduced slow-wave sleep is associated with tau pathology early in the trajectory of AD [54]. Indeed, early in the manifestation of cognitive changes in the trajectory of AD, e.g., when a patient may be classified as having mild cognitive impairment (MCI), sleep impairments are present [55]. Moreover, aspects of NREM sleep (e.g., SO-spindle coupling) are associated with regionally specific tau accumulation (medial temporal lobe) [52]. Thus, there appears to be a strong linkage of sleep changes to the known underlying pathological presentation of AD related brain changes. It has been suggested that these sleep features may serve as a cheaper (than PET) biomarker for the progression of AD [52].

Slow-wave sleep is critical in memory function [56]. Sleep impairments are associated acutely and chronically with measurable cognitive decrement and also with subjective cognitive decline in older adults [57, 58] and may also be predictive of the development of MCI/AD. Reduction in slow-wave sleep predicts cognitive decline in older people [57]. Sleep quality is associated with beta-amyloid clearance and may have a bidirectional association with the progression of AD [59], i.e., poor sleep may increase and accelerate the manifestation of AD pathology and, conversely, AD progression may worsen sleep quality. Changes in slow-wave sleep are evident in MCI and sleep quality is also further associated with APOE4 status [60].

Understanding these changes is important as current treatments (e.g., benzodiazepines and Z-drugs) are also associated with the eventual emergence of neurodegenerative disease [61].

3.5 CAP and Neurogenerative Disease

Low amounts of CAP rate have been reported in patients with neurodegenerative diseases, including multiple system atrophy (21.9 ± 11.7) [62] and Alzheimer's disease (29.1 ± 8.6) [25]. Thus, it is not clear whether low CAP rates are a negative or positive phenomenon, and their interpretation cannot be exhaustive without considering other aspects of the complex phenomenon of sleep instability and, in particular, the relative composition of subtypes (A1, A2, and A3).

In a sample of 27 patients with idiopathic Parkinson's disease and 13 healthy controls, sleep micro- and macrostructure were compared, as well as noradrenaline transporter density. CAP rate and A index were both lower in patients with Parkinson's disease than in healthy controls. Further, CAP metrics were significantly related to diminished noradrenaline transporter density in the raphe and locus coeruleus [41]. While not clear if degeneration in this network is causal, the linkage between noradrenaline transporter density and CAP is notable in that early synuclein pathology is evident in the locus coeruleus and degeneration of this structure has a relationship to treatment response [63].

Studies of patients with AD have provided experimental evidence that the LC is also one of the earliest sites of AD pathology [64]. Activation of the neurons of the LC modulates several processes that are altered in brains of patients at risk for AD including synaptic plasticity, inflammation, metabolism, and blood-brain-barrier permeability. Further, NE deficiency increases beta-amyloid deposition in the brain [65]. Thus, if LC degeneration and more broadly noradrenergic decline is causal in the presentation of changes in CAP, CAP rate may be a useful index of brain change in patients with neurodegenerative affective these circuits. And, in fact, in a longitudinal study of conventional polysomnography and quantitative microstructure approach of 19 patients with amnestic MCI and 11 cognitively normal healthy older adults followed over 2 years with ambulatory PSG, there was no difference in conventional PSG metrics. But, CAP rate was significantly lower in those with MCI who converted to AD [66], which has also been previously reported in cross sectional analysis [25].

3.6 CAP and Healthy Cognition

The relationship of CAP rates to healthy cognition is understudied. This presents a problem in evaluating the normative appearance of CAP and limits its utility in studies of populations with pathological conditions. There appears to be dissociation between CAP subtypes in their relationship to different cognitive functions. This may be in part due to the origin of the subtypes. There are data that suggest that different CAP subtypes may be generated by different brain networks such that A1 subtypes are generated by the frontal cortex and CAP A2 and A3 subtypes arise from the parietal–occipital areas. In a small n study we conducted on healthy adults ($n = 8$), two PSG studies and a series of next morning neuropsychological tests during the morning and afternoon of the first day and on the morning of the second day were performed. CAP A1 subtypes were correlated with better performances on verbal fluency, working memory, and both delayed recall and recognition of words. These same neuropsychological test results were found to be negatively correlated with CAP A2 subtypes. CAP A3 subtypes were negatively correlated with processing speed and set-shifting performances [26]. In a follow-up study, again in eight healthy adults, we demonstrated that CAP rates, namely the ostensibly frontally mediated A1, were related to participants' ability to perform divergent reasoning tasks, a critical component of creativity [67].

CAP rates have also been demonstrated to be related to implicit learning performance in 10 healthy young normal subjects (mean age 25.8 ± 1.8 years). Participants were administered a motor learning task prior to sleep. Sleep stages and CAP were quantified in the first hour of each recording. There was a significant increase in the number of CAP A1 subtypes per hour of NREM sleep on the night following the learning task. Also, the relationship of change in A1 and post-sleep performance of the task was positive.

CAP rate also been shown to be related to fluid ability in children ($n = 42$ mean age 7.6 ± 2.7) such that, controlling for age and SES, CAP rate in SWS, and A1 index in SWS explained 24% and 22% of the variance in nonverbal fluid reasoning test scores, respectively. Fluid abilities, in healthy older aging decline in the context of preserved crystallized function, and these fluid abilities are dependent on intact frontally mediated networks. Discrepancies in fluid and crystallized ability may serve as a marker of older aging related cognitive decline [68]. Future research examining the relationship of CAP rates to this discrepancy in healthy older adults may be useful to clarifying understanding of what CAP rates reflect in brain network functions in lifespan development and healthy and unhealthy brain aging.

4 Conclusions, Limitations, and Future Directions

CAP rates may be sensitive indicators of brain function and have been associated with cognitive performance, psychiatric phenomena, lifespan development, and neurodegenerative diseases. Further, some studies suggest that CAP rate may be more sensitive than conventional PSG evaluations to important change in brain function and health including in the trajectory of decline associated with neurodegenerative diseases; CAP rates are associated with subjective sleep quality, and CAP rates may be responsive to sleep targeted treatments. Largely, the available data quality is low. These studies have mostly been completed in small sample size studies and frequently in convenience samples. There are many reasons for this.

Polysomnography studies are expensive. Sleep clinics are novel environments and electrodes and wiring contribute to the novelty and discomfort to sleeping in a polysomnography clinic. Adapting to a polysomnography clinic has a well-established effect on results [69], further increasing the expense of using polysomnography in well designed and well controlled studies, as studies may require more than one night to control for this effect. Further, psychiatric conditions are heterogeneous. Complicating matters, different conditions and populations may have different responses to first night exposures [70].

Those who have symptoms sufficient to warrant undergoing a PSG are often already medicated and these medications may have effects on sleep architecture. Ethics and medical concerns limit the ability to modify treatment regimens to assess PSG for research purposes and thus larger sample sizes to control for medication effects are necessary. Because of the nature of PSG being most often performed in clinic, it is a limited resource, which is a rate limiting factor for the further development of AI classification models. Research may be competing for clinic time with clinical caseloads. Further, ambulatory equipment continues to be expensive and unwieldy. The expense, participant burden, and technical requirements of studies of CAP tend to result in very small sample sizes and poor controls, resulting in currently poor-quality research data, despite the identification of possible importance of CAP many decades prior.

Further, for research purposes, enrolling both patients and healthy populations may pose challenges that affect the generalizability of data acquired due to systematic biases. Those who agree to participate in sleep studies for research purposes do so at low rates per contact and may agree explicitly because of more prominent subjective issues with sleep quality. The success of AI methods in the development of accurate and useful classification tools would be greatly aided by larger datasets, more generalizable datasets (e.g., datasets which are fully representative of populations of interest), and normative data (e.g., lifespan healthy control data).

Quantitative methods of polysomnography analysis frequently require additional time and expertise and thus are not often used in clinical environments. Increasing integration of AI tools to automate quantitative analytic outputs in polysomnography and increasing the portability, usability, and cost of wearable technologies is critical to the furthering of and translation of research on the relationship of analytic approaches like CAP to clinical questions. In this chapter, we have reviewed recent developments in automation of CAP approaches via the use of AI driven mathematical approaches. Studies on the role of CAP in neurophysiological process and behavioral outcomes are limited by sample size. Use of automation approaches will likely accelerate accessibility and scientific literature on CAP subtypes and relationship to systemic and brain outcomes. Moving forward, wearable sophistication, cost, and availability may allow for more generalizable and less technically intensive access to polysomnography methods in research and clinical applications. Integration of analytic tools in these technologies such as CAP may be useful in clinical diagnostic and intervention evaluation.

References

1. Berry RB, Brooks, R., Gamaldo, C.E., Harding, S.M., Marcus, C. Vaughn, B.V.. The AASM manual for the scoring of sleep and associated events. Rules, Terminology and Technical Specifications, Darien, Illinois, American Academy of Sleep Medicine. American Academy of Sleep Medicine. 2012;12.
2. Chokroverty S. Overview of Normal Sleep. Chokroverty S, editor: Springer; 2017.
3. Phelps AJ, Kanaan RAA, Worsnop C, Redston S, Ralph N, Forbes D. An Ambulatory Polysomnography Study of the Post-traumatic Nightmares of Post-traumatic Stress Disorder. Sleep. 2018;41(1).
4. Leung AKC, Leung AAM, Wong AHC, Hon KL. Sleep Terrors: An Updated Review. Curr Pediatr Rev. 2020;16(3):176–82.
5. Sarilar AC, Ismailogullari S, Yilmaz R, Erdogan FF, Per H. Electroencephalogram abnormalities in patients with NREM parasomnias. Sleep Med. 2021;77:256–60.
6. Ferri R, Cosentino FI, Pizza F, Arico D, Plazzi G. The timing between REM sleep behavior disorder and Parkinson's disease. Sleep Breath. 2014;18(2):319–23.
7. Muzet A. Alteration of sleep microstructure in psychiatric disorders. Dialogues Clin Neurosci. 2005;7(4):315–21.
8. Parrino L, Ferri R, Bruni O, Terzano MG. Cyclic alternating pattern (CAP): the marker of sleep instability. Sleep Med Rev. 2012;16(1):27–45.
9. Terzano MG, Gatti PL, Manzoni GC, Formentini E, Mancia D. Is the EEG cyclic alternating pattern a true autonomous entity? Analytic study in a case of post-traumatic coma with good prognosis. Eur Neurol. 1982;21(5):324–34.
10. Terzano MG, Mancia D, Salati MR, Costani G, Decembrino A, Parrino L. The cyclic alternating pattern as a physiologic component of normal NREM sleep. Sleep. 1985;8(2):137–45.
11. Parrino L, Miloli, G., Melpignano, A., Tripp, I. The cyclic alternating pattern and the brain-body-coupling during sleep. Epileptologi. 2016;33:150–60.
12. Hartmann S, Baumert M. Automatic A-Phase Detection of Cyclic Alternating Patterns in Sleep Using Dynamic Temporal Information. IEEE Trans Neural Syst Rehabil Eng. 2019;27(9):1695–703.
13. Ferri R, Bruni O, Miano S, Smerieri A, Spruyt K, Terzano MG. Inter-rater reliability of sleep cyclic alternating pattern (CAP) scoring and validation of a new computer-assisted CAP scoring method. Clin Neurophysiol. 2005;116(3):696–707.
14. Terzano MG, Parrino L, Sherieri A, Chervin R, Chokroverty S, Guilleminault C, et al. Atlas, rules, and recording techniques for the scoring of cyclic alternating pattern (CAP) in human sleep. Sleep Med. 2001;2(6):537–53.
15. Terzano MG, Parrino L, Fioriti G, Spaggiari MC, Piroli A. Morphologic and functional features of cyclic alternating pattern (CAP) sequences in normal NREM sleep. Funct Neurol. 1986;1(1):29–41.
16. Berres S, Erdfelder E. The sleep benefit in episodic memory: An integrative review and a meta-analysis. Psychol Bull. 2021;147(12):1309–53.

17. Verleger R, Rose M, Wagner U, Yordanova J, Kolev V. Insights into sleep's role for insight: Studies with the number reduction task. Adv Cogn Psychol. 2013;9(4):160–72.
18. Drews HJ, Wiesner CD, Bethke-Jaenicke C, Weinhold SL, Baier PC, Goder R. Slow-wave sleep predicts long-term social functioning in severe mental illness. PLoS One. 2018;13(8):e0202198.
19. Li Y, Liu H, Weed JG, Ren R, Sun Y, Tan L, et al. Deficits in attention performance are associated with insufficiency of slow-wave sleep in insomnia. Sleep Med. 2016;24:124–30.
20. Ferrarelli F, Kaskie R, Laxminarayan S, Ramakrishnan S, Reifman J, Germain A. An increase in sleep slow waves predicts better working memory performance in healthy individuals. Neuroimage. 2019;191:1–9.
21. Djonlagic I, Rosenfeld A, Shohamy D, Myers C, Gluck M, Stickgold R. Sleep enhances category learning. Learn Mem. 2009;16(12):751–5.
22. Huber R, Ghilardi MF, Massimini M, Tononi G. Local sleep and learning. Nature. 2004;430(6995):78–81.
23. Moldofsky H, Rothman L, Kleinman R, Rhind SG, Richardson JD. Disturbed EEG sleep, paranoid cognition and somatic symptoms identify veterans with post-traumatic stress disorder. BJPsych Open. 2016;2(6):359–65.
24. Zhou Y, Li H, Jia Y, Wu J, Yang J, Liu C. Cyclic alternating pattern in non-rapid eye movement sleep in patients with vestibular migraine. Sleep Med. 2023;101:485–9.
25. Maestri M, Carnicelli L, Tognoni G, Di Coscio E, Giorgi FS, Volpi L, et al. Non-rapid eye movement sleep instability in mild cognitive impairment: a pilot study. Sleep Med. 2015;16(9):1139–45.
26. Arico D, Drago V, Foster PS, Heilman KM, Williamson J, Ferri R. Effects of NREM sleep instability on cognitive processing. Sleep Med. 2010;11(8):791–8.
27. Migueis DP, Lopes MC, Ignacio PSD, Thuler LCS, Araujo-Melo MH, Spruyt K, et al. A systematic review and meta-analysis of the cyclic alternating pattern across the lifespan. Sleep Med. 2021;85:25–37.
28. Ohayon MM, Shapiro CM. Sleep disturbances and psychiatric disorders associated with posttraumatic stress disorder in the general population. Compr Psychiatry. 2000;41(6):469–78.
29. Spoormaker VI, Montgomery P. Disturbed sleep in post-traumatic stress disorder: secondary symptom or core feature? Sleep Med Rev. 2008;12(3):169–84.
30. Kobayashi I, Boarts JM, Delahanty DL. Polysomnographically measured sleep abnormalities in PTSD: a meta-analytic review. Psychophysiology. 2007;44(4):660–9.
31. Svetnik V, Ferri R, Ray S, Ma J, Walsh JK, Snyder E, et al. Alterations in cyclic alternating pattern associated with phase advanced sleep are differentially modulated by gaboxadol and zolpidem. Sleep. 2010;33(11):1562–70.
32. Parrino L, Spaggiari MC, Boselli M, Di Giovanni G, Terzano MG. Clinical and polysomnographic effects of trazodone CR in chronic insomnia associated with dysthymia. Psychopharmacology (Berl). 1994;116(4):389–95.
33. Parrino L, Boselli M, Buccino GP, Spaggiari MC, Di Giovanni G, Terzano MG. The cyclic alternating pattern plays a gate-control on periodic limb movements during non-rapid eye movement sleep. J Clin Neurophysiol. 1996;13(4):314–23.
34. Williamson JB, Porges EC, Lamb DG, Porges SW. Maladaptive autonomic regulation in PTSD accelerates physiological aging. Front Psychol. 2014;5:1571.
35. Simor P, Bodizs R, Horvath K, Ferri R. Disturbed dreaming and the instability of sleep: altered nonrapid eye movement sleep microstructure in individuals with frequent nightmares as revealed by the cyclic alternating pattern. Sleep. 2013;36(3):413–9.
36. Melpignano A, Parrino L, Santamaria J, Gaig C, Trippi I, Serradell M, et al. Isolated rapid eye movement sleep behavior disorder and cyclic alternating pattern: is sleep microstructure a predictive parameter of neurodegeneration? Sleep. 2019;42(10).
37. Ferri R, Manconi M, Arico D, Sagrada C, Zucconi M, Bruni O, et al. Acute dopamine-agonist treatment in restless legs syndrome: effects on sleep architecture and NREM sleep instability. Sleep. 2010;33(6):793–800.

38. Chouvarda I, Mendez MO, Rosso V, Bianchi AM, Parrino L, Grassi A, et al. Cyclic alternating patterns in normal sleep and insomnia: structure and content differences. IEEE Trans Neural Syst Rehabil Eng. 2012;20(5):642–52.
39. Parrino L, Milioli G, De Paolis F, Grassi A, Terzano MG. Paradoxical insomnia: the role of CAP and arousals in sleep misperception. Sleep Med. 2009;10(10):1139–45.
40. Simor P, Kormendi J, Horvath K, Gombos F, Ujma PP, Bodizs R. Electroencephalographic and autonomic alterations in subjects with frequent nightmares during pre-and post-REM periods. Brain Cogn. 2014;91:62–70.
41. Doppler CEJ, Smit JAM, Hommelsen M, Seger A, Horsager J, Kinnerup MB, et al. Microsleep disturbances are associated with noradrenergic dysfunction in Parkinson's disease. Sleep. 2021;44(8).
42. Kraus T, Hosl K, Kiess O, Schanze A, Kornhuber J, Forster C. BOLD fMRI deactivation of limbic and temporal brain structures and mood enhancing effect by transcutaneous vagus nerve stimulation. J Neural Transm (Vienna). 2007;114(11):1485–93.
43. Capone F, Assenza G, Di Pino G, Musumeci G, Ranieri F, Florio L, et al. The effect of transcutaneous vagus nerve stimulation on cortical excitability. J Neural Transm (Vienna). 2015;122(5):679–85.
44. Bottari SA, Lamb DG, Porges EC, Murphy AJ, Tran AB, Ferri R, et al. Preliminary evidence of transcutaneous vagus nerve stimulation effects on sleep in veterans with post-traumatic stress disorder. J Sleep Res. 2023:e13891.
45. Bottari SA, Trifilio ER, Janicke DM, Porges EC, Cohen RA, Jaffee MS, et al. Effects of sleep disturbance on trauma-focused psychotherapy outcomes in posttraumatic stress disorder: A systematic review. Ann N Y Acad Sci. 2023;1526(1):30–49.
46. Healy NA, Vujanovic AA. PTSD symptoms and suicide risk among firefighters: The moderating role of sleep disturbance. Psychol Trauma. 2021;13(7):749–58.
47. Sesso G, Bat-Pitault F, Guyon A, Plancoulaine S, Banfi T, Milioli G, et al. Electrophysiological and microstructural features of sleep in children at high risk for depression: a preliminary study. Sleep Med. 2017;36:95–103.
48. Farina B, Della Marca G, Grochocinski VJ, Mazza M, Buysse DJ, Di Giannantonio M, et al. Microstructure of sleep in depressed patients according to the cyclic alternating pattern. J Affect Disord. 2003;77(3):227–35.
49. Lopes MC, Quera-Salva MA, Guilleminault C. Non-REM sleep instability in patients with major depressive disorder: subjective improvement and improvement of non-REM sleep instability with treatment (Agomelatine). Sleep Med. 2007;9(1):33–41.
50. Scharf MB, McDannold M, Zaretsky N, Spinner O, Stover R, Berkowitz DV, et al. Evaluation of sleep architecture and cyclic alternating pattern rates in depressed insomniac patients treated with nefazodone hydrochloride. Am J Ther. 1999;6(2):77–82.
51. Vitiello MV, Borson S. Sleep disturbances in patients with Alzheimer's disease: epidemiology, pathophysiology and treatment. CNS Drugs. 2001;15(10):777–96.
52. Winer JR, Mander BA, Helfrich RF, Maass A, Harrison TM, Baker SL, et al. Sleep as a Potential Biomarker of Tau and beta-Amyloid Burden in the Human Brain. J Neurosci. 2019;39(32):6315–24.
53. Mander BA, Marks SM, Vogel JW, Rao V, Lu B, Saletin JM, et al. beta-amyloid disrupts human NREM slow waves and related hippocampus-dependent memory consolidation. Nat Neurosci. 2015;18(7):1051–7.
54. Lucey BP, McCullough A, Landsness EC, Toedebusch CD, McLeland JS, Zaza AM, et al. Reduced non-rapid eye movement sleep is associated with tau pathology in early Alzheimer's disease. Sci Transl Med. 2019;11(474).
55. Peters ME, Rosenberg PB, Steinberg M, Tschanz JT, Norton MC, Welsh-Bohmer KA, et al. Prevalence of neuropsychiatric symptoms in CIND and its subtypes: the Cache County Study. Am J Geriatr Psychiatry. 2012;20(5):416–24.
56. Moyano MD, Diekelmann S, Pedreira ME, Forcato C. Sleep accelerates re-stabilization of human declarative memories. Neurobiol Learn Mem. 2019;162:1–8.
57. Taillard J, Sagaspe P, Berthomier C, Brandewinder M, Amieva H, Dartigues JF, et al. Non-REM Sleep Characteristics Predict Early Cognitive Impairment in an Aging Population. Front

Neurol. 2019;10:197.
58. Bubbico G, Di Iorio A, Lauriola M, Sepede G, Salice S, Spina E, et al. Subjective Cognitive Decline and Nighttime Sleep Alterations, a Longitudinal Analysis. Front Aging Neurosci. 2019;11:142.
59. Wang C, Holtzman DM. Bidirectional relationship between sleep and Alzheimer's disease: role of amyloid, tau, and other factors. Neuropsychopharmacology. 2019.
60. Hita-Yanez E, Atienza M, Gil-Neciga E, Cantero JL. Disturbed sleep patterns in elders with mild cognitive impairment: the role of memory decline and ApoE epsilon4 genotype. Curr Alzheimer Res. 2012;9(3):290–7.
61. DeKosky ST, Williamson JB. The Long and the Short of Benzodiazepines and Sleep Medications: Short-Term Benefits, Long-Term Harms? Neurotherapeutics. 2020;17(1):153–5.
62. Vetrugno R, D'Angelo R, Cortelli P, Plazzi G, Vignatelli L, Montagna P. Impaired cortical and autonomic arousal during sleep in multiple system atrophy. Clin Neurophysiol. 2007;118(11):2512–8.
63. Zhou C, Guo T, Wu J, Wang L, Bai X, Gao T, et al. Locus Coeruleus Degeneration Correlated with Levodopa Resistance in Parkinson's Disease: A Retrospective Analysis. J Parkinsons Dis. 2021;11(4):1631–40.
64. Mravec B, Lejavova K, Cubinkova V. Locus (coeruleus) minoris resistentiae in pathogenesis of Alzheimer's disease. Curr Alzheimer Res. 2014;11(10):992–1001.
65. Kalinin S, Gavrilyuk V, Polak PE, Vasser R, Zhao J, Heneka MT, et al. Noradrenaline deficiency in brain increases beta-amyloid plaque burden in an animal model of Alzheimer's disease. Neurobiol Aging. 2007;28(8):1206–14.
66. Carnicelli L, Maestri M, Di Coscio E, Tognoni G, Fabbrini M, Schirru A, et al. A longitudinal study of polysomnographic variables in patients with mild cognitive impairment converting to Alzheimer's disease. J Sleep Res. 2019;28(5):e12821.
67. Drago V, Foster PS, Heilman KM, Arico D, Williamson J, Montagna P, et al. Cyclic alternating pattern in sleep and its relationship to creativity. Sleep Med. 2011;12(4):361–6.
68. O'Shea DM, Fieo R, Woods A, Williamson J, Porges E, Cohen R. Discrepancies between crystallized and fluid ability are associated with frequency of social and physical engagement in community dwelling older adults. J Clin Exp Neuropsychol. 2018;40(10):963–70.
69. Hu S, Shi L, Li Z, Ma Y, Li J, Bao Y, et al. First-night effect in insomnia disorder: a systematic review and meta-analysis of polysomnographic findings. J Sleep Res. 2023:e13942.
70. Toussaint M, Luthringer R, Schaltenbrand N, Carelli G, Lainey E, Jacqmin A, et al. First-night effect in normal subjects and psychiatric inpatients. Sleep. 1995;18(6):463–9.

Deep Learning with Electrocardiograms

Wesley Chorney, Haifeng Wang, and Lir-Wan Fan

1 Electrocardiograms

The human heart undergoes a number of distinct pressure changes as it pumps blood throughout the body. These pressure changes are stimulated by electrochemical changes in the heart that cause contraction of the cardiac muscle [1]. An electrocardiogram (often abbreviated ECG or EKG, though we will use the former) is a medical test that measures the electrical activity of the heart over several cardiac cycles. Various types of ECGs exist: ECGs may be recorded at rest, during exercise, or worn over longer periods of time to record rarer cardiac events (called a *Holter monitor* or *ambulatory ECG*).

As a medical test, ECGs are valuable for two principle reasons. Firstly, ECGs are a *noninvasive assessment*: That is, they do not involve tools that break the skin or enter the body [2]. ECGs are recorded via electrodes that measure the electrical activity of the heart, which are placed on the skin for the duration of the test. Therefore, they are a fairly simple test to administer, with minimal discomfort to the patient. Secondly, ECGs can detect a wide variety of cardiovascular conditions, such as atrial fibrillation [3] and Wolff–Parkinson–White syndrome [4].

W. Chorney
Computational Engineering, Mississippi State University, Mississippi State, MS, USA
e-mail: wwc102@msstate.edu

H. Wang (✉)
Industrial and Systems Engineering, Mississippi State University, Mississippi State, MS, USA
e-mail: wang@ise.msstate.edu

L.-W. Fan
Pediatrics/Newborn Medicine, University of Mississippi Medical Center, Jackson, MS, USA
e-mail: lwfan@umc.edu

R. B. Berry et al. (eds.), *Handbook of AI and Data Sciences for Sleep Disorders*,
Springer Optimization and Its Applications 216,
https://doi.org/10.1007/978-3-031-68263-6_9

In addition, ECGs can also detect many noncardiac events [5]. The sympathetic and parasympathetic nervous systems act on the sinoatrial node to modulate the rhythm of the heart; therefore, the ECG provides information on autonomic functioning, which is useful for the diagnosis of sleep disorders [7]. ECGs are key components in polysomnography, which is a current standard for the diagnosis of sleep disorders [6]. In addition, recent research has demonstrated that the ECG itself is sufficient to detect a range of sleep disorders. Indeed, ECGs have been used to diagnose sleep apnea [9], insomnia, sleep-disordered breathing, and rapid eye movement behaviour disorder [8]. Therefore, this chapter presents different deep learning models to solve two common problems when working with ECG data. In particular, we discuss denoising ECGs in Sect. 2 and automated diagnosis of ECGs in Sect. 3.

2 Denoising ECGs

When measured by an ECG, the cardiac cycle has some recognizable patterns, which together can be used to diagnose different diseases. Figure 1 shows a simplified representation of the cardiac cycle. The P-wave represents atrial depolarization, whereas the QRS complex represents ventricular depolarization. Finally, the T-wave reflects ventricular repolarization. The length of time in between each of these events also carries important information (see, for instance, [10]).

Unfortunately, ECG monitoring is an imperfect procedure. Different types of noises can contaminate an ECG, masking the true signal contained therein and making accurate diagnosis a difficult task. For example, *baseline wander* is caused by varying electrode–skin impedance, patient movement, and breathing [11]. ECGs affected by baseline wander move consistently downwards or upwards in time, instead of adhering to a constant baseline, as shown in Fig. 1. Other types of noise are more complicated and do not follow a reliable pattern. Muscle artefact is an instance of complicated noise, which is caused by skeletal muscle activity that is recorded by an electrode [12]. Electrode motion can also obfuscate the signal contained in an ECG and is caused by changes in electrode–skin impedance or changes in skin potential [13]. Finally, noise can also be caused by operator error,

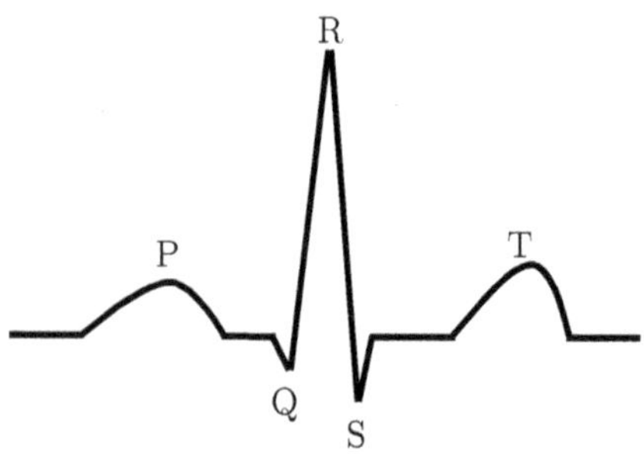

Fig. 1 The typical cardiac cycle as recorded by an ECG. P- and T-waves, as well as the QRS complex, are labelled

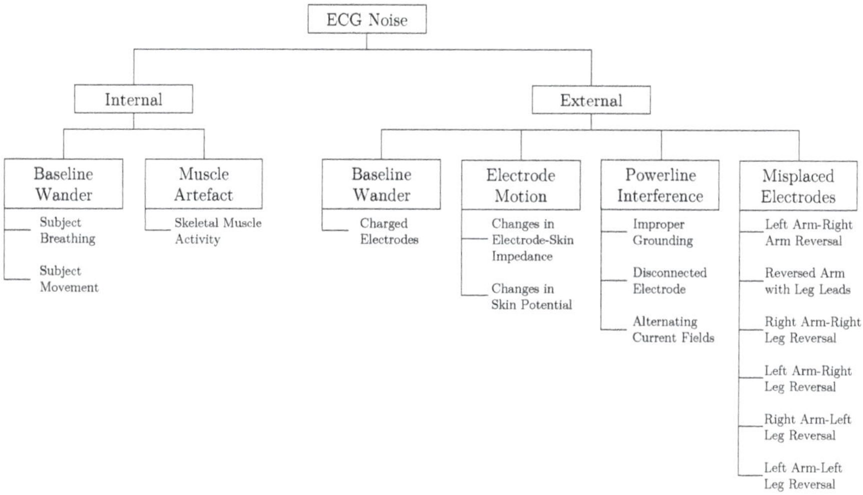

Fig. 2 A taxonomy of different types of noise that can affect ECG signals

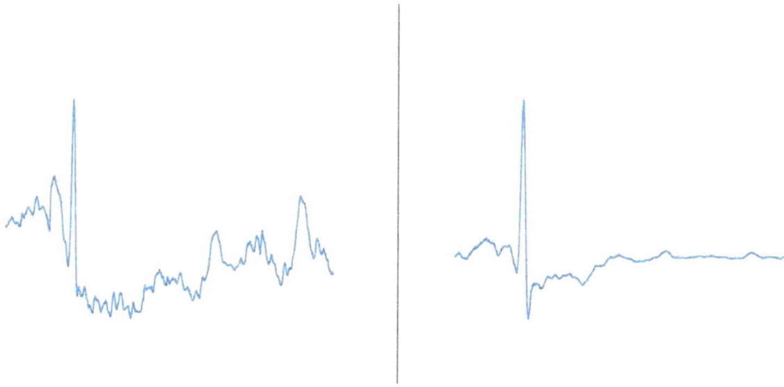

Fig. 3 An example of an ECG contaminated by noise (left), alongside its noiseless counterpart (right)

such as powerline interference [14] and misplaced electrodes [15]. Figure 2 gives a classification of these types of noise, based on the information in [11–15].

Noise in an ECG is a serious problem. For instance, a confusing signal was recorded in an ECG in 2005. It was initially hypothesized that the large T-waves in every lead except lead II were the result of abnormal left ventricular motion. The pattern was only resolved as noise due to a misplaced electrode 6 years later [16]. Figure 3 shows a noisy ECG signal alongside the same signal without noise. Observe in particular that the P- and T-waves, as well as the QRS complex, are indistinguishable in the noisy signal, but clear in the noiseless signal.

From the perspective of the automated diagnosis of sleep disorders, noise in an ECG is a problem that should be addressed as well. For example, because skeletal muscles maintain some level of activity during sleep, it is possible to record muscle artefact on the ECG of a polysomnogram. The recording of baseline wander and electrode motion is also possible when a patient is asleep due to the nature of the noise. Because noise obscures the signal contained in data, it renders any automated diagnosis more difficult. In particular, this includes sleep disorders that can be diagnosed via ECG analysis, including sleep apnea, insomnia, sleep-disordered breathing, and rapid eye movement behaviour disorder [8, 9]. Therefore, the following techniques can be readily applied to improve automated methods of sleep disorder diagnosis.

This section describes methods of denoising ECGs, beginning with standard denoising autoencoders (Sect. 2.2), then looking at convolutional and fully convolutional denoising autoencoders (Sect. 2.3), before describing a convolutional denoising autoencoder with block attention module (Sect. 2.5).

2.1 Autoencoders

Dimensionality reduction techniques such as principal component analysis (PCA) attempt to find a more efficient representation of input data. Given a dataset $D = \{x_i\}_{i=1}^N$, where $x_i \in \mathbb{R}^n$, PCA projects data onto a new set of coordinate axes such that the covariance of features along the new axes is minimized. Machine learning practitioners typically remove the m axes that contain the least variance ($m < n$), to obtain a modified dataset $D' = \{x_i'\}_{i=1}^N$, where $x_i' \in \mathbb{R}^{n-m}$. If the original dataset contained labels, the unaltered labels can be associated with the transformed data as well.

As methods in deep learning often mirror classical techniques, a natural question to ask is whether dimensionality reduction (or more generally, learning an efficient representation of input data) is possible with deep learning. *Autoencoders* [17] answer this question affirmatively. Suppose that $f_\theta : \mathbb{R}^n \to \mathbb{R}^n$ is a neural network with parameters θ (we omit the θ subscript when the context is clear). The goal for an autoencoder is to reconstruct its input data. That is, for a perfect autoencoder, we would have

$$f_\theta(x) = x. \tag{1}$$

While Eq. (1) is trivially achieved by an identity function, this would be rather pointless from the point of view of efficiently representing data. An autoencoder can be separated into two parts: the *encoder*, e_θ, which takes $x \in \mathbb{R}^n$ and maps it to some $\tilde{x} \in \mathbb{R}^{n-m}$, where $m < n$, and the *decoder*, d_θ, which takes $\tilde{x} \in \mathbb{R}^{n-m}$ and maps it back to $\hat{x} \in \mathbb{R}^n$. We refer to $\tilde{x}$ as the *encoded* or *latent representation* of x. For any input x, we may write the autoencoder more explicitly as

$$f_\theta(x) = d_\theta(e_\theta(x)) = \hat{x}. \tag{2}$$

We can think of $\hat{x}$ as the attempt by the autoencoder to recover the original signal x after it has been mapped into a lower dimensional space. In order to quantify how good this representation is and in order to train the model, we need a loss function. Typically, mean-squared error is used. Given $\hat{x}$ and x, the squared error between the two is written

$$L(\hat{x}, x) = \sum_{i=1}^{n} \left(\hat{x}_i - x_i\right)^2 = ||\hat{x} - x||^2, \tag{3}$$

where x_i is the ith component of x, and $||\cdot||$ is the L_2-norm on $\mathbb{R}^n$. The mean-squared error is the average of the squared errors for each pair of output $\hat{x}$ and input x in the dataset D.

As is typical for machine learning models, given a dataset D and a loss function L, we can perform some form of stochastic gradient descent in order to train the model.

2.2 Densely Connected Autoencoders

Conceptually, the simplest autoencoder is a densely connected autoencoder. In this model, each layer is a densely connected layer with activation σ, so that the entire autoencoder can be written as a series of simple matrix equations. Let W_i be the weights matrix for the ith layer of the model, $\mathbf{b}_i$ the corresponding bias vector, and σ_i the activation function. Then

$$e(x) = \sigma_j \left(W_j \left(\cdots \sigma_1 \left(W_1 x + \mathbf{b}_1\right) \cdots\right) + \mathbf{b}_j\right), \tag{4}$$

where $W_i \in \mathbb{R}^{d_i \times d_{i-1}}$, $\mathbf{b}_i \in \mathbb{R}^{d_i}$, and typically $d_j \leq d_{j-1} \leq \cdots \leq d_1 \leq d_0 = n$ where at least one of these inequalities is strict.[1] The decoder often mirrors the encoder, though this is not always the case. However, we do have that $d : \mathbb{R}^{d_j} \to \mathbb{R}^n$. Therefore, we write the decoder as

$$d(x) = \sigma_{k'} \left(W_{k'} \left(\cdots \sigma_{1'} \left(W_{1'} x + \mathbf{b}_{1'}\right) \cdots\right) + \mathbf{b}_{k'}\right), \tag{5}$$

where we use the prime notation to emphasize that weights are not shared between the encoder and the decoder. Figure 4 gives a visual representation of the densely connected autoencoder.

The discussion above does not relate directly to denoising ECGs. In fact, the autoencoder as described above would learn only an effective representation for ECGs, which would encode the noise and the signal. Suppose instead that we took

[1] There is also the notion of an *overcomplete* autoencoder, though this is far less common. We refer the interested reader to [18].

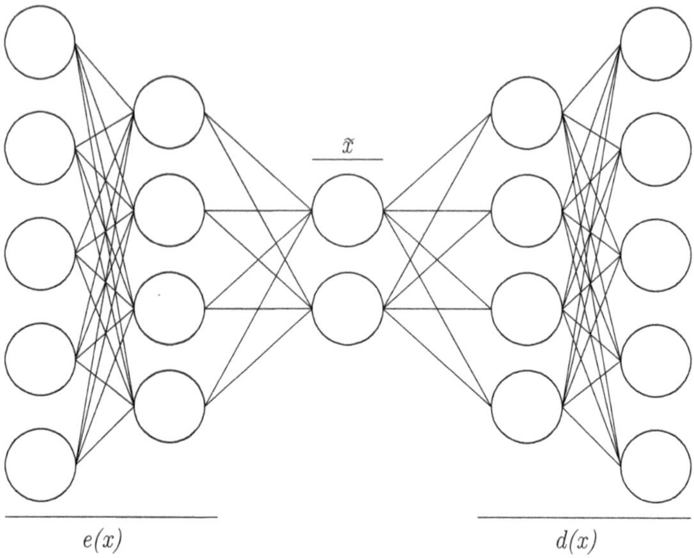

Fig. 4 A visual representation of the densely connected autoencoder, with the encoder, decoder, and latent representation labelled

our dataset $D = \{x_i\}_{i=1}^{N}$ and added Gaussian noise to each sample. That is, suppose we created a new dataset

$$\tilde{D} = \{x_i + \nu\}_{i=1}^{n}, \tag{6}$$

where ν is a random variable such that $\nu \sim \mathcal{N}(\mu, \sigma^2)$, where $\mathcal{N}(\mu, \sigma^2)$ is a normal distribution with mean μ and variance σ^2. $\tilde{D}$ has input that is masked by Gaussian noise, and a *denoising autoencoder* [19] f_θ attempts to remove this noise. Although the input to the denoising autoencoder (or DAE) is the corrupted input, it is evaluated on its ability to recover the noiseless signal. That is, for $x \in D$, the loss between the autoencoder output and x is written as

$$L(f_\theta(x + \nu), x) = \sum_{i=1}^{n} (f_\theta(x + \nu)_i - x_i)^2 = ||f_\theta(x + \nu) - x||^2. \tag{7}$$

While the denoising autoencoder described above uses Gaussian noise, other versions of denoising autoencoders exist. For example, some denoising autoencoders use dropout to randomly mute the input to (or output of) a neuron. Others corrupt samples with noise other than Gaussian noise. For denoising ECGs, we may use samples of noises such as baseline wander, electrode motion, or muscle artefact in order to corrupt samples with more realistic noise—this was done in Fig. 3.

Similar to the multilayer perceptron, the densely connected autoencoder is well suited to some types of data but is not suitable to others. For instance, densely connected autoencoders are typically not able to handle image data very well, mirroring the multilayer perceptron's inability to adequately handle image data. Because ECGs are a time series with many local features, densely connected layers are not suited to capture important features that vary in their exact placement and shape.

2.3 Convolutional Autoencoder

Classical approaches to detecting cardiac conditions from ECGs relied on hand-crafted features based on expert knowledge [20]. Different local features can give great insight into different cardiac conditions. For example, a patient with Wolff–Parkinson–White syndrome will typically have a short PR interval (the time from the onset of the P-wave to the start of the QRS complex) and a prolonged QRS complex with an initial upstroke showing on their ECG. Therefore, being able to capture local features is important when searching for an efficient representation of an ECG or when trying to denoise an ECG.

Convolutional layers are often thought of as feature detectors; thus, the convolutional layer would be a useful component in an autoencoder meant to work with ECG data. The convolutional layer uses a *kernel* to extract local features from its input. The kernel functions as a sliding window, where everything in the window is multiplied entry-wise and then summed together. Writing x_i for the ith entry of x and $x_{i:j}$ for entries i through j, we write each value of the convolution as

$$(x \star k)_j = \langle x_{j:j+L_k}, k \rangle, \tag{8}$$

where $k \in \mathbb{R}^{L_k}$ is the kernel, and $\langle \cdot, \cdot \rangle$ is the inner product on $\mathbb{R}^{L_k}$. $x \star k$ is then the convolution of x with k, which we may occasionally write as $C(x, k)$. Typically, padding is used to ensure that $x \star k$ and x have the same dimensions. Figure 5 gives a visual depiction of the convolution operation without padding. In the case of multiple channels (for instance, an ECG with different leads), the kernel is broadcast across the channels. Convolutions can also involve multiple kernels, to get an output with multiple channels. As convolutional layers are stacked in sequence, they are able to capture higher level features.

Ideally, convolutions are able to capture local features from an input. However, if the input is shifted, the output of the convolution will be affected. Therefore, *maximum* or *average pooling* is typically applied to the output of a convolution. Given $x \in \mathbb{R}^n$, we write maximum and average pooling, respectively, as

$$maxpool(x) = \max(x) \tag{9}$$

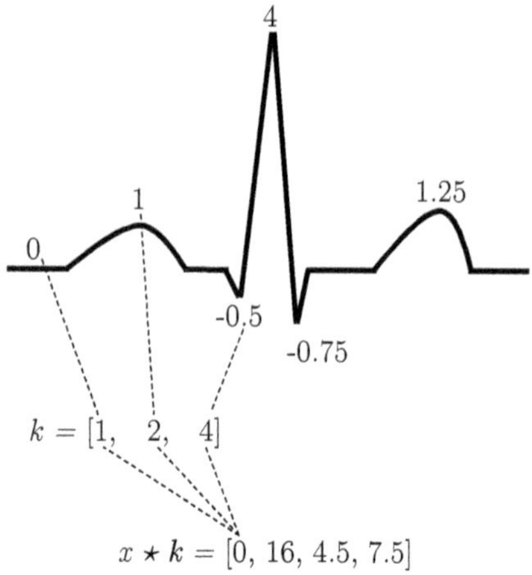

Fig. 5 An example of the convolution operation on a simplified ECG signal with a kernel in $\mathbb{R}^3$

$$avgpool(x) = \frac{1}{n}\sum_{i=1}^{n} x. \tag{10}$$

These are often computed using a sliding window of a given stride, in order to reduce the size of the input. For example, if $x \in \mathbb{R}^{2m}$, using maximum pooling with a window size of 2 and a stride of 2 would give an output $x' \in \mathbb{R}^m$.

How are these ideas used to create an autoencoder? In particular, it seems that using convolutions and pooling would serve only to decrease the dimension of a signal. In the best case scenario, the input would retain its original dimension, in which case we have not exactly created an autoencoder at all. While we could create an encoder with a series of convolutional layers and pooling operations, we need the opposite notion of a convolution, called a *convolutional transpose*, to create a decoder.[2]

We will fix a stride length of 2 so that the following discussion is more clear. Suppose $x \in \mathbb{R}^n$, and let k be a kernel in $\mathbb{R}^{L_k}$. Assuming j is divisible by 2, we define

$$(x * k)_j = x_{j/2} \cdot k. \tag{11}$$

That is, $(x * k)_j$ is the constant $x_{j/2}$ multiplied by the vector k. $(x * k)_j$ is extended to $\mathbb{R}^{2n}$ by setting indices that are not in $\{j/2, j/2 + 1, \ldots, j/2 + L_k\}$ to have zero value. Then we may define the convolutional transpose operation as

[2] Technically, a deconvolution reverses the process of a convolutional layer, while a convolutional transpose layer reverses the downsampling techniques applied to the input of the convolutional layer.

Fig. 6 A convolutional transpose operation between $x = [1, 2, 3, 4]$ and $k = [0, 1]$, using a stride of 2

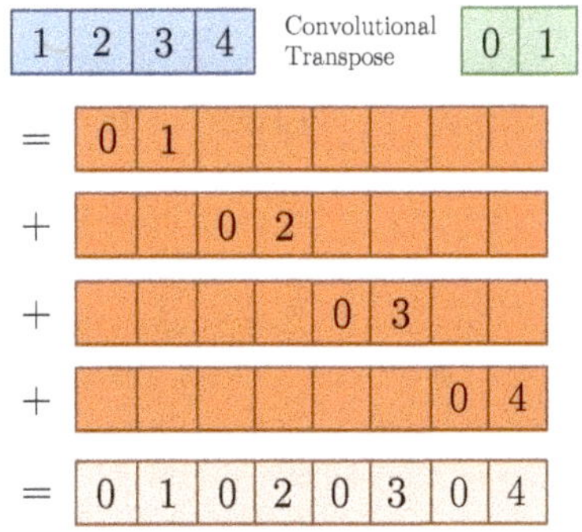

$$T(x, k) = \sum_{j=1}^{n} (x * k)_{2j}. \tag{12}$$

Note in particular that $T(x, k) \in \mathbb{R}^{2n}$, since we used a stride of 2. Figure 6 also demonstrates this operation visually.

Using a stride of 2, the convolutional transpose operation restores the dimensionality that would be reduced with a convolution layer followed by maximum pooling with a window of length 2 and a stride of 2. Based on the previous discussion, it is clear that we can stack convolutions and pooling operations to reduce the dimension of an input. By doing so, we can create an encoder. Now, we may stack convolutional transpose layers to recover the dimensionality lost and create a decoder.

Let $C_{M,\sigma}(x, k, r)$ denote a convolutional layer with r filters $k = \{k_1, \ldots, k_r\}$ where the activation σ is applied to the output, followed by maximum pooling (where the subscript M denotes maximum pooling). Similarly, let $T_\sigma(x, k, s)$ denote a convolutional transpose with s filters and the activation σ applied to the output. With this setup, we will assume that the dimension reduction achieved by $C_{M,\sigma}(x, k, r)$ is reversed by $T_\sigma(x, k, s)$, which can be achieved by choosing the appropriate stride length. Then, for a convolutional autoencoder, we define our encoder with c layers as

$$e(x) = C_{M,\sigma_{r_c}}(C_{M,\sigma_{r_{c-1}}}(\cdots C_{M,\sigma_1}(x, k_1, r_1), \ldots k_{c-1}, r_{c-1}), k_c, r_c), \tag{13}$$

and similarly, our decoder with t layers is defined as

$$d(x) = T_{\sigma'_{s_t}}(T_{\sigma'_{s_{t-1}}}(\cdots T_{\sigma'_1}(x, k'_1, s'_1), \ldots k'_{t-1}, s'_{t-1}), k'_t, s'_t), \tag{14}$$

where we again make use of the prime notation to emphasize that weights are not shared between any layers of the encoder and decoder.

Densely connected layers can be inserted between convolutional and convolutional transpose layers at any point in the above equations. If no densely connected layers are used, we refer to the autoencoder as a fully convolutional denoising autoencoder (FCDAE); otherwise, we refer to it as a convolutional denoising autoencoder (CDAE). Typically, the decoder is created with the same number of layers as the encoder, so that it essentially reverses the operations done by the encoder in order to recover the signal. That is, in Eqs. (13) and (14), $r_i = s_i$, so that the number of filters in corresponding layers is the same, and $\sigma_{r_i}, \sigma_{s_i}$ are the same type of activation function. While this is standard practice, it is not a requirement, and the notion of an *asymmetric* autoencoder exists [21].

Convolutional layers are powerful feature extractors and allow deep learning models to learn local features that vary in their positions. However, features captured by a certain kernel might be more relevant than those captured by other kernels. Similarly, a feature captured in one location of the signal might be made more or less relevant by features captured in other locations—for instance, in second-degree atrioventricular block, Mobitz type II, an ECG will show normal cardiac cycles with intermittent non-conducted P-waves [22]. If a kernel in a convolution captures several normal cycles with intermittent non-conducted P-waves, the latter are far more important with respect to accurately diagnosing the signal.

2.4 Block Attention

The attention mechanism is inspired by the fact that when our minds are presented with an image, we place more emphasis on certain parts of the image. For example, when looking at a portrait, we place more emphasis on the subject as opposed to the background of the image. Similarly, we can use matrices to weight different elements of a deep learning model's output [25]. Although it is a simple principle, the technique itself is extremely powerful. Most transformer models are based on some form of attention, and these models often perform exceptionally well in the domain for which they were designed [23, 24].

Feature detectors are able to extract many different types of features, but the salient information in the output of a convolutional layer is not evenly distributed. Therefore, different parts of the output should be weighted differently. These weightings could affect *channels*, which are the feature maps extracted by different kernels, or they could affect the spatial information across all channels. The former notion is *channel attention*, while the latter is *spatial attention*.

2.4.1 Spatial Attention

The output of a convolutional layer contains different high-level features across multiple channels, similar to how digital images are commonly stored with red, green, and blue channels. At times, regardless of the channel, certain locations in an image will be more important than others. Figure 7 shows an image of a sailboat. Regardless of the channel, the subject of the photograph is in the same location,

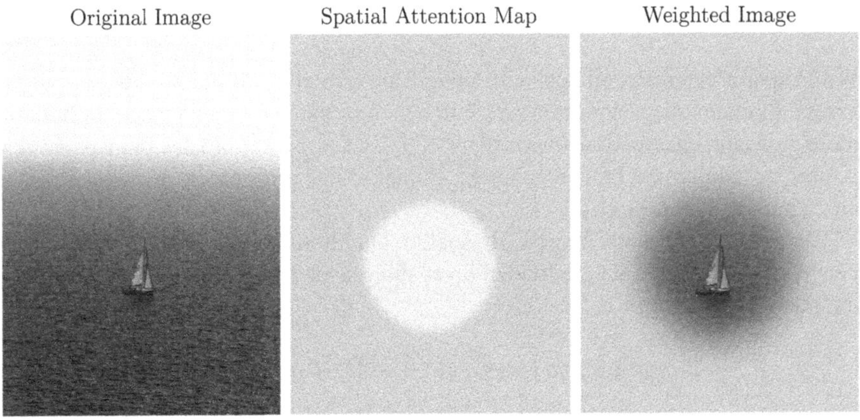

Fig. 7 A simplified example of spatial attention. An attention map is used to focus on the subject of the image. Photo taken by Alexandros Giannakakis; it is used here with permission

and a spatial attention map could help focus on the subject, deemphasizing the surroundings.

Focusing on ECGs, suppose that $x \in \mathbb{R}^{n \times c}$ is the output of a convolutional layer (or an ECG itself). Spatial attention uses the notion of *global average pooling* and *global maximum pooling*, as well as convolutional layers, to create a spatial attention map $A_s \in \mathbb{R}^n$.

Global maximum and global average pooling extend the notion of maximum and average pooling, as seen in Eq. (9), over an entire set of channels or input features. For example, given $x \in \mathbb{R}^{n \times c}$, global maximum pooling with respect to channels yields a vector $x_C \in \mathbb{R}^n$ where the ith entry of x_C is the maximum value across the channels.

We write $maxpool_{G,c}(x)$ for global maximum pooling over the c channels of x and $maxpool_{G,n}(x)$ for global maximum pooling over the n timesteps of x and analogously for global average pooling. Spatial attention uses both global maximum and global average pooling to obtain two maps $\mu_m, \mu_a \in \mathbb{R}^n$, which are then concatenated to form $\mu_m \oplus \mu_a \in \mathbb{R}^{n \times 2}$ (where we use $\oplus$ to represent concatenation). A convolutional layer f is then used with a sigmoid activation function to obtain $A_s \in \mathbb{R}^n$. Note in particular that because the activation function is sigmoidal, any entry a_{ij} of A_s satisfies $0 < a_{ij} < 1$, so that A_s can selectively mute or emphasize features in x. In the original paper, f has a kernel size of 7×7 (since f is used on image data), although in principle any kernel size can be used. Using σ to represent the sigmoid activation function, we may write the spatial attention map as

$$A_s = \sigma(f(\mu_m \oplus \mu_a)) \tag{15}$$

or a little more explicitly as

$$A_s = \sigma(f(maxpool_{G,c}(x) \oplus avgpool_{G,c}(x))). \tag{16}$$

2.4.2 Channel Attention

While spatial attention allows us to selectively attend to different parts of a signal across all channels, it does not take into account that certain channels might carry more relevant information than others. Channel attention creates a map A_c that is used to emphasize or deemphasize channels (as opposed to A_s, which works analogously for timesteps).

Channel attention is similar to spatial attention, except that in place of a convolutional layer, a single hidden layer multilayer perceptron (MLP) is used on the pooling layer outputs. We write

$$\begin{aligned} A_c &= \sigma(MLP(maxpool_{G,n}(x)) + MLP(avgpool_{G,n}(x))) \\ &= \sigma(W_1(W_0(maxpool_{G,n}(x))) + W_1(W_0(avgpool_{G,n}(x)))), \end{aligned} \tag{17}$$

where addition between vectors is done element-wise. The MLP is designed with a reduction factor r, so that $W_0 \in \mathbb{R}^{c/r \times c}$ and $W_1 \in \mathbb{R}^{c \times c/r}$.

Because densely connected layers are computationally expensive, a more efficient alternative has been proposed, called efficient channel attention [26]. Efficient channel attention formulates the channel attention map differently:

$$A_c = \sigma(f_\psi(avgpool_{G,n}(x))), \tag{18}$$

where f again denotes a convolutional layer. However, the authors propose using an adaptive kernel size based on the number of channels. The kernel size is given by

$$\psi(c) = \left| \log_2\left(\frac{c}{\gamma}\right) + \frac{b}{\gamma} \right|_{odd}, \tag{19}$$

where $|t|_{odd}$ denotes the nearest odd number to t, and b and γ are constants. The adaptive kernel size allows high-dimensional channels to have longer range interactions. Note that in their experiments, the authors fix the number of channels to be 3 and still obtain good results. Therefore, it is possible to use efficient channel attention with a constant kernel size in place of ψ.

Given attention maps A_s and A_c, how are they combined with the input x? Given the input x, the output of convolutional block attention is

$$y = A_s \odot (A_c \odot x), \tag{20}$$

where $\odot$ is the Hadamard product. Note that $x \in \mathbb{R}^{n \times c}$, $A_s \in \mathbb{R}^n$, and $A_c \in \mathbb{R}^c$, so that A_s is copied c times so that the Hadamard product can be taken with x and analogously for A_c.

The general nature of the convolutional block attention module means that it can be used between many different layers, and as such, it is often employed in computer vision tasks. A natural question to ask is how we can employ convolutional block attention in our denoising autoencoder.

2.5 *Convolutional Denoising Autoencoder with Block Attention Module*

Given our discussion on convolutional denoising autoencoders followed by a block attention module, perhaps the reader will not be surprised to find out that in this section, we combine the two concepts. The model we describe will be based on the convolutional denoising autoencoder described earlier but will incorporate the block attention we described in the previous section. Therefore, we will refer to the model as a convolutional denoising autoencoder with block attention module or more simply as CBAM-DAE.

Both the encoder and decoder blocks of CBAM-DAE make use of attention, and the encoder block will make use of a convolutional layer followed by batch normalization, LeakyReLU activation, dropout, and maximum pooling with a stride of 2 (in order to reduce its output size by a factor of 2). We will denote this layer by $C'(\cdot)$. Similar to the encoder block, the decoder block will begin with a convolutional transpose layer with a stride of 2 (reversing the reduction in size caused by an encoder block), followed by batch normalization, a LeakyReLU activation function, and dropout. We will denote this layer by $T'(\cdot)$. Both layers are followed by a block attention module. Figure 8 describes the proposed architecture visually.

Similar to the convolutional denoising autoencoder we described earlier, CBAM-DAE uses a sequence of encoder blocks and decoder blocks to remove noise from an

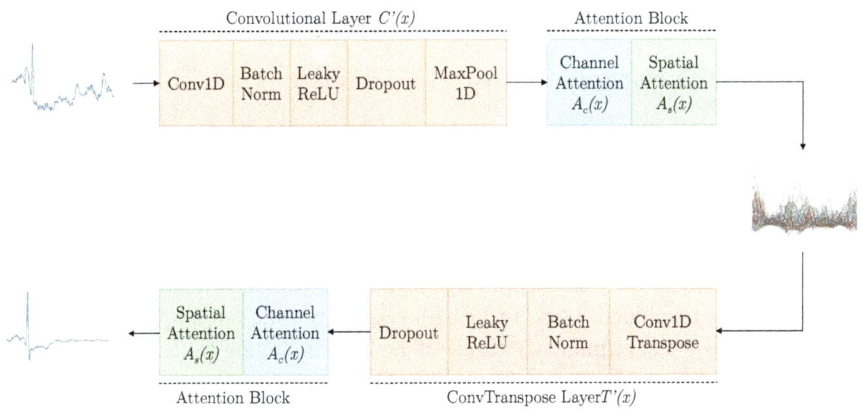

Fig. 8 The encoder and decoder block architecture, along with sample inputs and outputs. CBAM-DAE ultimately removes noise from a contaminated ECG signal

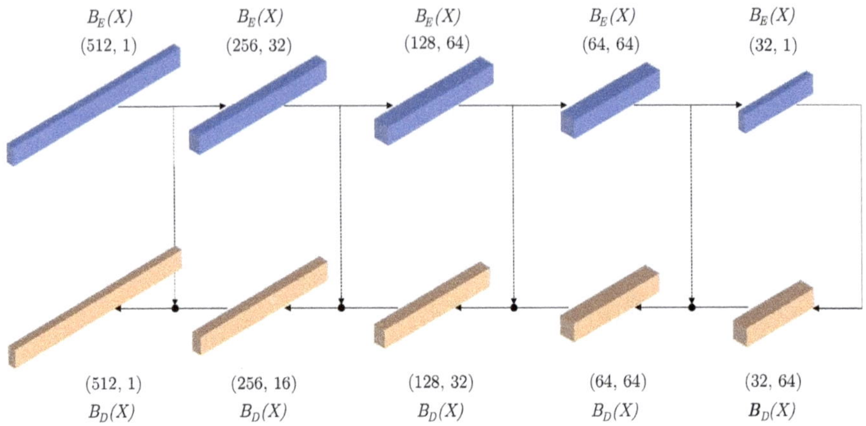

Fig. 9 Architecture of CBAM-DAE with five blocks. Blue layers are encoder blocks, and beige layers are decoder blocks. Filled circles denote element-wise addition, and dashed arrows show residual connections between different blocks

ECG signal. However, CBAM-DAE also uses residual connections between encoder and decoder blocks. Residual connections allow for better gradient flow, making backpropagation more effective, and are commonly used in computer vision tasks. They are well known for their use in the ResNet architecture [27].

In a residual connection, the output x' of an earlier layer is added element-wise to the output x of a later layer. For an autoencoder, residual connections must be made between layers with the same output dimension. Assume that we have a single-channel, noisy ECG with 512 timesteps. Denoting an encoder block as $B_E(\cdot)$ and a decoder block as $B_D(\cdot)$, Fig. 9 shows the architecture of CBAM-DAE with five blocks, with dashed arrows denoting residual connections.

2.6 *Model Performance*

With a lengthy discussion on different model architectures and their use in denoising ECGs, it would be remiss to not include how these models perform on actual data. In this section, we use ECG signals from the MIT-BIH QT database and add noise from the MIT-BIH Noise Stress Test database to contaminate the ECG. Both of these databases are freely available from PhysioNet [28]. Random samples of BW, EM, and MA noise are added to the ECG with randomly sampled amplitudes between 0.2 and 2 times the maximum amplitude of the ECG. A signal from the QT database is on the right side of Fig. 3, and the version contaminated with noise from the stress test database is on the left.

This gives us a database of the form $D = \{x_i, y_i\}_{i=1}^N$, where $y_i = x_i + \nu$, and ν represents the randomly sampled noise from the Noise Stress Test database. We segment the ECGs into sections with 512 timesteps, sampled at 250Hz (so that $x_i \in \mathbb{R}^{512}$). Each model is trained on about 87% of the data (and 30% of the training set is used as a validation set), using the rest as a test set. Models in the following experiments are trained with the Adam optimizer, with a batch size of 32 and a learning rate of 10^{-3}. Each model has five encoding blocks, followed by five decoding blocks. The learning rate is reduced by a factor of 2 if there are no improvements on the validation set after two epochs, with 10^{-10} being the minimum learning rate. Training is run until there are no improvements on the validation set loss after 10 epochs. We use a custom loss function:

$$L(y, \hat{y}) = \sum_{i=1}^{L} (y_i - \hat{y}_i)^2 + \lambda \cdot \max_i |y_i - \hat{y}_i|, \tag{21}$$

where again y_i denotes the ith entry of y. Note that this loss function is based on mean-squared error and *mean absolute error*: the greatest distance between corresponding points in the reconstructed signal and the noiseless signal. It creates a balance in faithfully constructing the entire noiseless signal, while ensuring important cardiac events, such as the peaks of QRS complexes, are not ignored. This loss function was designed in [29] and seems to give good performance when $\lambda = 50$.

We evaluate the trained models on a variety of evaluation metrics, in order to get a holistic view of the performance of each model.

Maximum Absolute Distance (MAD) This metric measures the maximum absolute difference between aligned points in the original and filtered signal. It is used in [30] in the context of compressing and then recovering ECG signals. It is a useful metric because it penalizes a model for not capturing significant but short cardiac events, such as the peak of a QRS complex. The formula is given by

$$MAD(y, \hat{y}) = \max_i |y_i - \hat{y}_i| \qquad 1 \leq i \leq n, \tag{22}$$

where $y, \hat{y}$ are signals in $\mathbb{R}^n$. In our specific case, y is the original signal and $\hat{y}$ is the denoised signal, and i is the signal index. We make the same assumptions for the sum of squared distances and percentage root-mean-square difference.

Sum of Squared Distances (SSD) While the MAD metric measures the point of maximum disparity, the SSD metric instead measures how similar two signals are across their entire length. Note that this is equivalent to the squared error described in Eq. (3). The formula is given by

$$SSD(y, \hat{y}) = \sum_{i=1}^{n} (y_i - \hat{y}_i)^2. \tag{23}$$

Percentage Root-Mean-Square Difference (PRD) This metric measures how different the point-wise representation of the filtered signal is to the original versus its difference from the best constant approximation of the original signal. A smaller value corresponds to a better representation. The formula is given by

$$PRD(y, \hat{y}) = \sqrt{\frac{\sum_{i=1}^{n} \left(y_i - \hat{y}_i\right)^2}{\sum_{i=1}^{n} \left(\overline{y} - \hat{y}_i\right)^2}} \cdot 100\%, \tag{24}$$

where by $\overline{y}$ we denote the mean of y.

Cosine Similarity The cosine similarity metric can be easily derived from the dot product. The dot product is the canonical inner product in $\mathbb{R}^n$ and can be written as

$$\langle y, \hat{y} \rangle = ||y||||\hat{y}|| \cos\theta = \sum_{i=1}^{n} y_i \hat{y}_i. \tag{25}$$

Since $-1 \leq \cos\theta \leq 1$ and normalizing the vectors by their L_2 norm means that $\cos\theta$ is the angle between the points represented by the vectors on the unit sphere, rearranging Eq. (25) gives us an effective measure of similarity:

$$CosSim(y, \hat{y}) = \frac{\langle y, \hat{y} \rangle}{||y||||\hat{y}||}. \tag{26}$$

Table 1 displays the experimental results. Note that the CBAM-DAE performs better than the other tested models on three of the four evaluation metrics (SSD, MAD, and Cosine Similarity). However, according to research in [31], SSD and MAD are better indicators for signal quality after compression than PRD, so the strengths of CBAM-DAE outweigh its weaknesses.

We note further that for each beat in the test set, a corresponding value is calculated (for each evaluation metric), and since the beats can vary drastically in their values, so too does the standard deviation in Table 1. Nevertheless, using a Wilcoxon sign-rank test on the model output confirms that they are significantly different, with $p < 0.01$.

Figure 10 shows a case study of each model's performance, where we use a sample ECG signal from the test set contaminated with noise and observe each

Table 1 Summary of experimental results. Values are written mean plus or minus standard deviation

Model	SSD	MAD	PRD	Cosine similarity
DAE	19.951 ± 31.276	0.752 ± 0.484	$\mathbf{76.083} \pm 28.962$	0.685 ± 0.239
CDAE	19.441 ± 28.970	0.762 ± 0.524	77.624 ± 35.236	0.699 ± 0.257
FCDAE	28.268 ± 45.102	0.849 ± 0.595	77.755 ± 34.454	0.660 ± 0.287
CBAM-DAE	$\mathbf{10.650 \pm 14.795}$	$\mathbf{0.596 \pm 0.379}$	77.041 ± 36.244	$\mathbf{0.795 \pm 0.200}$

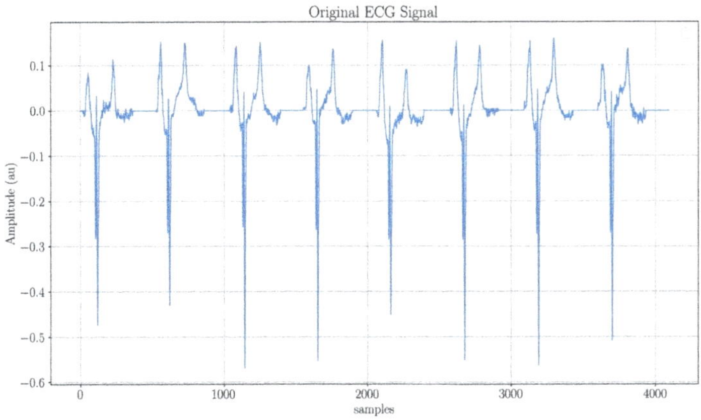

(a)

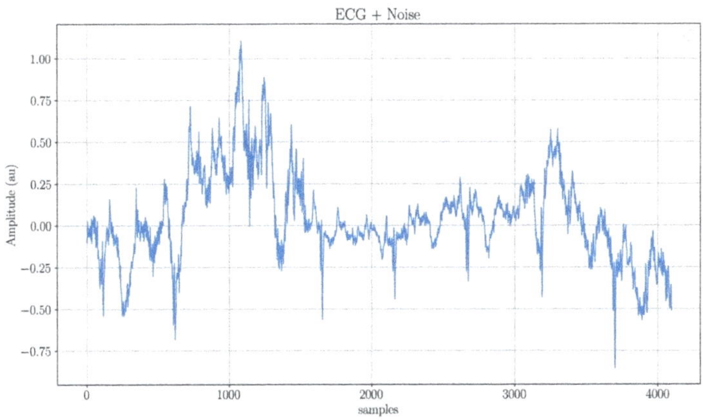

(b)

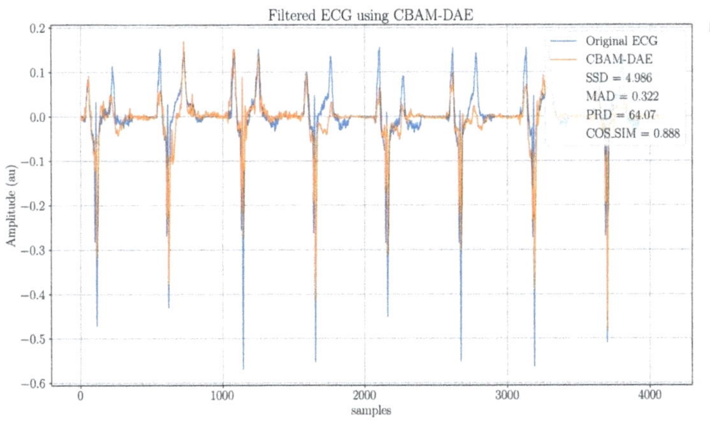

(c)

Fig. 10 Original and noisy ECGs, along with filtered ECGs from each models. (**a**) Original ECG signal. (**b**) ECG signal with noise. (**c**) Filtered ECG signal using CBAM-DAE. (**d**) Filtered ECG signal using FCDAE. (**e**) Filtered ECG signal using CDAE. (**f**) Filtered ECG signal using DAE

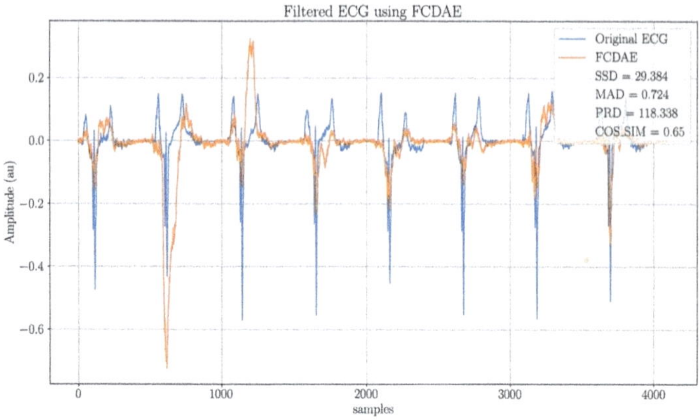

(d)

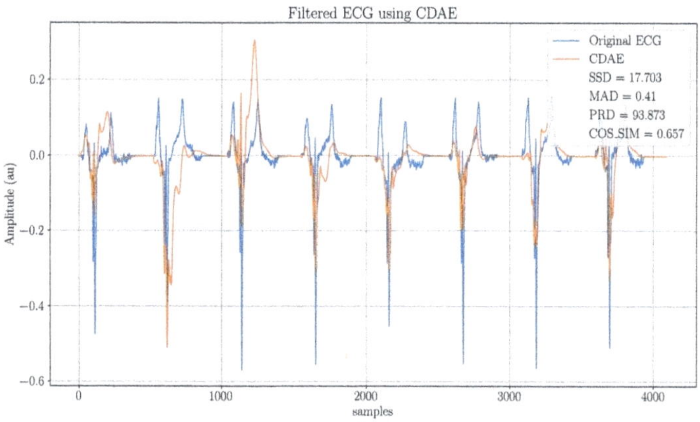

(e)

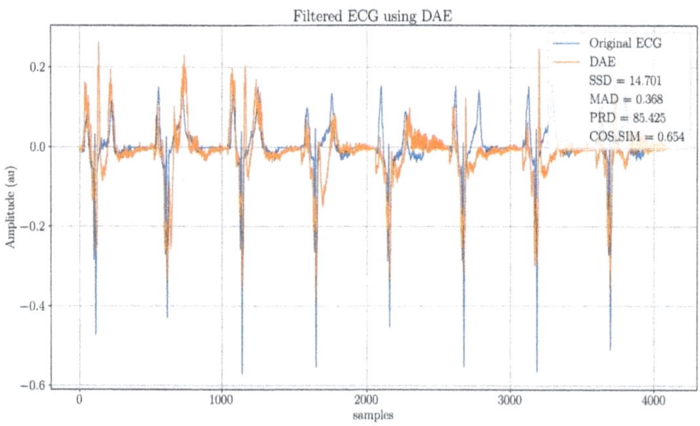

(f)

Fig. 10 (continued)

model's denoised output. We visually compare the model output to the true signal in order to judge its quality. Notably, CBAM-DAE performs significantly better than the others, with an output much closer to the true signal than the other models. It does a better job of capturing cardiac events and does not mistake the direction of the peak of the QRS complex, unlike the other tested models. Each subfigure in Fig. 10 also gives the value of each performance metric discussed above. For the given signal, CBAM-DAE outperforms all other models on each metric.

3 Diagnosing ECGs

While denoising ECGs is an important application of machine learning, diagnosing ECGs is another interesting way in which machine learning can be applied to ECGs. The ability to automatically diagnose ECGs is useful since it could save doctors' time, allowing it to be spent on more challenging tasks, thus leading to better patient care overall.

Because ECG diagnosis relies primarily on feature detection, as discussed in the previous section, similar methods can be used to detect different disorders, provided there is adequate information to train a model to diagnose a disorder. Therefore, the information in the following section can be broadly applied to automated ECG diagnosis and, in particular, to diagnosing sleep disorders from ECGs.

In this section, we introduce an automated ECG diagnosis model based on the principles described in the previous section. We evaluate this model on how well it can distinguish ECGs recorded from healthy patients versus those with COVID-19. Although the cause-and-effect relationship between sleep disorders and COVID-19 is unknown, it has been shown that poor sleep is related to greater COVID-19 susceptibility, as well as a poorer clinical course compared to patients with good sleep [32]. Therefore, the specific classification task we study is also very relevant to sleep disorders.

3.1 ECGs as Images

Previously, we focused on ECGs as signals in $\mathbb{R}^{n \times c}$, where n represented the timesteps and c the channels—for instance, a 12-lead ECG recorded for 10 seconds at 360Hz would produce a signal $x \in \mathbb{R}^{3600 \times 12}$. However, ECG data can also be consumed in other formats. For example, when interpreted by doctors or displayed to patients, ECGs are presented in image format. Figure 11 shows two different 12-lead ECG recordings from a dataset described in [33].

The dataset in question contains ECG images of patients with various conditions, including healthy patients, those with COVID-19, and patients who have a history of myocardial infarction. Interestingly, patients with COVID-19 have notable changes in their ECG, such as ST-T changes, conduction defects, and arrhythmias [34].

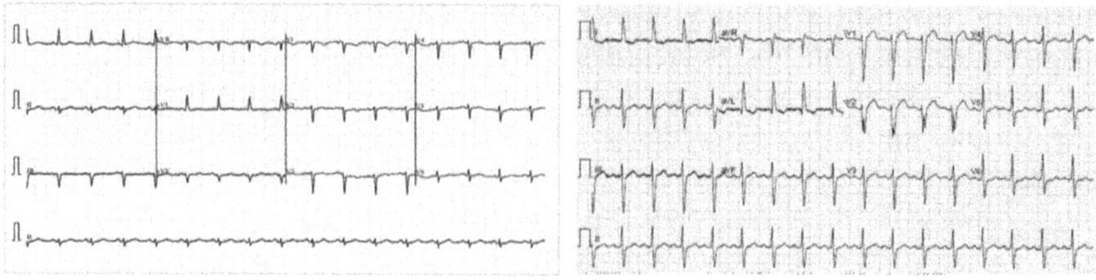

Fig. 11 Two ECG images from [33]. The left image is a normal ECG, while the right is an ECG of a patient with COVID-19

In principle, we should be able to build a model that diagnoses different ECG diseases using this dataset. However, the techniques that we have described thus far are only applicable to data in $\mathbb{R}^{n\times c}$. The data we would be working with is in $\mathbb{R}^{h\times w\times c}$. Fortunately, there is a natural way to extend the techniques we described above, so that they can be applied to the current data.

3.2 *Two-Dimensional Convolutions*

Convolutional layers are a natural choice for working with image data. Because features in an image might differ slightly in their location, it is of paramount importance to capture *local* features rather than global features. For example, a shortened PR interval can occur in ECGs of patients with Wolff–Parkinson–White syndrome; however, the location of this shortened PR interval may vary in its precise location. Therefore, the ability to extract features locally is very important.

Fortunately, two-dimensional convolutional layers (and convolutional transpose layers) work very similarly to their one-dimensional counterparts. Let $\mathbf{1}$ be the column vector with entries all 1s. In the two-dimensional case, $k \in \mathbb{R}^{k_1\times k_2}$ is a kernel, and the ijth entry in the convolution of $x \in \mathbb{R}^{h\times w}$ with k is

$$(x \star k)_{ij} = \mathbf{1}^T \left(x_{i:i+k_1, j:j+k_2} \odot k\right) \mathbf{1}. \tag{27}$$

Equation (27) simply expresses that we will take the Hadamard product of $x_{i:i+k_1, j:j+k_2}$ and k and then the sum over all the entries to get the ijth element of the convolution between x and k.

Two-dimensional convolutions extend to channels identically to the one-dimensional case, and their output can be extended to an arbitrary number of channels by including multiple kernels. Figure 12 also gives a visual example of the convolutional operation in two dimensions.

What about the convolutional transpose? This layer can also be extended to two dimensions, analogous to the convolutional layer. However, since diagnosing ECGs is an image classification task, which relies on the ability to extract features from images, we do not need them. When denoising ECGs, we were using autoencoders, which compress the input to a smaller dimension and then decompress the input.

Fig. 12 A simple example of a two-dimensional convolution, with the input on the left, the kernel on the right, and the output below

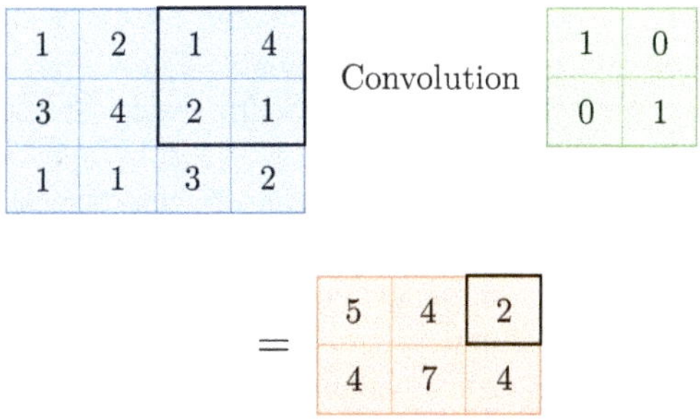

Therefore, we needed both convolutions and convolutional transpose layers. In the diagnosis case, we are interested in extracting features, which can be done with stacked convolutional layers. Therefore, we leave describing the convolutional transpose in two dimensions as an exercise to the reader.

Convolutional block attention also extends intuitively to two dimensions. In this case, the spatial attention map is a matrix A_s in $\mathbb{R}^{h \times w}$ and is able to emphasize or deemphasize elements at any position in the two-dimensional image. The channel attention map is still an element $A_c \in \mathbb{R}^c$.

In order to use attention in two dimensions, we must be able to compute global maximum and global average pooling. $maxpool_{G,c}$ and $avgpool_{G,c}$ are identical to the introduction in Sect. 2.4.1: The aggregation operations are performed along the channel operation to map an element x from $\mathbb{R}^{h \times w \times c} \to \mathbb{R}^{h \times w}$. A_s is obtained as described in Eq. (15).

The operations $maxpool_{G,h \times w}$ and $avgpool_{G,h \times w}$ map an element x from $\mathbb{R}^{h \times w \times c} \to \mathbb{R}^c$. If we think of x as a collection of c matrices with dimensions $h \times w$, this means that for every matrix, we retain only one value, to obtain c values. Besides using these pooling operations across two dimensions, the channel attention map is obtained identically to how it is introduced in Sect. 2.4.2. That is,

$$A_c = \sigma(W_1(W_0(maxpool_{G,h \times w}(x))) + W_1(W_0(avgpool_{G,h \times w}(x)))) \quad (28)$$

for channel attention, or, for efficient channel attention,

$$A_c = \sigma(f_\psi(avgpool_{G,h \times w}(x))). \quad (29)$$

In the case of Eq. (29), $\psi(c)$ is used to determine the $\psi(c) \times \psi(c)$ kernel of f_ψ. Finally, given the input x, the output of convolutional block attention in two dimensions is identical to Eq. (20).

3.3 *COVID-19 Diagnosis from ECGs*

Now that we have extended the notion of a convolutional layer, as well as convolutional block attention, to two dimensions, we may consider how to use these layers to build a model to diagnose COVID-19 from ECGs. At the time of writing, the dataset in question is relatively new, and few studies have been performed using it. We will focus on an existing model that is most relevant to this data and build another model making use of the techniques we described in the previous section.

The authors in [33] propose using a model with six convolutional layers. The first two layers are in sequence and followed by maximum pooling, while the next eight layers alternate between convolutional layers and maximum pooling. Finally, the output is flattened, and two densely connected layers are used. ReLU activations are used for all convolutional and dense layers (except the first convolutional layer, which has no activation function, and the last dense layer, which uses a softmax activation function). All convolutional layers have a 3×3 kernel. The authors name this model *ECG-COVID*. Figure 13 depicts the proposed architecture visually.

We will also compare a model that uses the spatial and channel attention we described in the previous subsection. Because our dataset is small, we will use a model with four blocks $C_B(\cdot)$. Each block will include a convolutional layer, followed by batch normalization, a LeakyReLU activation, dropout, maximum pooling, and attention. Figure 14 shows a single convolutional block. Finally, the

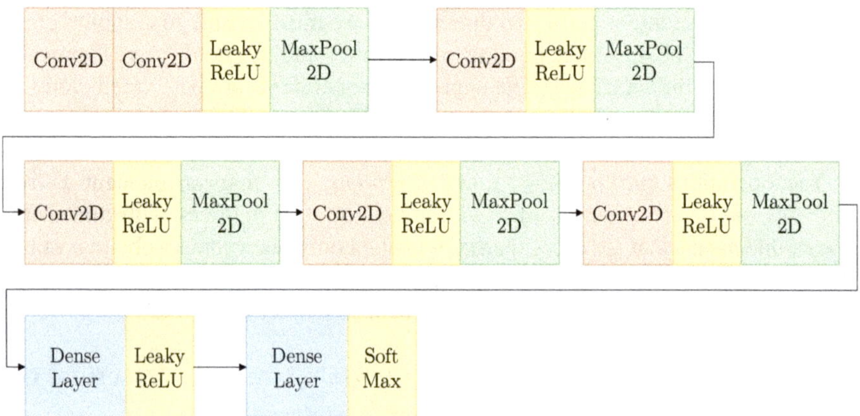

Fig. 13 The model architecture proposed in [33]. The model makes use of convolutional and dense layers

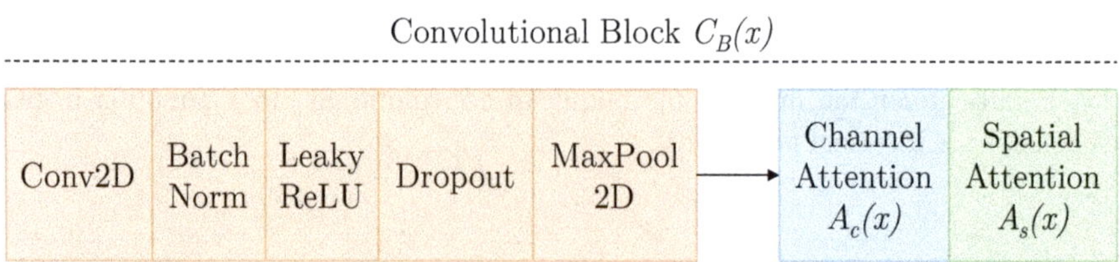

Fig. 14 A convolutional block $C_B(x)$ of the proposed model. The block is similar in structure to the encoder block of CBAM-DAE

output is flattened and fed into two dense layers, similar to ECG-COVID. In our experiments, we also use a 3 × 3 kernel size for convolutional layers.

Denoting the densely connected layers as d_1 and d_2, a LeakyReLU activation as σ_1, a softmax activation as σ_2, and adopting the convention that $C_B^n(x)$ represents n applications of $C_B(\cdot)$ with separate parameters, then we may represent this model, *Attention-ECG-COVID*, as

$$f(x) = \sigma_2(d_2(\sigma_1(d_1(C_B^4(x))))). \tag{30}$$

We use ECG images from healthy patients and patients with COVID in our experiments. Because the dataset is small (there are about 1000 images in total), we use fivefold cross validation and represent any results as the average over the five folds. We use binary cross-entropy loss to train our models and perform training identically to our previous experiment (with learning rate decay and a callback to halt training).

In order to evaluate the performance of each model, we use four evaluation metrics: accuracy, precision, recall, and F1-score. We will denote true positives by TP, false positives FP, true negatives TN, and false negatives FN. Then, the above metrics can be defined as

$$Accuracy = \frac{TP + TN}{TP + TN + FP + FN} \tag{31}$$

$$Precision = \frac{TP}{TP + FP} \tag{32}$$

$$Recall = \frac{TP}{TP + FN} \tag{33}$$

$$F1\text{-}Score = 2\frac{Precision \cdot Recall}{Precision + Recall}. \tag{34}$$

Because the dataset in question is imbalanced (250 ECGs from COVID-19 patients versus 859 from healthy patients), observing precision, recall, and F1-Score alongside accuracy allows us to more holistically view model performance. For example, a trivial classifier (always reporting a patient as healthy) would have approximately 77.5% accuracy, but an F1-Score of 0.

Table 2 gives an overview of the experimental results. Notably, although we removed two convolutional layers from ECG-COVID, adding convolutional block attention seems to have improved the overall performance of the model. Based on our previous discussion, we assume this is because attention allows the model to focus on more important cardiac events that present in COVID-19 patients, such as ST-T changes and conduction defects. Revisiting the example of second-degree atrioventricular block, Mobitz type II, spatial attention might emphasize elements such as non-conducted P-waves, which would then help achieve a more reliable output from a classifier.

Table 2 Summary of experimental results using fivefold cross validation. Results are presented as means of the results on each fold plus or minus standard deviation

Model	Accuracy	Precision	Recall	F1-score
ECG-COVID	98.83 ± 2.36	0.9896 ± 0.0213	0.9883 ± 0.0236	0.9889 ± 0.0253
Attention-ECG-COVID	**99.00** ± 2.24	**0.9908** ± 0.0206	**0.9900** ± 0.0224	**0.9904** ± 0.0238

While we restricted our focus to models that used the types of layers we described earlier in the chapter, other authors have proposed interesting models using other techniques. While the dataset, at the time of writing, is relatively new, we refer the interested reader to [35] and [36], both of which use different techniques than the ones discussed here.

4 Conclusion

In this chapter, we discussed two critical applications of deep learning to electrocardiograms—denoising and diagnosis. Both applications are relevant for the automated diagnosis of sleep disorders. In particular, we discussed how convolutional block attention can improve current methods in denoising ECGs, and we showed further that convolutional block attention can be successfully employed to improve ECG diagnosis methods.

Deep learning with ECGs is a rich field with a wealth of ongoing research. While we have described two methods of working with ECGs, both denoising and diagnosing, the interested reader can find many more applications in the literature.

While we focused on signal processing techniques, viewing the ECG as either a signal or an image, other authors propose different approaches. The field is enriched by the variety of models and techniques that are constantly evolving, and we encourage the interested reader to look further into the literature to keep up with current trends.

Besides being an interesting area of research in its own right, advancements in deep learning with ECGs can also benefit the medical field by enabling doctors to focus on more involved tasks, while machines handle simpler ones. The authors hope that this will lead to better patient care, more accessible doctors, and more equitable healthcare for everyone.

References

1. Pollock, Joshua D., and Amgad N. Makaryus: Physiology, cardiac cycle. StatPearls [Internet]. StatPearls Publishing (2022)
2. Vorvick, Linda: Noninvasive. Medline Plus Medical Encyclopedia (2011).
3. Platonov, Pyotr G: Atrial conduction and atrial fibrillation: what can we learn from surface ECG? Cardiology journal **15**:5, 402–407 (2008)

4. Berkman, Norman L., and Lawrence E. Lamb: The Wolff–Parkinson–White electrocardiogram: a follow-up study of five to twenty-eight years. New England Journal of Medicine **278**:9, 492–494 (1968)
5. Van Mieghem, Carlos, Marc Sabbe, and Daniel Knockaert: The clinical value of the ECG in noncardiac conditions. Chest **125**:4, 1561–1576 (2004)
6. Penzel, Thomas, et al.: Modulations of heart rate, ECG, and cardio-respiratory coupling observed in polysomnography. Frontiers in physiology **7**, 460 (2016)
7. Stein, Phyllis K., and Yachuan Pu.: Heart rate variability, sleep and sleep disorders. Sleep medicine reviews **16**:1, 47–66 (2012)
8. Widasari, Edita Rosana, Koichi Tanno, and Hiroki Tamura: Automatic sleep disorders classification using ensemble of bagged tree based on sleep quality features. Electronics **9**:3, 512 (2020)
9. Xu, Shuting, et al.: A review of automated sleep disorder detection. Computers in Biology and Medicine, 106100 (2022)
10. Kwok, Chun Shing, et al.: Prolonged PR interval, first-degree heart block and adverse cardiovascular outcomes: a systematic review and meta-analysis. Heart **102**:9, 672–680 (2016)
11. Jacek M Leski and Norbert Henzel: ECG baseline wander and powerline interference reduction using nonlinear filter bank. Signal processing, **85**:4, 781–793 (2005)
12. Victor de Pinto. Filters for the reduction of baseline wander and muscle artifact in the ECG. Journal of electrocardiology, **25**, 40–48 (1992)
13. Michael Johannes Rooijakkers, Shuang Song, Chiara Rabotti, S Guid Oei, Jan WM Bergmans, Eugenio Cantatore, and Massimo Mischi: Influence of electrode placement on signal quality for ambulatory pregnancy monitoring. Computational and mathematical methods in medicine (2014)
14. Sarang L Joshi, Rambabu A Vatti, and Rupali V Tornekar. A survey on ECG signal denoising techniques. In 2013 International Conference on Communication Systems and Network Technologies, IEEE, 60–64 (2013)
15. Andrés Ricardo Pérez-Riera, Raimundo Barbosa-Barros, Rodrigo Daminello-Raimundo, and Luiz Carlos de Abreu: Main artifacts in electrocardiography. Annals of Noninvasive Electrocardiology, **23**:2, e12494 (2018)
16. Aslanger, Emre, and Preben Bjerregaard: Mystery of "bizarre electrocardiogram" solved. Journal of electrocardiology **44**:6, 810–811 (2011)
17. Rumelhart, David E., Geoffrey E. Hinton, and Ronald J. Williams: Learning internal representations by error propagation. California Univ San Diego La Jolla Inst for Cognitive Science (1985)
18. Jiang, Yihan, et al.: Turbo autoencoder: Deep learning based channel codes for point-to-point communication channels. Advances in neural information processing systems **32** (2019)
19. Vincent, Pascal, et al.: Extracting and composing robust features with denoising autoencoders. Proceedings of the 25th international conference on Machine learning (2008)
20. Parvaneh, Saman, et al.: Cardiac arrhythmia detection using deep learning: A review. Journal of electrocardiology **57**, S70-S74 (2019)
21. Majumdar, Angshul, and Aditay Tripathi: Asymmetric stacked autoencoder. 2017 International Joint Conference on Neural Networks (IJCNN). IEEE (2017)
22. Mangi, Muhammad Asif, et al.: Atrioventricular block second-degree. StatPearls [Internet]. StatPearls Publishing (2021)
23. Yuan, Li, et al.: Volo: Vision outlooker for visual recognition. IEEE Transactions on Pattern Analysis and Machine Intelligence (2022)
24. Vaswani, Ashish, et al.: Attention is all you need. Advances in neural information processing systems **30** (2017)
25. Woo, Sanghyun, et al.: Cbam: Convolutional block attention module. Proceedings of the European conference on computer vision. (2018)
26. Wang, Qilong, Banggu Wu, Pengfei Zhu, Peihua Li, Wangmeng Zuo, and Qinghua Hu: ECA-Net: Efficient channel attention for deep convolutional neural networks. In Proceedings of the

IEEE/CVF conference on computer vision and pattern recognition, pp. 11534–11542. IEEE (2020)
27. He, Kaiming, Xiangyu Zhang, Shaoqing Ren, and Jian Sun: Deep residual learning for image recognition. In Proceedings of the IEEE conference on computer vision and pattern recognition, pp. 770–778. IEEE (2016)
28. Moody, George B., Roger G. Mark, and Ary L. Goldberger: PhysioNet: a web-based resource for the study of physiologic signals. IEEE Engineering in Medicine and Biology Magazine 20, **3**, 70–75 (2001)
29. Romero, Francisco P., David C. Piñol, and Carlos R. Vázquez-Seisdedos: DeepFilter: An ECG baseline wander removal filter using deep learning techniques. Biomedical Signal Processing and Control **70**, 102992 (2021)
30. Nygaard, Ranveig, Gerry Melnikov, and Aggelos K. Katsaggelos: A rate distortion optimal ECG coding algorithm. IEEE Transactions on biomedical engineering **48**(1), 28–40 (2001)
31. Němcové, A., Smíšek, R., Maršánová, L., Smital, L., and Vítek, M: A comparative analysis of methods for evaluation of ECG signal quality after compression. BioMed research international (2018)
32. Bhat, Sushanth, and Chokroverty, Sudhansu: Sleep disorders and COVID-19. Sleep medicine **91**(1), 253–261 (2022)
33. Khan, A. H., Hussain, M., and Malik, M. K.: ECG Images dataset of Cardiac and COVID-19 Patients. Data in Brief **34**, 106762 (2021).
34. Kaliyaperumal D, Bhargavi K, Ramaraju K, Nair KS, Ramalingam S, and Alagesan M.: Electrocardiographic Changes in COVID-19 Patients: A Hospital-based Descriptive Study. Indian J Crit Care Med. **26**(1), 43–48 (2022)
35. Rahman, Tawsifur, et al.: COV-ECGNET: COVID-19 detection using ECG trace images with deep convolutional neural network. Health Information Science and Systems **10**(1) (2022)
36. Attallah, Omneya. ECG-BiCoNet: An ECG-based pipeline for COVID-19 diagnosis using Bi-Layers of deep features integration. Computers in biology and medicine **142**, 105210 (2022)

Machine Learning Automated Analysis Applied to Mandibular Jaw Movements During Sleep: A Window on Polysomnography

Jean-Benoit Martinot, Nhat-Nam Le-Dong, and Jean-Louis Pépin

1 Introduction

The application of data science and artificial intelligence (AI) to bio-signal analysis is not necessarily a revolutionary process, but rather follows on from studies in medical physiology. Thus, the use of data science and AI in bio-signal analysis is just one step further along the journey of studying the physio-pathological processes captured by bio-signals such as electrocardiogram (ECG), electroencephalogram (EEG), and electromyogram (EMG).

Most machine learning experiments on bio-signals have been conducted by a shortcut, where data scientists have direct access to a public or experimental bio-signal dataset and then attempt to find the optimal solution for a special classification task, such as sleep staging identification or apneas and hypopneas detection during sleep. Using this approach, the physiological relationship between the signal under investigation and the targeted outcomes is implicitly accepted. In contrast, the application of mandibular jaw movements (MJM) as a surrogate bio-signal in sleep medicine is a special case. MJM is a completely new type of bio-signal and therefore

J.-B. Martinot (✉)
Sleep Laboratory, CHU Université Catholique de Louvain (UCL) Namur Site Sainte-Elisabeth, Namur, Belgium

Institute of Experimental and Clinical Research, UCL Bruxelles Woluwe, Brussels, Belgium
e-mail: martinot.j@respisom.be

N.-N. Le-Dong
Sunrise, Namur, Belgium

J.-L. Pépin
HP2 Laboratory, Inserm U1300, University Grenoble Alpes, Grenoble, France

R. B. Berry et al. (eds.), *Handbook of AI and Data Sciences for Sleep Disorders*, Springer Optimization and Its Applications 216,
https://doi.org/10.1007/978-3-031-68263-6_10

a solid foundation about its physiological significance and clinical utility in sleep-disordered breathing (SDB) needed to be established first.

Several clinical and experimental studies were conducted between 2014 and 2021 to answer the following three important questions:

1. Association between MJM bio-signal properties and physiological and pathological processes during sleep: Is there a relationship between the change in the MJM bio-signal during sleep and similar effects on reference signals such as esophageal pressure (PES) or diaphragmatic EMG?
2. Feasibility of the machine learning classification task: Are the target events associated with specific MJM bio-signal patterns? Could these patterns be identified, at least manually by human visual perception?
3. Compatibility with the conventional framework: The agreement between the MJM bio-signal derived metrics and conventional polysomnography (PSG) indices needs to be determined, along with the diagnostic value of the MJM surrogate indices.

2 Question 1: Association Between MJM Bio-Signal Properties and Clinical Features of Respiratory Disturbances During Sleep

The upper airway muscles are involved in complex interactions that allow prioritization or combination of breathing, swallowing, speech, and/or masticatory activities. The mandibular jaw plays a central role in all these oro-facial functions [1]. As a result of these different activities, awake MJM are highly variable, often fast, and unpredictable in amplitude and frequency [2, 3] (Fig. 1). During sleep, the upper airway patency depends on a delicate dynamic balance and, from a mechanics standpoint, this is a "critically stable" system where the mandibular jaw is leveraged for strengthening the pharyngeal walls [4, 5]. During sleep, MJM occur at the breathing frequency in the range of 0.15–0.60 Hz [6]. This strongly suggests that MJM become primarily driven by the brainstem, specifically by the motor nucleus of the motor branch of the trigeminal nerve located in the mid pons [7]. This branch of the fifth cranial nerve provides motor nerves to the agonist and antagonist muscles of the mandible. The drive from these motor nerves generates cyclical breathing MJM as soon as non-rapid eye movement (NREM) stage N1 light sleep is scored on the EEG, based on a specific ratio of theta/alpha waves [8] (Fig. 1). A tight connectivity between the motor trigeminal nerves and the respiratory centers in the brainstem explains these observations. Similar connectivities are well known between the hypoglossal nucleus for tongue movements during sleep and the spinal nuclei for activity of the diaphragm or other accessory respiratory muscles [7]. It is essential that the pharynx stiffens before diaphragmatic contraction because this is accompanied by a decrease in airway pressure that can destabilize pharyngeal caliber. This negative pressure reflex is likely involved in the recruitment

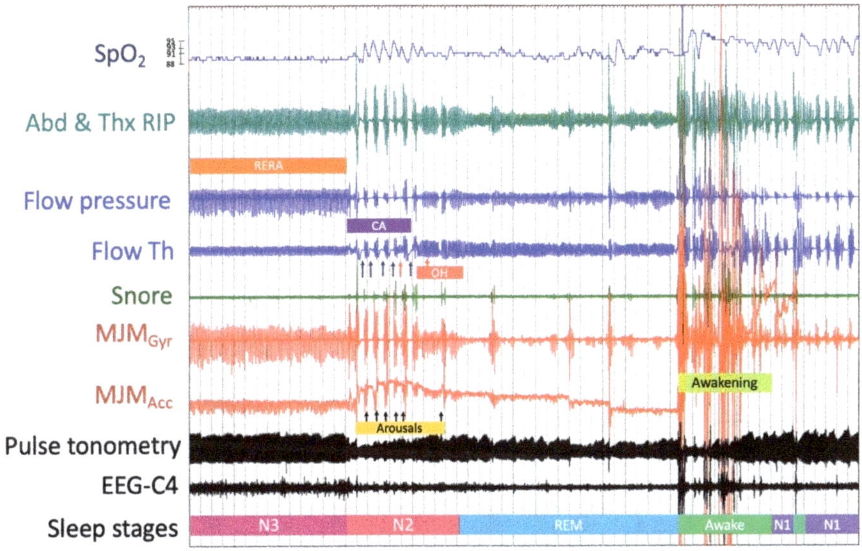

Fig. 1 A 30-minute fragment of polysomnography (PSG) including the mandibular jaw movement (MJM) bio-signal. This fragment shows a long period of respiratory effort related arousal (RERA) and then successive episodes of apneas, a period of REM sleep followed by awakening, and finally N1 sleep stage where mandibular jaw movements (MJM) oscillate at the breathing frequency. The period of RERA is highlighted by high MJM amplitudes measured by the gyroscope (MJM_{Gyr}). The following apneas are of central nature (CA) with a decrease in the respiratory drive. Then, obstructive hypopneas occur (OH). The REM sleep stage exhibits irregular frequencies and changing amplitudes of MJM that are on average smaller compared to non-REM sleep MJM amplitudes. Awakening is marked by larger mandibular displacements at a non-predictable frequency. Arousals scored based on EEG/EMG channels are depicted by the black arrows on the MJM_{Acc} channel. From the top to the bottom: SpO_2: peripheral oxygen saturation; rib cage and abdominal movements captured by respiratory inductive plethysmography (RIP); nasal airflow pressure captured by the canulae; oral nasal thermistor; snore monitored by a microphone; mandibular jaw movements (MJM) recorded by the gyroscope (MJM_{Gyr}) and accelerometer (MJM_{Acc}) included in the inertial unit of the Sunrise technology; pulse tonometry captured by photoplethysmography (PPG); sleep/wake states and sleep stages based on EEG, EOG, EMG scoring (only EEG-C4 channel is shown)

of trigeminal motoneurons and the resulting MJM, and this is enabled by brainstem inter-connectivity [1, 9–11]. While many of the pharyngeal muscles are attached to the mandible directly, or indirectly via the hyoid bone, the central drive utilizes the lower jaw as a fine-tuning lever to stiffen the upper airway musculature and safeguard the patency of the pharynx.

While the PSG is still the conventional method for diagnosis and management of SDB, recent progresses in bio-signal computing technology led to the development of an alternative solution, with the possibility of using a single point of contact sensor and AI for personalized sleep test at home. The overall concept is to simulate the PSG manual scoring process by using a machine learning algorithm (Fig. 2). The algorithm can identify typical patterns in surrogate MJM bio-signals

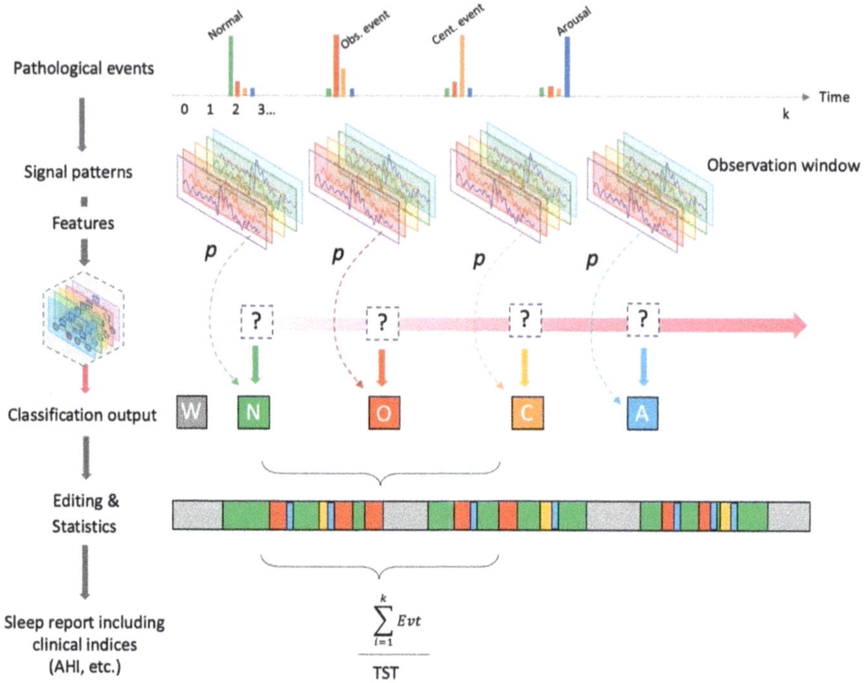

Fig. 2 Machine learning–based procedure to estimate clinical indices from mandibular jaw movement (MJM) bio-signals. The automated analysis procedure aims to evaluate sleep structure and to identify the occurrence of pathological events during sleep, including respiratory disturbance events and respiratory disturbance induced arousals. Since target events are associated with specific patterns of MJM bio-signals, the classification task can be handled by a machine learning algorithm. The outputs generated by the machine model allow estimation of the clinical scores for clinical decision-making. Cent. central, Obs. obstructive, TST total sleep time. N = normal; O = obstructive event; C = central event; A = arousal

which are related to physiological or pathological events such as sleep stages [6], arousals, apneas, hypopneas [12], respiratory effort-related arousals (RERAs), or other masticatory muscle activities [13, 14]. Then, the output of the classification task can be transformed into clinical scores.

Basic research on the physiological mechanisms of MJM signaling in SDB is of great importance. Published studies have provided strong evidence for the specific association between the MJM bio-signal and pathological events, such as SDB characterized by a change in RE [15]. Studying time-series data of bio-signals allows to determine the mechanism and the origin of the changes in signal patterns, and whether these changes are directly associated with the event, are just a coincidence, or a secondary effect following the event.

For example, it is commonly observed in the clinical setting that a displacement of the lower jaw is associated with an arousal at the end of a period of obstructive apnea or hypopnea during sleep, especially in presence of gasping and choking episodes. The underlying mechanism of this observation has been investigated in the past by many physiologists [16–20]. However, a causal relationship between those events has only been conclusively established in 2020 by Martinot et al. [21]. In their experiment on raw signals of MJM, nasal airflow pressure and concurrent surface EMG activity of the masseters were recorded before, during, and after increased respiratory effort (RE) induced arousals. Based on a descriptive sequence analysis, they found that vertical mandibular displacements were directly associated to the EMG-masseteric activity while mandibular displacement always occurred before the effective change in nasal airflow. By using the Brodersen's causal impact model [22], the authors also demonstrated a significant causal impact of the vertical mandibular displacement on the airflow amplitude. Vertical mandible depression (mouth opening) was associated with a median (95% CI) reduction in nasal airflow of 40.9% (14.6–71.3%), while vertical mandible elevation (mouth closure) was associated with a median (95% CI) relative increase in airflow after arousal of 52.6% (17.9–56.2%).

Such findings contributed to the evidences of rationality and reliability of the machine learning solution involving the MJM bio-signal. On the other hand, the lack of causality between sleep/awake status and wrist actigraphy signals can explain why the sleep/awake detection algorithms based on this type of signal are less accurate than implied EEG signals [23]. The use of explainable AI is also key to convince clinicians of the robustness of the findings and to facilitate dissemination in routine clinical care.

The capturing technology and bio-signal preprocessing are other important factors. The earliest studies validating the clinical use of MJM relied on a magnetometry sensor (Nomics, Liège, Belgium) [2, 3, 6, 12, 24–27]. For example, physiologists demonstrated in 2017 a significant correlation between MJM amplitudes and the reference endo-esophageal diaphragmatic EMG (EMG-d) signal to estimate changes in RE during sleep [3]. Variations in MJM amplitudes indicated similar patterns to those observed with EMG-d activity with a clear contrast between normal breathing, obstructive, mixed, and central apnea periods. MJM amplitudes approximately increased by 0.28 mm for each 10 μV of increase in EMG-d activity.

Since 2017, MJM can also be captured by a single point of contact sensor attached to the patient's chin (in the mentolabial sulcus) (Sunrise, Namur, Belgium) [8, 15, 28]. Compared with magnetometry, this coin-sized, tri-axial sensor including a gyroscope and an accelerometer has some advantages, including a higher signal resolution and the ability to record MJM in three dimensions (rather than only vertical movements). Even though there are similarities between the two types of sensors in terms of signal frequency during normal or disordered breathing characterized by changes in RE level and common specific patterns related to arousals, data processing is different. The machine learning algorithm of the magnetometry device utilizes only one channel, whereas the Sunrise algorithm uses six channels of raw data (x, y, z components of the gyroscope and accelerometer) providing different information at a given time, one channel being more informative than another (better reflecting the pattern associated with the target event) depending on the head position. Moreover, a strict parallelism between the two magnets is required with the magnetometry device in order to optimize the signal/noise ratio and can be difficult to obtain during self-setting up at home.

A study published in 2021 established a clear relationship between signals recorded by the tri-axial chin sensor and PES, which is the gold-standard signal for quantitative measurement of RE [15]. This analysis was based on 8042 data blocks extracted from the PES and simultaneous MJM recordings of 38 patients. These sequences included periods of normal breathing, obstructive apnea/hypopnea or central apnea/hypopnea, RERAs, and mixed apnea. The results showed that the amplitude of both the PES and MJM bio-signals provided statistically efficient differentiation between central and obstructive events, and between apneas and hypopneas. Obstructive events were characterized by higher values of MJM amplitudes across all quartiles and a wider range of MJM amplitudes compared with central events. There was also a proportional relationship between PES and MJM amplitudes in obstructive hypopneas and obstructive apneas. In addition, there was a high level of synchronization between PES and MJM signal sequences, with median similarity scores of 0.82–0.99.

3 Question 2: Solving a Machine Learning Task with the MJM Bio-Signal

The potential application of MJM bio-signals in the field of sleep medicine has been extensively studied. As early as 2007, the MJM bio-signal was integrated into PSG recordings in some sleep laboratories as a surrogate signal for monitoring respiratory movements. Through observational studies and manual scoring process, physiologists have recognized the polyvalence of the MJM bio-signal. It has been showed that the MJM bio-signal allows to identify wake/sleep states [2, 25], arousals, apnea, and hypopnea events [12, 29]. Naturally, advances in science and technology led to a higher level of expectation: building a computed analysis tool for this new bio-signal. However, the process from observational findings to a complete machine learning–based solution was not straightforward. Some important technical issues impacting the success of machine learning model development on MJM bio-signals are discussed below.

3.1 Constructing a Good Machine Learning Task

Setting-up a good machine learning task has a significant impact on the performance of the solution and its suitability for clinical application. First, a balance between practical application, complexity, and feasibility of the task needs to be achieved. A good example is the sleep stage classification task, which could be approached at different levels of complexity. The simplest task would consist of a binary classifier to differentiate sleep from wake state. Adopted by many actigraphy-based sleep trackers, this model would be sufficient to estimate the most basic parameters, including total sleep time (TST), sleep efficiency (SE), awake after sleep onset (WASO), and sleep onset latency (SOL). However, it would not allow differentiation between sleep stages.

A three-class classification task would target three sleep stages: awake, non-REM sleep (including stages N1, N2, and N3), and REM sleep. This model would allow determination of REM latency (with application in individuals with narcolepsy) or rate of apnea-hypopnea events specifically associated with REM sleep.

Ideally, the perfect model should handle the classification of all five sleep stages, including N1, N2, N3, REM, and awake. This would allow a standard hypnogram to be established, equivalent to the PSG outcome. Tasks of this complexity have usually been applied to EEG signals but might be impossible for a mono-signal-based sleep tracker.

An alternative approach that provides a compromise between the level of complexity and clinical utility is a four-class sleep staging model. By combining N1 and N2 as "light sleep" and separating deep sleep (N3) and REM sleep, conventional clinical indices can be achieved using the MJM bio-signal. This approach was used in 2021 to develop a sleep staging classification task using only MJM bio-signals recorded with the Sunrise device [8]. This study was conducted in a large dataset of 1026 adults with suspected obstructive sleep apnea (OSA). Using the extreme gradient boosting (XGBoost) classifier as the core algorithm, a machine learning sleep staging algorithm was trained using overnight PSG data and simultaneous MJM recordings from 800 participants. The algorithm automatically classified each 30-second epoch of MJM patterns as wake, light non-REM (N1 + N2), deep non-REM (N3), or REM stage sleep. Validated on unseen data from 226 subjects, the algorithm classified sleep epochs with substantial qualitative agreement to manual PSG scorers (Kappa = 0.71 and accuracy = 78.3%).

It should be noted that the target labels are mutually exclusive. This is why certainty is needed about the specificity and uniqueness of a pathophysiological event compared with other potential outcomes when considering that event as an output of the machine learning model. Sometimes, several events could be integrated into a composite group if those events have highly similar signal patterns. Eventually, introducing a label beyond the scope of the task must be considered to optimize the specificity of classification. For example, a classifier task that handles the detection of an apnea or hypopnea event should also target arousals because an arousal is associated with a specific MJM signal pattern that could be recaptured within the sampling window. Differentiating arousals from an adjacent respiratory event would improve the model's accuracy during the transition from a respiratory disturbance to normal breathing during sleep.

In another machine learning experiment which aimed to identify the rhythmic masticatory muscles activities (RMMA) in patients with sleep bruxism by using MJM bio-signals [30], the authors demonstrated that the target RMMA label should be isolated from arousals and baseline breathing pattern, rather than applying a simple binary classification task. Indeed, the model validation showed that $F1$

scores were 0.83, 0.82, and 0.95 for RMMA events, arousals, and MJM at the breathing frequency, respectively. Thus, adding the arousal label would improve the classification performance for RMMA events.

3.2 Sampling Window

The size of the sampling window is an important factor that determines the measurement precision for time-based clinical indices. For example, the optimal size of a sampling window should be 30 seconds for the sleep staging classification task to allow the precision of TST, SOL, WASO, SE, or REM latency measurements to be equivalent to that of PSG scoring. The sampling window size has also an important impact on the feasibility and performance of the model. In the respiratory event classification task, the window size should be sufficiently long to recapture the specific signal pattern of every target event, including obstructive/central hypopneas, apneas, and RERAs. The length of those events could vary from 8 seconds to several minutes. Practically, the optimal window length should ensure that the target event can still be visually identified after data segmentation. However, if the window is too long, this could bias the analysis by mixing the signal pattern of interest with noise and adjacent components. Conversely, if the window is too short, a long event may be fragmented into multiple shorter events, which would result in overestimation of the corresponding index. A shorter window also limits the data sampling space and does not allow the model to recognize all characteristics determining the target event. The window size is also an optimizing factor for computation cost when classification is handled in real time. For all these reasons, the size of sampling windows should be carefully determined based on a rational analysis rather than on an arbitrary decision. Based on visual explorations and statistical analysis, it has been determined that a sampling window of 10 seconds would be optimal for the classification of arousals, obstructive and central events using the tri-axial chin sensor capturing MJM bio-signals.

3.3 Selecting a Machine Learning Algorithm

Different approaches for the classification task have been applied in sleep medicine. The earliest solutions consisted of simple threshold-based decision rules. Later, machine learning algorithms became mainstream. The most popular algorithms include linear discriminant (LDA), probabilistic models like Hidden Markov model (HMM), Support Vector machine (SVM), and Random Forest (RF). Recently, some authors also used deep learning (long short-term memory (LSTM), one-dimensional or two-dimensional convolutional neural networks (CNNs) and hybrid structure). The use of machine learning algorithms has significantly improved the ability to obtain insights from raw signals or high dimensional features sets. These models have clear advantages over the earlier threshold-based decision rules.

However, the efficiency of the model for a specific task depends on multiple factors including the signal composition, feature set, and data structure (but not on the algorithm alone). Based on the reported data, it is not clear yet whether any specific algorithm is superior to another. Based on machine learning on MJM bio-signals, once the problem is clearly defined and the corresponding signal patterns are well established, the algorithm alone is not a key factor because the handcrafted feature extraction and structured data-driven algorithms (e.g., RF and XGBoost) perform as well as, or even better, than a deep learning model. The handcrafted feature extraction procedure allows also better control and understanding of input data compared with black-box models such as a CNN. The XGBoost is a good choice because this algorithm dominates the classification tasks on structured data and offers several advantages over classical methods (e.g., SVM, RF) including high efficiency in computation and resources, and allowing a very fast training and execution speed.

4 Question 3: Agreement Between MJM Bio-Signal Derived Metrics and Conventional PSG Indices

Achieving a high performance for the classification task is not the end of the road because the goal is not only to classify among defined labels but also to accurately produce conventional clinical scores, such as those provided by the PSG. Ultimately, all validations must imply a quantitative agreement analysis and a diagnostic performance analysis. A 2020 review on diversity in study designs and statistical analytic methods in validation studies for OSA testing devices proposed requirements that should be considered for a high-quality clinical validation study [31]. The study population should include both healthy subjects and individuals diagnosed with SDB to some extent. The clinical condition would determine both the application and measurement ranges for a specific index. For example, validation on a mixed population including individuals with insomnia or hypersomnia would require a longer measurement scale of TST (200–1000 minutes), which is much greater than that in a standard population of OSA patients (TST of 250–500 minutes). In addition, outcomes should cover at least the primary indices such as TST, SE, apnea-hypopnea index (AHI), and respiratory disturbance index (RDI). A Bland-Altman analysis is recommended as the main analytic method for evaluating the agreement with AHI sensitivity and specificity at conventional cutoffs (i.e., at 5, 15, and 30 events/h) determining the utility for clinical diagnosis, which is independent of the prevalence of OSA in the study sample.

The clinical validation of a machine learning–based home sleep test based on MJM recording (Sunrise, Namur, Belgium) was published in 2020 [20]. The structure of this system is described in Fig. 3. The core algorithm implied a

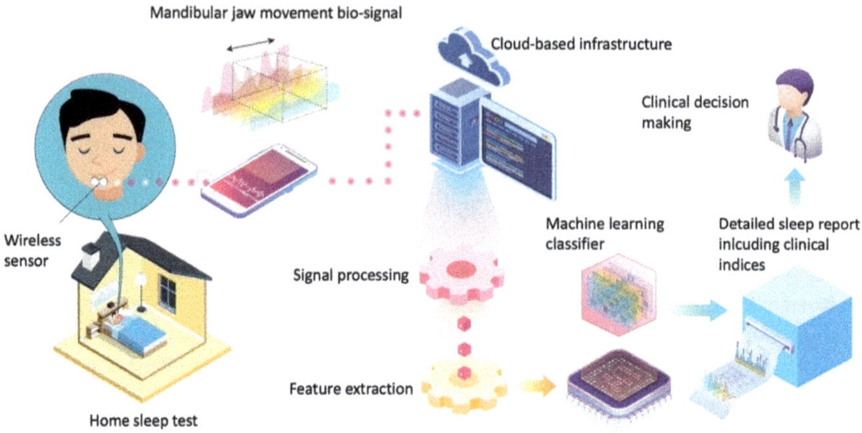

Fig. 3 Overview on structure of a machine learning–based home sleep test utilizing the mandibular jaw movement (MJM) bio-signal. The system consists of three elements: (1) A compact, wireless, single point of contact sensor placed on the chin of the tested subject; (2) a smartphone user interface; (3) a cloud-based infrastructure for data storage and analysis. The sleep test is carried out at home. During sleep, the sensor acquires MJM bio-signals that are transferred to the smartphone application via Bluetooth for external control. At the end of the night, raw data is transferred via wireless connection to the cloud-based platform that has a certified protocol to ensure security and confidentiality of medical data. Raw data is passed through a preprocessing algorithm, then a feature extraction algorithm generates specific input data for the machine learning analysis. This procedure performs at least two classification tasks: (1) sleep staging identification with ability to classify four sleep stages including wake, light non-REM (N1 + N2), deep non-REM (N3), and REM stage sleep, and (2) sleep disturbances detection including obstructive/central apneas, hypopneas, and arousals. Finally, the output of these machine learning tasks is integrated and automatically converted into a clinical score provided in a detailed report, available for clinicians via a secure portal within minutes after the test

RF multiclass classifier and statistical features. The agreement between the new MJM-based technology and reference in-laboratory PSG for determination of the obstructive RDI (ORDI) was evaluated in 376 adults with suspected OSA. The results showed a reliable agreement between PSG-ORDI and MJM-ORDI in subjects without OSA ($n = 46$; mean difference of 1.31 events/h; 95% confidence interval [CI] −1.05, 3.66) and in patients with a PSG-ORDI of at least 5 events/h and symptoms of OSA ($n = 107$; mean difference of −0.69 events/h; 95% CI −3.77, 2.38). In patients with the most severe OSA, the MJM-based system was found to underestimate ORDI compared with PSG (difference of −11.74 events/h; 95% CI −20.83, −2.67). At the two optimal cutoff values of 7.63 and 12.65 events/h, the MJM-ORDI had an accuracy of 0.92 (95% CI 0.90–0.94) and 0.88 (95% CI 0.86–0.90); post-test probabilities were 0.99 (95% CI 0.99–0.99) and 0.89 (95% CI 0.88–0.91) when the PSG-ORDI was at least 5 events/h and at least 15 events/h, respectively. This corresponds to positive likelihood ratios of 14.86 (95% CI 9.86–30.12) and 5.63 (95% CI 4.92–7.27), respectively.

In another study, the agreement and diagnostic capabilities of the MJM-ORDI were validated against in-laboratory PSG in 140 pediatric patients (aged 3–17 years) referred for clinically suspected OSA [32]. According to the International Classification of Sleep Disorders, Third Edition (ICSD-3), OSA diagnosis and severity in pediatric patients are defined as an obstructive AHI (OAHI) of $\geq$1 event/h (mild), $\geq$5 events/h (moderate), and $\geq$10 events/h (severe). A Bland-Altman analysis showed a median measurement bias of 1.57 events/h (95% CI −2.49, 8.11) between MJM-ORDI and PSG-ORDI. At optimal thresholds of 5.75, 9.61, and 13.07 events/h, MJM-ORDI detected individuals with PSG-based OAHI of $\geq$1, $\geq$5, and $\geq$10 events/h with an accuracy of 68%, 85%, and 94%, respectively. These rules allowed the detection of mild OSA with a good sensitivity (82%), moderate OSA with very good balanced sensitivity (90%) and specificity (80%), and showed excellent performance for the detection of severe OSA (sensitivity 100%, specificity 88%). Based on this data, the MJM-based simplified diagnosis framework is highly reliable for the detection of moderate-to-severe OSA in pediatric patients, a group where therapeutic intervention is clearly indicated.

The latest publication directly related to the Sunrise MJM-based system consists of a machine learning experiment for detecting phasic sleep bruxism using only the MJM bio-signal [18]. The study included 67 individuals with suspected OSA. The classification task was to detect stereotypical MJM associated with RMMA. A XGBoost multiclass classifier was trained on 79,650 10-second epochs of MJM data from 39 subjects with a history of sleep bruxism targeting three labels: RMMA episodes (n = 1072), arousals (n = 1311), and baseline MJM at the breathing frequency (n = 77,267). Validated on unseen data from 28 subjects, the model showed very good epoch-by-epoch agreement (Kappa = 0.799) and balanced accuracy of 86.6%. The RMMA episodes were detected with a sensitivity of 84.3%. There was good agreement between the MJM analytic model and manual EMG signal scoring of RMMA (median bias of −0.80 events/h, 95% CI –9.77, 2.85). These results support the reliability of the Sunrise MJM-based device for detecting sleep bruxism.

5 Clinical Case Report

In this section, we present a real-life case study (from which raw data are available upon reasonable request) where we applied automated analysis of the MJM bio-signal. We were able to identify typical patterns of the MJM bio-signal that correspond to various breathing disturbances, including changes in RE and arousal, compared to conventional PSG signals. Additionally, we demonstrated that a machine learning–based estimator can accurately estimate manual PSG scoring derived indices from input data that includes only MJM bio-signals.

The case involves a 54-year-old male patient with typical OSA symptoms, such as loud snoring and morning headaches, and an Epworth Sleepiness Scale (ESS) score of 7. The patient had been treated with bisoprolol (5 mg once a day) for systemic arterial hypertension for 10 years. On physical examination, the patient weighed 77 kg, had a body mass index (BMI) of 27.3 kg/m^2, and a neck circumference of 41 cm. The oropharyngeal examination was normal, with no tonsils.

The patient underwent a type 1 PSG in a laboratory setting (Somnoscreen Plus type-I acquisition system (Somnomedics, Randersacker, Germany)). This system included EEG recordings from Fz−A+, Cz−A+, and Pz−A+, as well as right and left electro-oculogram (EOG), submental EMG, respiratory motion measurements via respiratory inductance plethysmography (RIP) bands (SLP Inc., Elgin, USA), and measurements of nasal and oral airflow using a pressure transducer and thermistor, respectively. Additionally, oxygen saturation levels were monitored using a digital oximeter that displayed pulse waveform (Nonin Medical Inc., Plymouth, USA). PSG data was scored by two experienced investigators, following the recommended criteria established by the American Academy of Sleep Medicine (AASM) manual for the scoring of sleep and associated events [33, 34].

During the sleep study, MJM was simultaneously monitored using a wireless tri-axial single point of contact sensor attached to the chin (Sunrise, Namur, Belgium). At the end of the night, recorded MJM data was automatically transferred to a cloud-based infrastructure. A dedicated machine learning algorithm was used for data analysis, which was conducted blindly to the manual PSG scoring process.

Figure 4a presents a 10-minute excerpt of PSG, incorporating MJM channels after manual PSG scoring. During this period, changes in respiratory drive level are depicted by the MJM_{Gyr} and MJM_{Acc} bio-signals recorded by the gyroscope and accelerometer of the capturing technology, respectively, in relation to the corresponding changes in the pressure flow waveform (especially the high-frequency oscillations on the plateau of the curve). This fragment includes central apneas (A) during N1 stage, followed by obstructive hypopneas (H) where the respiratory drive increases. This is well illustrated by the increasing amplitude of MJM (MJM_{Gyr}) until an arousal occurs to peak the airflow (also marked on the RIP bands signal), while the pharynx is not fully re-open (as observed through the nasal pressure curve oscillations). RE is also highlighted by the occurrence of snoring. Interestingly, the RE level is changing from one cycle to another during the obstructive hypopnea as emphasized by the red horizontal arrow, showing an opening of the mouth along a distance of 1.2 mm (see the black arrow on the MJM_{Acc} channel) before an arousal occurs. This example illustrates how well RE is depicted through the changes in MJM amplitudes in relation to the other PSG routine signals.

Figure 4b shows the overnight trends of the different signals. The temporal association is well depicted between the mandibular displacements calculated from the rotational speed measured by the gyroscope, and the scored events (respiratory disturbances and arousals) as well as periods of oxygen desaturations and snoring. RERAs are highlighted by a sustained increase in the respiratory drive (illustrated by the MJM_{Gyr} channel reflecting the rotational speed of the mandible). Concomitantly, changes in the position of the mandible are well depicted by the accelerometer (MJM_{Acc} channel). REM sleep stage is marked by a contrasted mandibular behavior

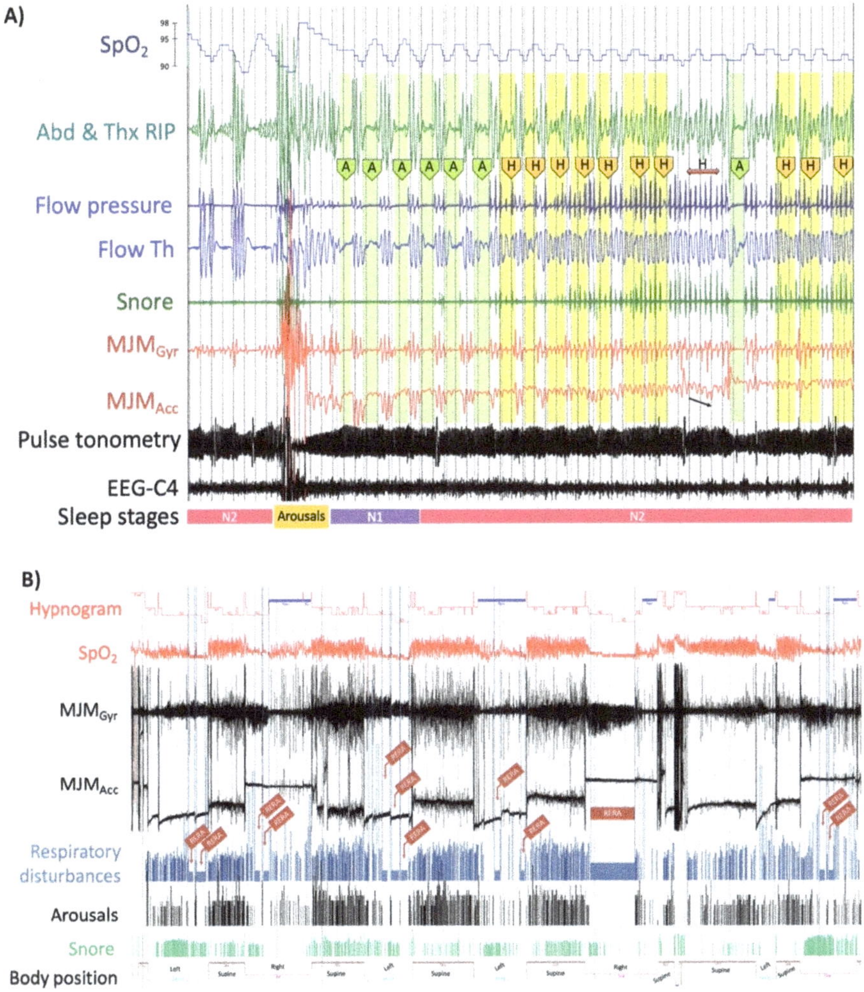

Fig. 4 Case report illustration. From the top to the bottom: SpO_2: peripheral oxygen saturation; rib cage and abdominal movements captured by respiratory inductive plethysmography (RIP); nasal airflow pressure captured by the canulae; oral nasal thermistor; snore monitored by a microphone; mandibular jaw movements (MJM) recorded by the gyroscope (MJM_{Gyr}) and accelerometer (MJM_{Acc}) included in the inertial unit of the Sunrise technology; pulse tonometry captured by photoplethysmography (PPG); sleep/wake states and sleep stages based on EEG, EOG, EMG scoring (only EEG-C4 channel is shown). **(a)** A 10-minute excerpt of PSG recording with MJM channels incorporated. Explored channels, from top to bottom: peripheral oxygen saturation (SpO_2); rib cage and abdominal movements captured by respiratory inductive plethysmography (RIP); nasal airflow pressure captured by the canulae; oral nasal thermistor; snoring monitored by a microphone; mandibular jaw movements (MJM) recorded by the gyroscope (MJMGyr) and accelerometer (MJMAcc) included in the inertial unit of the Sunrise technology; pulse tonometry captured by photoplethysmography (PPG); electroencephalogram (EEG, only C4 channel is shown). Event labelling: A = central apneas; H = obstructive apneas. Sleep staging was based on EEG, EOG, EMG manual scoring. **(b)** Overnight trends of the different signals including MJM bio-signals. Explored channels, from top to bottom: hypnogram; peripheral oxygen saturation (SpO_2); mandibular jaw movements (MJM) recorded by the gyroscope (MJMGyr) and accelerometer (MJMAcc); sleep respiratory disturbances; arousals; snoring; and body positions

Table 1 Comparison of the sleep test outcome between the two techniques (PSG and Sunrise MJM-based technology)

Parameters	Unit	True value (PSG scoring)	Machine learning–based estimation
Total sleep time	Minutes	452.50	450.00
Light sleep	%	74.14	73.23
Deep sleep	%	6.19	5.02
REM sleep	%	19.67	21.75
Sleep efficiency	%	92.81	92.30
SOL	Minutes	9.52	12.25
WASO	Minutes	25.02	25.28
Awakening index	n/h	2.78	2.60
REM latency	Minutes	83.00	75.50
AHI	n/h	65.40	67.33
OAHI	n/h	60.30	65.48
CAHI	n/h	5.10	1.85
RDI	n/h	78.00	74.29
ArI	n/h	71.40	74.29

with, in mean, a reduced signal amplitude on the MJM_{Gyr} channel. In this patient, OSA is positional.

As showed in Table 1, there is a clinically acceptable agreement between results obtained by manual PSG scoring and those estimated from the automated analysis of MJM. Results from both methods confirmed that this patient had severe OSA with an AHI of 65.4 and 67.3 events/hour, respectively, and required continuous positive airway pressure (CPAP) therapeutic intervention.

6 Conclusion

A strong and specific comprehensive physiological association has been documented between the MJM bio-signal and related periods of normal or disturbed breathing, arousals, and different sleep stages. The robust inertial unit included in the capturing technology and overnight positional stability of the sensor provide a bio-signal that can be used in algorithmic analysis. Moreover, and independently to the algorithmic analysis, the MJM bio-signal can be displayed on the screen as a function of time like any standard PSG signal (e.g., airflow, oxygen saturation) and interpreted in the context of the target period of breathing and its associated RE level. These fundamental characteristics of the MJM bio-signal contrast with photoplethysmography (PPG), airflow, or oxygen saturation signals that report more about the consequence of the disturbed breathing than about the event itself.

References

1. Bianchi, A. L., & Gestreau, C. (2009). The brainstem respiratory network: an overview of a half century of research. Respiratory Physiology & Neurobiology, 168(1–2), 4–12.
2. Senny F., Destiné J., Poirrier R., Midsagittal jaw movements as a sleep/wake marker, IEEE Trans Biomed Eng. 2009; 56: 303–9.
3. Senny F, Destiné J, Poirrier R. (2008). Midsagittal jaw movement analysis for the scoring of sleep apneas and hypopneas. IEEE Trans Biomed Eng, 55 (1), 87–95.
4. Isono Shiroh. Contribution of obesity and craniofacial abnormalities to pharyngeal collapsibility in patients with obstructive sleep apnea. Sleep and Biological Rhythms 2004; 2:17–21.
5. Indu Ayappa, David M Rapoport. The upper airway in sleep: physiology of the pharynx. Sleep Med Rev. 2003;7(1):9–33. https://doi.org/10.1053/smrv.2002.0238.
6. Martinot, J. B., Borel, J. C., Cuthbert, V., Guénard, H. J. P., Denison, S., Silkoff, P. E., ... & Pepin, J. L. (2017). Mandibular position and movements: suitability for diagnosis of sleep apnoea. Respirology, 22(3), 567–574.
7. Leszek Kubin. Neural Control of the Upper Airway: Respiratory and State-Dependent Mechanisms. Compr Physiol. 2016 Sep 15;6(4):1801–1850. https://doi.org/10.1002/cphy.c160002.
8. Le-Dong NN, Martinot JB, Coumans N, Cuthbert V, Tamisier R, Bailly S, Pépin JL. (2021) Machine Learning-based Sleep Staging in Sleep Apnea Patients Using a Single Mandibular Movement Signal. Am J Respir Crit Care Med. 204 (10): 1227–1231
9. Berquin, P., Bodineau, L., Gros, F., & Larnicol, N. (2000). Brainstem and hypothalamic areas involved in respiratory chemoreflexes: a Fos study in adult rats. Brain research, 857(1–2), 30–40.
10. Moore, J. D., Kleinfeld, D., & Wang, F. (2014). How the brainstem controls orofacial behaviors comprised of rhythmic actions. Trends in neurosciences, 37(7), 370–380.
11. Isono, S., Tanaka, A., Tagaito, Y., Ishikawa, T., & Nishino, T. (2004). Influences of head positions and bite opening on collapsibility of the passive pharynx. Journal of Applied Physiology, 97(1), 339–346.
12. Martinot, J. B., Le-Dong, N. N., Cuthbert, V., Denison, S., Borel, J. C., Gozal, D., & Pépin, J. L. (2019). Respiratory Mandibular Movement Signals Reliably Identify Obstructive Hypopnea Events During Sleep. Frontiers in neurology, 10, 828.
13. Jean-Benoît Martinot, N Nam Le-Dong, Stéphane Denison et al. Persistent respiratory effort after adenotonsillectomy in children with sleep-disordered breathing. Laryngoscope. 2018;128(5):1230–1237. https://doi.org/10.1002/lary.26830.
14. Martinot JB, Le Dong NN, Malhotra A. et al. Respiratory effort during sleep and prevalent hypertension in obstructive sleep apnoea. European Respiratory Journal 2023 61: 2201486; https://doi.org/10.1183/13993003.01486-2022.
15. Pepin, J. L., Le-Dong, N. N., Cuthbert, V., Coumans, N., Tamisier, R., Malhotra, A., & Martinot, J. B. (2022). Mandibular Movements are a Reliable Noninvasive Alternative to Esophageal Pressure for Measuring Respiratory Effort in Patients with Sleep Apnea Syndrome. Nature and Science of Sleep, 14, 635.
16. Miyamoto K., Ozbek M.M., Lowe A.A., Sjöholm T.T., Love L.L., Fleetham J.A., Ryan C.F., Mandibular posture during sleep in patients with obstructive sleep apnoea, Arch Oral Biol. 1999; 44: 657–64.
17. Miyamoto K., Ozbek M.M., Lowe A.A., Sjöholm T.T., Love L.L., Fleetham J.A., Ryan C.F., Mandibular posture during sleep in healthy adults, Arch Oral Biol. 1998; 43: 269–75.
18. Hollowell D.E., Suratt P.M., Mandible position and activation of submental and masseter muscles during sleep, J Appl Physiol. 1991; 71: 2267–73.
19. Hollowell D.E., Suratt P.M., Activation of masseter muscles with inspiratory resistance loading, J Appl Physiol. 1989; 67: 270–5.
20. Kato J, Katase T, Yamashita S et al. Responsiveness of Jaw Motor Activation to Arousals during Sleep in Patients with Obstructive Sleep Apnea Syndrome. Clin Sleep Med 2013;9(8):759–765.

21. Jean-Benoit Martinot, Nhat Nam Le-Dong, Valérie Cuthbert et al. The key role of the mandible in modulating airflow amplitude during sleep. Respir Physiol Neurobiol. 2020;279:103447. https://doi.org/10.1016/j.resp.2020.103447.
22. Brodersen, K.H., Gallusser, F., Koehler, J., Remy, N., Scott, S.L., 2015. Inferring causal impact using Bayesian structural time-series models. Ann. Appl. Stat. 9 (1), 247–274.
23. Rachel Danzig, Mengxi Wang, Amit Shah, Lynn Marie Trotti. The wrist is not the brain: Estimation of sleep by clinical and consumer wearable actigraphy devices is impacted by multiple patient- and device-specific factors. J Sleep Res. 2020 Feb;29(1):e12926. https://doi.org/10.1111/jsr.12926. Epub 2019 Oct 17. PMID: 31621129.
24. Maury G, Cambron L, Jamart J, Marchand E, Senny F, Poirrier R. (2013). Added value of a mandible movement automated analysis in the screening of obstructive sleep apnea. J Sleep Res. 22 (1), 96–103.
25. Senny F, Maury G, Cambron L, Leroux A, Destiné J, Poirrier R. (2012). The sleep/wake state scoring from mandible movement signal. Sleep Breath. 16 (2), 535–542.
26. Martinot JB, Denison SJ, Senny FH, Robillard TA, Khatwa U, Guenard H. (2014). Mandibular Movements Identify Respiratory Efforts Due to Obstructive Sleep Apnoea in a Pre-school Child. Open Sleep J. 7(1), 1–5.
27. Martinot JB, Le-Dong NN, Cuthbert V, Denison S, Silkoff PE, Guénard H, Gozal D, Pépin JL, Borel JC. (2017) Mandibular Movements As Accurate Reporters of Respiratory Effort during Sleep: Validation against Diaphragmatic Electromyography. Front Neurol. 8: 353. https://doi.org/10.3389/fneur.2017.00353. eCollection 2017.
28. Pépin JL, Letesson C, Le-Dong NN, Dedave A, Denison S, Cuthbert V, Martinot JB, Gozal D. (2020). Assessment of Mandibular Movement Monitoring With Machine Learning Analysis for the Diagnosis of Obstructive Sleep Apnea. JAMA Netw Open. 3 (1): e1919657.
29. Gisèle Maury, Frédéric Senny, Laurent Cambron et al. Mandible behaviour interpretation during wakefulness, sleep and sleep-disordered breathing. J Sleep Res. 2014 Dec;23(6):709–716. https://doi.org/10.1111/jsr.12180.
30. Jean-Benoit Martinot , Nhat-Nam Le-Dong , Valérie Cuthbert et al. Artificial Intelligence Analysis of Mandibular Movements Enables Accurate Detection of Phasic Sleep Bruxism in OSA Patients: A Pilot Study. Nat Sci Sleep. 2021 Aug 23;13:1449–1459. https://doi.org/10.2147/NSS.S320664. PMID: 34466045.
31. Tangudu V, Afrin K, Reddy S, Deutz NEP, Woltering S, Bukkapatnam STS. (2021). Toward standardizing the clinical testing protocols of point-of-care devices for obstructive sleep apnea diagnosis. Sleep Breath. 25 (2): 737–748.
32. Martinot JB, Cuthbert V, Le-Dong NN, Coumans N, De Marneffe D, Letesson C, Pépin JL, Gozal D. (2021). Clinical validation of a mandibular movement signal based system for the diagnosis of pediatric sleep apnea. Pediatr Pulmonol. 57 (8): 1904–1913.
33. Berry RB, Budhiraja R, Gottlieb DJ, et al; American Academy of Sleep Medicine; Deliberations of the Sleep Apnea Definitions Task Force of the American Academy of Sleep Medicine. Rules for scoring respiratory events in sleep: update of the 2007 AASM Manual for the Scoring of Sleep and Associated Events. J Clin Sleep Med. 2012;8(5):597–619. doi:https://doi.org/10.5664/jcsm.2172.
34. Berry RB, Brooks R, Gamaldo C, et al. AASM Scoring Manual updates for 2017 (version 2.4). J Clin Sleep Med. 2017;13(5):665–666. doi:https://doi.org/10.5664/jcsm.6576.

Nightmare Disorder: An Overview

Brian Robertson, Alexander Semenov, Tyler Skluzacek, Han Coburn, and Matthew Miller

1 Introduction

Nightmare disorder, characterized by the frequent occurrence of distressing and disruptive dreams, has emerged as a significant mental health concern, necessitating urgent attention and effective treatment strategies. The disorder not only impairs sleep quality but also adversely affects daytime functioning, contributing to a decline in overall well-being. Despite its drastic negative impacts to patients' well-being, Nightmare disorder remains under-diagnosed and under-treated, often overshadowed by co-occurring mental health conditions. Addressing nightmare disorder grows even more critical given its high prevalence in individuals with post-traumatic stress disorder (PTSD), wherein nightmares can act as nocturnal re-enactments of traumatic experiences, perpetuating the cycle of distress. It is estimated that 71% of trauma victims who have been diagnosed with PTSD experience frequent nightmares. This figure towers over the general population where 2–5% of people experience frequent nightmares [1]. Additionally, nightmare disorder has been shown to heighten patient risks of suicidality.

Given these severe impacts, finding effective treatments for nightmare disorder is not just a matter of individual health, but also of broader mental health management. Traditional therapeutic interventions have proven effective in managing mental

B. Robertson (✉) · T. Skluzacek · H. Coburn
NightWare, Inc., Washington, DC, USA
e-mail: brian@nightware.com; tyler@veselianalytics.com

A. Semenov
Department of Industrial and Systems Engineering, University of Florida, Gainesville, FL, USA
e-mail: asemenov@ufl.edu

M. Miller
US Navy, Radiology Department at Naval Medical Center San Diego, San Diego, CA, USA

R. B. Berry et al. (eds.), *Handbook of AI and Data Sciences for Sleep Disorders*,
Springer Optimization and Its Applications 216,
https://doi.org/10.1007/978-3-031-68263-6_11

health, but have thus far failed to reach strong levels of accessibility and patient adherence. For instance, Imagery Rehearsal Therapy (IRT) involves working with a mental health professional to create detailed benign endings to previously frightening recurring nightmares, discussing the new nightmares, and slowly learning to "control" one's own nightmares. In another case, Cognitive Behavioral Therapy (CBT) is a widely used form of psychotherapy that focuses on changing patterns of thinking and behavior to help people manage problems and improve their mental health. However, both IRT and CBT require regular, affordable access to mental health professionals, which introduces barriers of cost, the perceptions and stigma surrounding "attending therapy," and a consistent time commitment [2].

To avoid these barriers to access and adherence, digital therapeutics have emerged as a promising avenue, offering scalable, accessible, and user-friendly solutions to mitigate the impact of nightmare disorder. Digital therapeutics encompass a variety of technology-based interventions, ranging from mobile applications to virtual reality, tailored to provide individualized relief. Most importantly, these therapeutics are commonly designed to run on ubiquitous hardware—such as mobile phones, smartwatches, and other smart devices—to which users already have access, can be relatively low cost, and users already have some basic understanding as to how to use these devices. Furthermore, accelerating technical capabilities in artificial intelligence, battery life, and human-computer interaction have led to these devices being powerful foundations on which to build positively impactful digital therapeutics.

A notable digital therapeutic aimed at treating nightmare disorder is NightWare, which is built atop the Apple Watch. NightWare utilizes statistical learning algorithms to analyze sleep patterns and detect nightmares based on heart rate and body movement. Upon nightmare detection, the application employs gentle haptic feedback to disrupt the nightmare without awakening the user, facilitating a return to peaceful sleep. This intervention represents a significant advancement in the treatment of nightmare disorder. By harnessing the power of technology, NightWare offers a non-invasive, personalized, and accessible solution, potentially revolutionizing how we approach the management of sleep disturbances. Its use of real-time data analysis and intervention aligns with the growing trend of precision medicine, providing targeted treatment tailored to individual patient needs. Furthermore, the convenience and familiarity of wearable technology like the Apple Watch make such therapeutics more approachable and less stigmatized compared to traditional therapy sessions. The development of NightWare and similar applications signifies a hopeful future where effective management of nightmare disorder is within reach for a broader segment of the population, transcending the barriers of traditional mental health care. This shift toward digital therapeutics could pave the way for more innovative, accessible, and effective treatments for a variety of mental health conditions, reflecting a new era in psychological well-being and sleep health.

The remainder of this chapter is structured as follows: Section 2 presents background information for nightmare disorder, highlighting the co-occurring nature of nightmare disorder with PTSD. Section 3 discusses at a high level how traumatic nightmare detection can be framed as a machine learning problem and discusses how to convert automatically collected data into actionable features that can be used by applications and statistical learning models. Section 4 introduces digital therapeutics for nightmare disorder, including NightWare. Finally, Sect. 5 discusses future avenues of work at the intersection of traumatic nightmares and artificial intelligence.

2 Background of Nightmare Disorder

2.1 Introduction

Nightmare disorder is characterized by recurrent nightmares that are accompanied by awakenings, detailed dream recall, and emotional distress [3]. The term "nightmare disorder" is assigned when the repetition and intensity of nightmares and subsequent distress lead to the need for clinical attention [3]. Nightmare disorder is associated with disrupted sleep with nocturnal awakenings and increased sleep latency [4]. Untreated nightmare disorder can lead to insomnia, daytime somnolence, fatigue, and impaired quality of life [5, 6].

In the following sections, we summarize the current literature on nightmare disorder epidemiology, causes and risk factors of this condition. We also review available treatments and identify challenges in the evaluation of treatment efficacy and safety. Finally, we propose key aspects of effective treatment strategy and introduce a new digital therapy for nightmare disorder.

2.2 Epidemiology

Episodic nightmares are common in the general population, from children to adults. In children, approximately 50% experience occasional nightmares [7]. About 85% of adults reported having at least one nightmare per year [8], and 45% reported having at least one nightmare per 2 weeks [9]. A current large investigation of 69,813 Finnish general adults showed that 36.2% of men and 43.5% of women had occasional nightmares during the past 30 days [10]. With advancing age, occasional nightmares become more common among both men and women [10]. Infrequent nightmares, even disturbing ones, rarely require treatment and are considered a normal phenomenon that does not appear to have any effect on daytime functioning or sleep quality. On the other hand, clinically significant nightmares, typically defined as nightmares occurring one or more per week, affect from 0.9% to 6.8% of the adult population [11–16]. The discrepancy of the results is attributed to the diversity of methodology in defining nightmare and the nightmare frequency, in addition to the different study populations in various cultural settings, follow-up periods, retrospective versus dream logs review. Frequent nightmares are present in approximately 3% of men and 5% of women [10, 16]. However, increased prevalence of clinically significant nightmares is observed in men with advancing age, but not in women [10, 16]. Additionally, the prevalence of frequent nightmares is high among children, with 20% reported having recurrent nightmares [7].

In contrast to the general population, those with insomnia or psychiatric conditions such as anxiety, depression/mood disorders, and psychotic disorders have higher occurrences of nightmare disorders. In a large questionnaire study on 5622 French adults, Ohayon et al. [4] found that frequent nightmares were reported in 18.3% of insomniac subjects ($N = 1049$), compared to an average of 4% of the general population [11–16]. Those with insomnia and nightmare reported difficulties in initiating and maintaining sleep more frequently than non-nightmare insomniacs [4]. 16.7% of patients with major depressive disorder (MDD) suffer frequent nightmares, compared to 4.9% of healthy controls (mean of 44.6 nightmares per year versus 18 nightmares per year, respectively) [17]. Among patients with psychotic disorders, the prevalence of recurrent nightmares is found to be 9% of 338 schizophrenia-spectrum disorder patients [18]. Report from 40 psychotic patients (42.5% had PTSD) showed that 55% of them had recurrent nightmares [19]. One study found that 17% of patients with both MDD and schizophrenia have frequent nightmares, significantly more than 4.9% in healthy controls [17]. In older adults with clinically significant depressive and anxiety symptoms, 11.4%, and 17.1%, respectively, report having nightmares [20].

The comorbid disorders of sleep disturbances, sleep disorders, depression, PTSD, and anxiety were all associated with clinically significant nightmares. Complaints of frequent nightmares are often associated with disturbed sleeps, in which patients have multiple awakenings, increased sleep onset latency [4, 21, 22], and REM sleep latency [21]. Moreover, frequent nightmares are associated with difficulties staying asleep in about 52.9% of general adults, while it affects 90.7% of combat veterans with PTSD, 62.5% of combat veterans without PTSD, and 63.1% of era veterans, as reported in a study with 2062 subjects [22]. Following a nightmare, veterans reported more symptoms of insomnia, depression, and anxiety with repeated nightmares, compared to non-veterans [10]. It has been demonstrated that distress from frequent nightmares, possibly not the incidence of nightmares itself, is associated with poorer psychological functioning, especially anxiety and depression states [8, 23].

Nightmare Disorder is Under-recognized and Under-treated

Despite their high prevalence and serious affliction, nightmare disorder lacks recognition, and this continues to be a problem. Alarmingly, Creamer et al. [21] found that 31.2% of active-duty members that presented at a military sleep clinic had at least weekly nightmares with sleep disturbances, but only 3.9% complained about nightmares at the time of their visit. Moreover, these patients with traumatic-related nightmares had more severe insomnia symptoms than those without. The reasons why nightmares are underreported to clinicians are not clear. A report pointed out that 60% of patients with recurrent nightmares do not discuss it with their health care providers, only when the condition is clinically severe do patients seek help

[24]. Two-thirds of patients in this study suffering from nightmare disorder do not believe that it is treatable [24]. This stems from the lack of understanding of disease mechanisms as well as difficulty in the development of treatments for nightmare disorders.

Clinically unattended nightmare disorder can lead to serious consequences. Untreated nightmare disorder decreases sleep quality and increases patients' risk of developing insomnia and comorbid disorders of depression, PTSD, and anxiety [10, 21, 25]. Prolonged nightmare disorder can also exacerbate the symptoms of underlying psychological dysfunction in patients with depression and anxiety, leading to poor occupational and or social functioning [5, 6]. Importantly, in the general population, frequent nightmares constitute an independent risk factor for suicidal ideation, attempted as well as completed suicide [16, 26, 27]. People with chronic nightmares have a two- [16] to fivefold [27] increase risk for suicidality compared with people who had no nightmares at all. Nightmares were found to be associated with higher suicidality in patients with depression and mood disorders [28–32]. Female sexual assault survivors with PTSD and sleep disorders suffered from the most severe depression and suicidality [33]. Notably, a report showed that 72% of women who suffered depression with frequent nightmares, at least twice per week, were more suicidal than those without nightmares [34]. These converging evidence assert that treating nightmare disorder is an integral part of treating sleep disturbances to improve quality of life, especially in those that suffer PTSD and other psychiatric illnesses.

2.3 *Causes of Nightmare Disorder*

The causes of nightmares are multifactorial. The precipitating causes of nightmares can be idiopathic (without clinical signs of psychopathology) or emerge in association with a physical or emotional traumatic experience in the past, as in PTSD [5, 35]. Individuals with PTSD repeatedly re-experience the trauma typically as intrusive thoughts and nightmares, flashbacks, avoidance of trauma-related stimuli, and hyperarousal [5, 35–37]. Nightmares and PTSD are closely related [5, 35] and both show altered activity in the same brain regions [38], but the exact pathological mechanisms remain unclear. A postulated hypothesis is that disrupted REM sleep in PTSD can contribute to nightmares [37, 39–41], as increased REM sleep or REM rebound are associated with nightmares [42–44]. The combination of REM disruption and amygdala hyperactivity during sleep is a strong candidate mechanism for PTSD nightmares [8]. In addition, changes in NREM are recorded in nightmare sufferance [43–45], and PTSD-nightmares have been observed to emerge from non-REM (NREM) sleep [37, 39–41]. In a cohort of 35 patients that suffered from PTSD, an almost equal percentage of patients were documented to have NREM and REM-related nightmares [47]. Yet, other reports suggested a global increase in emotional and physical arousal whether expressed as leg movements [37], longer sleep latency, and nocturnal awakenings [4, 21, 22, 45], increased heart rate and respiratory rate arising from nightmares or PTSD-nightmares [47, 48].

Nightmare disorder also occurs along with stress and anxiety, and other psychiatric illnesses (depression, general anxiety disorder, bipolar disorder, and schizophrenia) [23, 49]. The exact pathophysiology of nightmares in patients with psychiatric disorders remains elusive. It has been postulated that nightmares and psychiatric symptoms represent a common domain with shared pathophysiology [50]. Nevertheless, further studies are necessary to better understand nightmare-specific physio-pathological mechanisms, since nightmares in the context of psychiatric disorders may have different pathways and causes.

A typical chronic or sustaining cause of nightmare disorder is sleep disturbances. A nightmare episode can cause restless sleep with disruptive awakenings. After each nightmare episode, it is often difficult for individuals to return to sleep because of fear or anxiety. Thus, frequent nightmares can lead to heightened physiologic and emotional arousal, prolonged sensation of fear going to sleep, longer sleep onset latency, and subsequent insomnia [3, 4, 10, 36, 37, 51]. On the other hand, sleep disturbances or sleep deprivation can worsen the trajectory of nightmare frequency and intensity [39].

2.4 *Diagnosis*

The third edition of the International Classification of Sleep Disorders (ICSD-3) [52] states the following minimum criteria for nightmare disorder:

1. Repeated occurrences of extended, extremely dysphoric, and well-remembered dreams that usually involved threats to survival, security, or physical integrity.
2. On awakening from the dysphoric dreams, the person rapidly becomes oriented and alert.
3. The dream experience, or the sleep disturbance produced by the awakening from it, causes clinically significant distress or mental impairment in social, occupational, or other important areas of functioning as indicated by the report of *at least one* of the following:

   (a) Mood disturbance (e.g., persistence of nightmares affects, anxiety, dysphoria).
   (b) Sleep persistence (e.g., bedtime anxiety, fear of sleep/subsequent nightmares).
   (c) Cognitive impairments (e.g., intrusive, nightmare imagery, impaired concentration, or memory.)
   (d) Negative impact on caregiver or family functioning (e.g., nighttime disruption).
   (e) Behavioral problems (e.g. bedtime avoidance, fear of the dark).
   (f) Daytime sleepiness.
   (g) Fatigue or low energy.

(h) Impaired occupational or educational function.
(i) Impaired interpersonal/social function.

The diagnosis of nightmare disorder is made by clinical history and examination. Laboratory tests are not routine unless there is suspicion of a drug use disorder. Sleep diagnostic testing using Polysomnography is not indicated for the diagnosis of nightmare disorder, as nightmares tend to occur less frequently in a clinical sleep laboratory setting [40]. This is presumed to be due to the "first night effect" in which patients' sleep architecture may be different than in their natural home sleep environment. Nightmares can be assessed using outpatient psychometric tools, including the Symptom Checklist-90 and Symptom Questionnaire [53, 54]. The Clinician-Administered PTSD Scale (CAPS), developed by the National Center for PTSD, is currently the gold standard diagnostic interview for PTSD and PTSD-related nightmare disorder [55].

2.5 Treatment

Pharmacological treatments Several medications have been studied for treating nightmare disorder: atypical antipsychotics, benzodiazepines, clonidine, cyproheptadine, fluvoxamine, gabapentin, nabilone, phenelzine, topiramate, trazodone, tricyclic antidepressants [56, 57]. The AASM position paper [58] recommended prazosin, nitrazepam, and triazolam as "may be used" for treating PTSD-associated nightmares. For a long time, prazosin has been used as the first choice of intervention [56, 57].

Prazosin

Prazosin is an α1-adrenergic receptor antagonist. This medication is FDA-approved for use as an antihypertensive, although the exact mechanism of the hypotensive action of prazosin is unclear [59]. Individuals with PTSD have elevated sympathetic outflow in the brain during sleep [56, 60]. It is believed that prazosin can be effective in treating the severity and frequency of PTSD-associated nightmares by reducing noradrenergic activity in the brain, hence reducing the sympathetic outflow [56, 60]. Nevertheless, multiple common side effects from prazosin that raise concern including dizziness, nausea, headache, morning cataplexy and sedation, lethargy, dry mouth, nocturnal urine incontinence, nasal congestion, and palpitations [56, 59, 61, 62]. Even more concerning is the risk of orthostatic hypotension and the potential for syncope-related injury; rebound hypertension with missed doses [59, 62]. Thus, the American Academy of Sleep Medicine suggests that clinicians monitor patients for potential orthostatic hypotension when prescribing prazosin for nightmares [56]. In addition, prazosin's interaction profile with other medications also limits use in clinical populations [60]. Interaction between prazosin and antidepressants, possibly from binding to the same site—α1-Acid Glycoprotein [63], was demonstrated across various studies [57].

Studies on the efficacy of prazosin in treating PTSD-nightmare disorder showed contradictory outcomes [57, 64–67]. Most data are limited by small study sizes, lack of diversified investigators and study regions [62, 65]. A large randomized placebo-controlled trial published on The New England Journal of Medicine in 2018 shed evidence opposing the mainstream [67]. The trial conducted on 304 veterans with chronic PTSD and nightmare disorder from 13 VA centers for 26 weeks showed no significant difference in any outcomes (CAPS-5, Pittsburgh Sleep Quality Index) after using prazosin. Concerning these mixed results, the AASM decided to downgrade the recommendation regarding prazosin use in 2018 [57]. Despite that, prazosin is still considered the first line for pharmacological therapy because many patients appear to respond well to this agent.

Non-pharmacological treatments Compared to pharmacological agents, non-pharmacological treatments are more favored by the AASM task force [57]. Image rehearsal therapy is recommended for the treatment of PTSD-associated nightmares and nightmare disorder. Although evidence was less clear, the following therapies may be used in the treatment of PTSD-associated nightmares: cognitive behavioral therapy (also for nightmare disorder), cognitive behavioral therapy for insomnia; exposure, relaxation, and rescripting therapies (also for nightmare disorder); eye-movement desensitization and reprocessing. Other therapies that may be used for nightmare disorders are hypnosis, lucid-dreaming therapy, and progressive deep-muscle relaxation techniques [56, 57].

Image Rehearsal Therapy

Image Rehearsal Therapy (IRT), a modified cognitive behavioral therapy technique, is a non-pharmacological approach that appears to be effective [68–72]. IRT conceives chronic nightmares as a learned behavior that can be modified via the mental imagery system during wakefulness [73]. During the therapy, the patient recalls a nightmare, then consciously imagines changes in the theme, storyline, ending, or any part of the dream, to a more positive and tolerable one. The intended outcome would be that when a patient has the rehearsed dream during sleep, they will replace the disturbing content with the positive and tolerable content imagined during the day. The patient will commonly practice the rehearsal of these dreams for 10–20 minutes per day.

While IRT has been demonstrated to be generally effective in the treatment of nightmare disorder in patients with PTSD [68–72], there are contradictory results [51], and IRT's extensive impact and practicality remain questionable. A randomized control trial with a higher number of group sessions on veterans with severe PTSD showed no improvement over credible placebo [74]. At the same time, there was an increased drop-out rate in the IRT group [74]. In fact, studies consistently demonstrate poor compliance with therapy with a dropout rate of approximately 30–50% [68–71, 74]. It is likely that rehearsing the nightmares immediately before bed carries the risk of re-exposing the patient to their traumatic nightmare and, thus, exacerbating the PTSD symptoms of nightmares, as well as increasing the frequency of nightmares [56]. Likewise, patients were reluctant to fill out the sleep logs to document the frequency and content of nightmares for fear of re-exposure [71]. For these reasons, not to mention the specialized staff training and time for repeated clinic visits, IRT has a low potential to have a large population-level impact on PTSD-related nightmares.

2.6 Nightmares Disorder and Suicidality

The connections between chronic recurrent nightmares and suicidal ideation, suicide attempts, and completed suicide have been increasingly described in an emerging body of literature. The impact of treating nightmares on subsequent suicidality has not been explored fully to date, which suggests the need for further investigation. Identification of the correlations between nightmare disorder, nightmares, and suicidal feelings and behaviors has been obscured due to the more established associations made between suicide and other mental health disorders. For example, McCall et al. found that while insomnia is a risk factor for suicide, the effects of insomnia on suicidal ideation are mediated through both dysfunctional beliefs about sleep and nightmares [75]. Their mediation analysis showed that if the effects of dysfunctional beliefs and nightmares were accounted for, insomnia itself had no significant effect on suicidal ideation. This study suggests that some, if not all, of the increased risk of suicide with insomnia was due to nightmares. Li et al. independently demonstrated that nightmares were at least as potent a risk factor as insomnia for suicide and were highly associated with nightmares in depressed patients (OR 8.40) [76].

History of a suicide attempt is a commonly cited and well-known risk factor for suicide; significant nightmare problems increased the risk for future suicidality. In a study of patients with a suicide attempt history, those with nightmares had an increased risk of suicidality (OR 3.7) independent of axis-I disorders, post-traumatic stress symptoms, and symptom intensity, compared to those with a suicide attempt history that did not have nightmares [27].

Another large-scale epidemiological study demonstrated the direct and graded association between nightmare frequency and death from suicide in general population. This was a prospective follow-up study in 36,211 Finnish patients starting in 1972, which discovered that the frequency of nightmares was directly related to the risk of suicide. The adjusted relative risk of suicide in subjects with occasional nightmares was 57% higher compared with subjects reporting no nightmares at all. Among those reporting frequent nightmares, this risk is 105% higher [16]. A 2-year prospective study of 165 patients with suicide attempts in Sweden demonstrated that frequent nightmares were the only sleep variable at baseline that was associated with a repeat suicide attempt [77].

A recent large-scale study of 11,740 Chinese college students demonstrated similar findings regarding suicide and nightmares as shown by studies in other countries [78]. In Shi et al., the authors found that frequent nightmares at baseline predicted both subsequent suicidal ideation and suicide attempts (adjusted OR 1.35–1.69 and 2.40, respectively). A study of 6932 Chinese adolescents found that suicidal thoughts, plans, and attempts were increased at 1 year in those with nightmares [79]. The association between nightmares and suicide in this group increased with both nightmare frequency and distress as a result of nightmare.

Three meta-analyses demonstrate the association between suicide and nightmares. Pigeon et al. conducted a meta-analysis in 2012 of sleep disturbances and suicidal thoughts and behaviors, which supported not only an association between suicidality and sleep disturbances, but also insomnia and nightmares individually [26]. In 2019, Wang et al. conducted a meta-analysis of 18 studies, which demonstrated that nightmares were more highly correlated with suicidal behavior (OR 4.47) than insomnia (OR 2.29) [80]. Another 2019 meta-analysis of longitudinal studies of sleep disturbances and suicidal behavior found that of the types of sleep disturbances, insomnia best predicted suicidal ideation (OR 2.10), and nightmares significantly predicted suicide attempt (OR 1.81) [81]. A systematic review of the literature in 2019 by Russell and colleagues also found that nightmares and insomnia were both highly associated with suicidality [82]. A review by Andrews and Harris in 2020 explores the possible mechanisms by which nightmares could lead, directly or indirectly, to suicidal behaviors [81]. The authors note that seeking help for nightmare disorder may be much more attractive to patients than seeking help for suicidal thoughts, and call for more research to better understand how nightmares could lead to suicidality.

2.7 Clinical Opinion

The key aspect of treating nightmare disorders involved early intervention. Patients suffering from nightmare disorder must initiate early discussions with their healthcare providers, who can refer patients to accredited sleep centers with board-certificated sleep physicians. Early assessments to identify the pathology, causes, and risk factors for nightmares can be made by sleep physicians. In the absence of clear guidance and evidence on treatments of nightmare disorder, developing effective treatment plans for nightmare disorders can be daunting. Therefore, the judgment and expertise of knowledgeable clinicians are essential to treatment success. The therapy benefits versus risks should be carefully weighted, as current therapies for nightmare disorder have considerable side effects as well as compliance burdens.

As firm proof for effective nightmare disorder treatment is lacking and that establishing therapies can be challenging for physicians, we herein propose several treatment strategies that may aid in mitigating nightmare disorder manifestation and concurrent distress.

Improve Sleep Quality

Sleep has an important role in the consolidation and modification of fear memories and their extinction. Specifically, both slow-wave sleep and REM sleep have been linked to the consolidation of extinction memory [83, 84]. REM sleep may enhance the consolidations of both emotional memory [85] and extinction learning [83, 84, 86, 87]. Thus, less slow-wave sleep and fragmentation of REM, as observed in PTSD [39–41, 88, 37], might block consolidation of extinction thus increasing expression of older traumatic memories [83, 84]. Intriguingly, the repetitive nightmares of PTSD could reinforce conditioned fear via re-traumatization or rehearsal [8]. Rehearsed fear memories became sufficiently reinforced (become resistant to extinction) and significantly contribute to PTSD symptomology [89]. Therefore, preserving REM sleep or general improvement of sleep quality may ameliorate nightmares by strengthening naturally acquired extinction. Moreover, preliminary data suggested that recovery sleep after sleep deprivation from long nocturnal awakenings almost abolishes dream recall, down to 75% decrease [90]. Restoring normal sleep architecture, whether by pharmacological and non-pharmacological interventions, could mitigate the expression of nightmares.

Improved sleep quality is beneficial to physical and mental well-being. In subjects with chronic nightmare disorder, reduction in nightmares was strongly associated with improved sleep [79]. Improved sleep quality can significantly decrease anxiety, depression, hostility, somatization, and total distress [79]. Short-term sleep deprivation is linked to poorer short-term memory, attention, and processing speed [91]; chronic sleep deprivation contributes to long-term cognitive decline and possibly the development of dementia [92]. On the other hand, longer sleep duration, better sleep quality, and greater sleep consistency were associated with better cognitive performance [93].

Preventive Intervention Post-trauma

Preventing nightmares before they cluster may decrease trauma re-exposure and the emergence of mental disorders. Attenuating the heightened fear response from nightmares in PTSD perhaps also prevents the formation of secondary depression. Interventions should be administered within a short window following trauma exposure, as memory consolidation appears particularly vulnerable to disruption in the 6 hours after trauma [94]. This method possibly reduces the initial consolidation and/or reconsolidation of conditioned fear memories [95] without affecting the distributed cortical representation of declarative memories [96], since conditioned fear has a distinct neural circuit localized in the amygdala [97]. Studies proposed that early pharmacologic interventions including morphine [97, 98], glucocorticoids [99, 100], propranolol (mixed results) [101, 102] can reduce the emergence of PTSD symptoms (of which nightmares are the manifestation) via limiting fear conditioning or enhancing fear memory extinction. In addition to pharmacologic agents, early post-trauma psychological interventions could also prevent PTSD symptoms. Psychotherapies administered to survivors of rape and sexual assault within 72 hours of the event were associated with lower PTSD symptomatology at a later time [103]. The Battlemind Psychological Debriefing intervention administered to soldiers post-deployment produced fewer post-traumatic stress, stigma, and depression symptoms [104, 105]. These converging results demonstrate that early post-trauma interventions potentially ameliorate trauma-related distress, even though it is not clear whether it helps to reduce nightmare frequency and severity. There are considerable safety and practicality concerns regarding current early interventions [106]. Up to date, the field still needs new types of therapies that "do no harm" and are easy to comply with, as patients with nightmare disorder have a plethora of physical and emotional burdens in life.

Adjunctive Therapies
The outcomes from current small studies on single treatment modalities are inconclusive and hard to reproduce. The disappointing results from a large randomized controlled trial on prazosin funded by the VA Cooperative Study Program [67] suggest that there may be no "one-size fits all" therapy for nightmare disorder. Since nightmare disorder is multicausal, it may not be plausible to rely on single therapy irrespective of the nature of triggering events. Selecting treatments should depend on a patient's background and preferences, and the clinician's expertise to deliver the therapy. Therefore, future strategies should focus on the adjunctive iteration of therapies tailored to an individual's experience of nightmares and socio-cultural background. Finally, concurrent management of sleep disturbances, psychiatric conditions (PTSD, depression, and anxiety), and suicidality should be aligned with treating nightmares.

3 Using Machine Learning to Detect and Treat Nightmare Disorder

Statistical models that monitor and identify patterns in sleep need advanced time series data—data of similar formats collected at regular intervals. Some learning models like neural networks might require vast amounts of data for training, whereas heuristic, clustering, or tree-based methods can provide meaningful insights with much less.

There is a growing body of literature recognizing the importance of applying machine learning to extract various insights from human physiological parameters. Recent examples include the supervised classification of sleep stages based on EEG data [107–110]. These studies classify sleep stages using datasets such as the sleep-edf database, which contains whole-night polysomnographic sleep recordings, including EEG, EOG, EMG, and other data, with manually labeled sleep patterns [111, 112]. Other applications of machine learning involve the classification of subjective sleep quality based on clinical, demographic, and EEG-based measures [113]. Additionally, some research treats sleep analysis as an unsupervised machine learning problem, applying anomaly detection methods to detect mouthbreathing in children [114]. Methodologically similar research focuses on detecting driver drowsiness through the analysis of drivers' faces using machine learning methods [115].

Identifying nightmares through biometric stress markers is a quintessential anomaly detection problem within the realm of medical data analysis. By leveraging wearable technology to continuously monitor physiological parameters such as heart rate and movement during sleep, a rich time series of biometric data is amassed by the software system. In the normal course of a restful sleep, these metrics maintain a relatively consistent pattern [110]. However, during nightmares, these biometric stress markers tend to exhibit irregular behavior, deviating significantly from the patient's established sleep patterns. The challenge lies in developing sophisticated algorithms capable of discerning these subtle yet critical variations in real-time, categorizing them as anomalies indicative of a nightmare episode. This task requires not just an accurate identification of the anomalous patterns, but also a nuanced understanding of the variability inherent in biometric data across different individuals. Addressing this anomaly detection problem is crucial for timely and effective interventions, aiming to alleviate the distress caused by nightmares and contribute to improved sleep quality and overall well-being.

In order to understand the relationship between biometric markers and nightmares, one must first define the key components of a nightmare. We define the following:

- A *sleep session* refers to a single instance of a patient falling asleep to awakening. Each sleep session $s \in S$ is a time series that can be represented as $\boldsymbol{X}^{(s)} = \left\{\boldsymbol{x}_t^{(s)}\right\}_{t=1}^{T_s}$, where T_s is a positive duration of the session.
- Each observation $\boldsymbol{x}_t^{(s)}$ at time t for session s is a vector of d *biometric markers (features)* $\boldsymbol{x}_t^{(s)} = \left(x_{t,1}^{(s)}, x_{t,2}^{(s)}, \ldots, x_{t,d}^{(s)}\right)$ and *environmental markers* that contain information about the patient's sleeping environment. For instance, $\boldsymbol{x}_t^{(s)}$could include heart rate, body temperature, or blink frequency and could include ambient temperature, light brightness, noise level, and derived features.
- Target variable (*nightmare events*) can be represented as $\boldsymbol{Y}^{(s)} = \left\{y_t^{(s)}\right\}$, where $y_t^{(s)}$ refers to a single nightmare event that happens at time t. Patients can have only one experience one nightmare event at a time but can have multiple nightmare events over the course of a sleep session.

For creating features, we use a sliding window approach of size w for session s: $\boldsymbol{X}_{\text{train}}^{(s)} = \left\{\boldsymbol{x}_{t-w+1:t}^{(s)}\right\}_{t=w}^{T_s}$, and introduce a machine learning model f that is trained on the aggregated training data from all sessions: $\hat{y}_t^{(s)} = f\left(\boldsymbol{x}_{t-w+1:t}^{(s)}, \boldsymbol{\theta}\right)$, where $\hat{y}_t^{(s)}$ is the predicted value at time t for session s, and $\boldsymbol{\theta}$ is the vector of parameters. In order to find the vector of optimal parameters $\boldsymbol{\theta}$, we need to choose a function f (such as a neural network or random forest) and minimize the loss function $L\left(\hat{y}_t^{(s)} y_t^{(s)}\right)$,between the actual and predicted classes.

Alternatively, we can define unsupervised model g that will return the anomaly score at time t, that is $\hat{a}_t^{(s)} = g\left(\boldsymbol{x}_{t-w+1:t}^{(s)}, \boldsymbol{\theta}\right)$, and then a threshold τ can be set to classify points as normal or anomalous.

3.1 *Selecting the Appropriate Machine Learning Model or Heuristic*

Introduction to Model and Heuristic Selection
The choice of machine learning model or heuristic is a pivotal decision in the analytics process, directly influencing the effectiveness and efficiency of the solution. While machine learning models can capture complex patterns in data, heuristic methods provide simplified, rule-based solutions that are often more interpretable and computationally efficient. Emphasizing the use of heuristic methods is crucial, especially when they outperform complex models, as they often encapsulate the inherent physiological or logical nature of the problem at hand, leading to more robust and reliable solutions.

Machine Learning Models—When and Why
Machine learning models, ranging from linear regression and decision trees to advanced ensemble methods and deep learning, offer a wide array of options for data analysis and prediction. The choice of model depends on various factors including the nature of the data, the problem type (classification, regression, clustering, etc.), and the requirement for interpretability.

For instance, linear models might be preferred when interpretability is crucial and the relationship between variables is approximately linear. On the other hand, ensemble methods like Random Forest or Gradient Boosting might be employed when the focus is on performance and the data encompasses complex, non-linear relationships.

Heuristic Methods—Simplicity and Efficiency
Heuristic methods provide an alternative approach, offering simpler, rule-based solutions that are often more interpretable and computationally efficient. In scenarios where domain knowledge is extensive, developing heuristic solutions based on this knowledge can yield highly effective results, bypassing the need for complex modeling and extensive data requirements.

The key advantage of heuristics is their ability to encapsulate the natural or logical rules governing the problem, reflecting the physiological or intrinsic nature of the scenario. This often results in solutions that are not only efficient but also robust and easily understandable, facilitating better adoption and trust among end-users.

Balancing Complexity and Simplicity
Balancing the trade-off between the complexity of machine learning models and the simplicity of heuristic methods is crucial. While machine learning models might

provide superior performance in terms of accuracy or other metrics, the additional complexity, computational cost, and potential for overfitting must be taken into consideration.

Furthermore, it is imperative to validate the performance of heuristic methods against machine learning models, ensuring that simpler, more interpretable solutions are not overlooked. When heuristic methods provide comparable or superior performance, they should be favored, aligning with the principle of Occam's razor, which advocates for the simplest solution that adequately solves the problem.

Selecting Hyperparameters for Machine Learning Models

Hyperparameters are external configurations for machine learning algorithms that need to be specified prior to training. They play a crucial role in the performance of machine learning models, as they govern the learning process. However, selecting the optimal set of hyperparameters can be a challenging task, given their impact on the model's ability to generalize from the training data to unseen data.

One of the primary methods for hyperparameter tuning is Grid Search, where a predefined range of values for each hyperparameter is set, and the model is trained and evaluated for every possible combination of these parameters. Although Grid Search is comprehensive, it can be extremely time-consuming and computationally expensive, especially when dealing with a large number of hyperparameters. A more efficient alternative is Random Search, where random combinations of hyperparameters are selected to train the model. This method is less exhaustive but can yield good results with significantly less computation time.

For more sophisticated needs, Bayesian Optimization can be employed. This probabilistic model-based optimization technique aims to reduce the number of function evaluations required to find the minimum or maximum of an objective function, making it more efficient for hyperparameter tuning. It works by constructing a posterior distribution of functions that best describes the function you want to optimize. As the number of observations grows, the model is updated to provide a better and more refined approximation of the objective function.

To summarize, selecting the appropriate machine learning model or heuristic, and its hyperparameters is a nuanced decision, requiring careful consideration of the problem context, data characteristics, and performance requirements. Emphasizing heuristic methods when they outperform or match the performance of complex models is paramount, as they often reflect the physiological nature of the problem, providing efficient, interpretable, and reliable solutions. Balancing the trade-off between complexity and simplicity and validating the performance of heuristic methods against machine learning models, ensures that the most effective and efficient solution is employed.

3.2 Data and Features Engineering

While it may seem obvious that more data is always better for modeling, our means of collecting it is constrained both by technology (e.g., battery life, sensor types) and human effort (e.g., survey fatigue). In this section, we discuss the breadth of data available, as well as strategies for determining what to use given patient needs.

When monitoring and treating nightmare disorder, practitioners and medical devices would ideally have maximum data available, such as second-by-second EKG readings, pulse oxygen data, and cortisol levels. While generating these data would be maximally valuable in treating nightmare disorder, collecting them is infeasible at best. Most patients do not have nightly access to EKG machines outside of their providers' facilities due to the cost and complexity in both operating the machine and both interpreting and processing its data outputs. Pulse oxygen data from a pulse oximeter, which can be collected by smart devices and fitness bands, can be further used in analysis. Finally, cortisol levels (customarily sampled through saliva or skin electroconductivity) provide a direct report of a patient's stress hormone. In sum, all of these data can help providers identify the period when patients have nightmares but are cumbersome to collect.

The measurement of alternative biometric markers can provide actionable insights about nightmares at a fraction of the complexity and cost. Fortunately, the recent and meteoric rise of the Internet of Things (IoT) has led to a diversity of lightweight and affordable sensor devices capable of streaming data to the cloud. To name a few, smart phones, smart watches, and wireless cameras and microphones represent a ubiquitous subset of these IoT devices that have not only received mainstream adoption by consumers, but also can present application programming interfaces (APIs) that enable software developers to—with permission—leverage user data as part of their own applications. As such, digital therapeutic developers now have a complete data warehouse that can be mined to create analytic dashboards based on features constructed from measured biometric data for further statistical or machine learning analysis.

Both are key to treating patients with traumatic nightmare disorder: the dashboards can help providers learn more about a patient's traumatic nightmares as they occur in their "normal" sleep environment, and the machine learning models can not only be used to derive more advanced indicators of sleep behaviors, but also be used in tandem with digital therapeutic technologies to "intervene" when certain learned conditions are met.

What dashboards and models can do with data depend largely on whether there is some underlying relationship between the data and the physical phenomenon we are trying to study—in this case, traumatic nightmares. Generally, the data science to find these relationships can go one of two ways:

1. Leveraging domain knowledge about the physical phenomenon, choose only features that are believed to solve the problem.
2. Try many combinations of features, regardless of any well-known links to the physical phenomenon.

Utilizing domain knowledge involves tapping into existing understanding and expertise about the problem at hand, which can lead to a more interpretable and efficient model. This method has the advantage of being grounded in proven principles, potentially leading to quicker convergence and more reliable results.

However, it may be limited by the extent of current knowledge and could potentially overlook novel or unexpected relationships within the data.

In the second case, the computational approach of "seeing what sticks" entails an exhaustive trial-and-error method, systematically testing numerous features to discern their impact on the model's performance. This method can be advantageous in uncharted or complex domains, where existing knowledge is sparse or non-existent, as it allows for the discovery of unexpected patterns and relationships. However, it often demands considerable computational resources and time, and it can lead to models that are difficult to interpret due to the sheer number of features considered. Moreover, without proper regularization or feature selection techniques in place, this approach can lead to overfitting, where the model becomes overly tailored to the training data and performs poorly on unseen data.

In essence, leveraging domain knowledge offers a more targeted and potentially efficient approach but may be constrained by the current state of knowledge, while the computational "seeing what sticks" method is more exploratory and unconstrained, but at the cost of increased resource demands and potential issues with model interpretability and overfitting. The choice between these two methods ultimately depends on the specific context of the problem, the availability of domain expertise, and the computational resources at hand.

In the contemporary landscape of digital health, smartwatches and smartphones stand out as potent tools for data collection and intervention in the treatment of traumatic nightmares. These devices harbor a wealth of sensors and capabilities that can be harnessed to gather pertinent information, aiding machine learning models in generating insights and delivering timely interventions.

3.2.1 Smartwatch-Based Features

3.2.1.1 Physiological Data

Smartwatches are equipped with an array of sensors capable of monitoring various physiological parameters. For treating traumatic nightmares, key features include the following:

- *Heart Rate*: Monitoring fluctuations and patterns in heart rate can help identify moments of distress potentially linked to nightmares.
- *Heart Rate Variability (HRV)*: As a marker of autonomic nervous system activity, HRV provides insights into the individual's stress and recovery levels.
- *Skin Conductance*: This feature measures the electrical conductance of the skin, which varies with moisture levels and can indicate arousal or stress.
- *Temperature*: Monitoring body temperature can contribute to understanding sleep cycles and identifying disturbances.
- *Accelerometer and Gyroscope*: These sensors detect movement and orientation, helping to identify restless sleep or physical responses to nightmares.

3.2.1.2 Sleep Analysis

- *Sleep Stages*: By analyzing motion and heart rate data, smartwatches can estimate sleep stages, helping to identify disruptions in sleep architecture.
- *Sleep Quality*: Aggregating various data points, smartwatches can provide an overall assessment of sleep quality.

3.2.1.3 Ambient Environment

- *Light Sensor*: Monitoring ambient light levels can contribute to understanding sleep conditions and potential disruptions.
- *Sound Sensor*: Detecting noises in the environment can aid in identifying external factors that might influence nightmares or sleep quality.

3.2.2 Smartphone-Based Features

3.2.2.1 Audio Analysis

- *Microphone*: Smartphones can record and analyze audio data, potentially identifying sounds that could trigger or coincide with nightmares.

3.2.2.2 User Input and Interaction

- *Self-Reported Data*: Users can input data regarding their dreams, sleep quality, and emotional state, providing valuable subjective insights.
- *Response Times*: Analyzing interaction times and response patterns can help assess the user's state of alertness and cognitive function.

3.2.2.3 Location and Movement Data

GPS and Accelerometer: These features can track movements and location, offering context that might relate to sleep patterns and nightmares.

Feature Selection for Models

Introduction to Feature Selection

The indiscriminate addition of features to a machine learning model can lead to overfitting, where the model performs well on the training data but fails to generalize to unseen data. This can result in decreased model interpretability, increased computational complexity, and reduced model performance on new data, highlighting the importance of feature selection and dimensionality reduction techniques in model development.

Feature selection is a critical step in the machine learning pipeline, where the goal is to identify and retain the most relevant variables from the dataset. This process not only helps in improving the model's performance but also in reducing computational costs and enhancing interpretability. The challenge lies in determining which features contribute significantly to the predictive power of the model, and which can be safely omitted.

Techniques for Feature Selection

There are various strategies for feature selection, broadly categorized into filter methods, wrapper methods, and embedded methods. Filter methods involve ranking features based on statistical tests (such as chi-square or ANOVA) and selecting the top-ranking features. They are computationally less expensive but might not capture all the dependencies between features and the target variable.

Wrapper methods, on the other hand, evaluate subsets of features based on the model performance. Common examples include forward selection, backward elimination, and recursive feature elimination (RFE). These methods provide a more accurate assessment of feature importance but are computationally intensive, especially with large datasets.

Embedded methods perform feature selection as part of the learning algorithm itself. Techniques such as L1 regularization (Lasso) add a penalty term to the cost function, encouraging the model to shrink the coefficients of less important features to zero, effectively performing feature selection during model training.

Best Practices and Considerations

When selecting features, it is crucial to consider the domain knowledge, as it can provide valuable insights into which features are likely to be important. Additionally, it is essential to be mindful of the risk of overfitting, especially when dealing with high-dimensional data. In such cases, dimensionality reduction techniques like Principal Component Analysis (PCA) can be employed.

Feature importance scores, obtained from tree-based models like Random Forest or Gradient Boosting, can also guide feature selection. These models provide a ranking of features based on their contribution to the model's performance, which can be used to eliminate less important variables.

Handling High-Dimensional Data and Conclusion

In scenarios involving high-dimensional data, where the number of features significantly exceeds the number of observations, feature selection becomes even more crucial. Techniques like Lasso or Elastic Net regularization can be particularly effective in these cases, as they not only help in feature selection but also in preventing overfitting.

In conclusion, feature selection is a vital step in optimizing machine learning models, aiding in performance improvement, reduction of computational costs, and enhancement of model interpretability. Employing a combination of filter, wrapper, and embedded methods, along with leveraging domain knowledge and being mindful of overfitting risks, can lead to a robust and efficient feature selection process. As machine learning continues to evolve, automated feature selection tools and algorithms are also becoming more prevalent, further streamlining and improving the feature selection process.

4 Smart Solutions for Treating Nightmare Disorder

The current section describes a number of implemented wearable devices and software systems aimed at improving sleep quality and preventing nightmares. Summary of leading digital therapeutics for treating traumatic nightmares is presented in Table 1.

Table 1 Summary of leading digital therapeutics for treating traumatic nightmares

Therapeutic name	Description
Smart headbands	The Dream Band, a specialized wearable designed for in-depth sleep analysis, offers significant potential for managing traumatic nightmares. Its precise sleep stage tracking and brainwave monitoring capabilities enable the identification of disturbances that may be linked to nightmares, offering a clear picture of sleep quality and patterns. The device's ability to detect REM sleep in real-time provides a unique avenue for immediate interventions during nightmares, such as gentle audio cues to alter dream content without waking the user. By offering personalized insights and recommendations based on the collected data, the Dream Band actively contributes to improving sleep hygiene and reducing the occurrence of nightmares. Additionally, its user-friendly interface ensures easy access to valuable sleep information and intervention options, making it a practical and effective tool for individuals seeking to manage traumatic nightmares
Smart rings	The Oura Ring, with its advanced sleep tracking and physiological monitoring capabilities, holds potential as a valuable tool in managing traumatic nightmares. By providing detailed insights into sleep patterns, heart rate variability, and body temperature, it helps in identifying disruptions associated with nightmares. The device's trend analysis and personalized insights, backed by long-term data tracking, offer a nuanced understanding of sleep disturbances, paving the way for tailored interventions. Furthermore, the integration of sleep hygiene tips and relaxation exercises directly through the app, combined with the option to share data with healthcare providers, enhances the potential for a comprehensive approach to mitigating the impact of traumatic nightmares
Virtual reality (VR)	Utilizing the immersive and interactive capabilities of VR, therapists can help patients recreate and re-experience their nightmares in a controlled environment, allowing them to confront and process their fears directly. Through a process called imagery rehearsal therapy (IRT), patients are encouraged to modify the nightmares into less threatening scenarios, promoting a sense of control and mastery over their traumatic dreams. By repeatedly engaging with and altering the nightmare content in the virtual space, patients can reduce the frequency and intensity of traumatic nightmares, leading to improved sleep quality and overall well-being
White noise machines	White noise machines can serve as a supportive tool by promoting better sleep quality and creating a calm and controlled auditory environment. The consistent background noise helps mask potential auditory triggers, providing a sense of safety and routine, which is particularly beneficial for individuals with PTSD who may experience disrupted sleep and heightened sensitivity to sudden or loud noises

The concept of a one-size-fits-all digital therapeutic, particularly in the context of managing sleep-related disorders, faces inherent challenges due to the vast diversity in individual physiologies and sleep profiles. People's sleep patterns, circadian rhythms, and responses to interventions can vary widely, influenced by a myriad of factors including age, genetic predispositions, lifestyle choices, and existing medical conditions. A digital therapeutic designed with a universal approach may not accommodate these variations, potentially leading to suboptimal outcomes or even adverse effects for certain user groups. Personalized adjustments and considerations are crucial to ensure that digital interventions are not only safe but also effective across the diverse spectrum of users, thereby maximizing their potential benefits and minimizing risks.

NightWare

Identifying and implementing effective treatments for nightmare disorder, particularly within the demographic of patients suffering from PTSD, cannot be overstated. Nightmare disorder is significantly under-diagnosed and under-treated, predominantly due to the prevailing misconceptions and diagnostic criteria outlined in the DSM-IV-TR, which stipulates that nightmares must not occur exclusively during the course of another mental disorder for a nightmare disorder diagnosis to be considered (*CITE*). This criterion potentially leads to a clinical oversight, wherein the severe and distressing nightmares experienced by PTSD patients may be overlooked or attributed solely to the PTSD, without recognizing the co-occurring nightmare disorder. This is a critical lapse in mental health care, as there is a well-established connection between Nightmare disorder and increased suicidality, further amplifying the risk in patients already vulnerable due to PTSD. Research indicates a high prevalence of nightmare disorder in individuals with PTSD, with some studies suggesting that up to 71–96% of PTSD patients experience frequent nightmares, compared to 2–8% in the general population. This underscores the urgent need for a paradigm shift in the assessment and treatment of nightmares that co-occur with PTSD, advocating for a more integrative and holistic approach that addresses both the PTSD and the nightmare disorder concurrently, to mitigate the associated risks and improve patient outcomes.

The origin of NightWare's "observe and respond" behavior stems from arguably the most natural treatment for nightmare disorder, and man's best friend—the service dog. Canine-assisted interventions, specifically involving service dogs trained for PTSD support, have emerged as an efficacious strategy to mitigate the distress associated with such episodes. These service dogs are trained to discern onset signs of nighttime distress in their handlers. Preliminary studies indicate that, upon detection, these canines can effectively rouse their handlers, thus curtailing the duration and potential physiological repercussions of the traumatic nightmare. Upon arousal, the immediate presence of the service dog serves a dual purpose: offering tactile comfort and anchoring the individual, minimizing episodes of post-awakening disorientation or heightened anxiety. The symbiotic bond cultivated between the patient and the service dog has been shown to engender an enhanced sense of security, which may subsequently contribute to a reduction in the overall frequency and severity of traumatic nightmares. This suggests that service dogs, in providing both anticipatory and responsive support, play an integral role in the holistic management of nocturnal PTSD manifestations.

Service dogs, *for those who can obtain them*, present a promising solution for nightmare disorder. Unfortunately, the demand for PTSD service dogs far exceeds the supply, leading to many patients being on years-long waiting lists and others having cases deemed too benign to even be considered for one. The shortage is due not only to the intricate and expensive training processes for these dogs, but also the strict criteria that service dogs must meet to ensure their reliability in diverse scenarios inevitably narrows the pool of potential canine candidates. As reported by Assistance Dogs International, an alliance of organizations dedicated to training and providing service animals, there are more than 9000 individuals currently on the waiting list for a dog trained to assist with various needs. This figure does not account for the countless others who might also reap the advantages of such support [116]. This shortage, coupled with the meteoric rise of digital therapeutic technologies, has led to the founders of NightWare to attempt to bridge the supply gap using alternative methods that leverage off-the-shelf wearable technology that seem, for now, to be in more-than-adequate supply.

NightWare functions as a digital counterpart to a service dog for individuals dealing with disruptive sleep caused by nightmares. Much like a service dog that is trained to detect and respond to signs of distress in its owner, NightWare continuously monitors the user's sleep through various metrics such as heart rate and movement. It constantly observes the patient, waiting for "anomalous" periods that could indicate a nightmare, emulating the trained attentiveness of a service dog. Upon detection, NightWare delivers a response in the form of gentle haptic feedback through the Apple Watch, aiming to mitigate the duration and intensity of the nightmare without fully awakening the user. NightWare can be compared as a digital service dog that, instead of kibble and walks, just requires a good daily charging to be ready for a night of watchful companionship.

Despite the allure of a fully automated solution, there are compelling reasons for individual practitioners to seek control over adjusting the parameters of how NightWare administers its treatment. As such, practitioners should have an interface to manually manage an array of patient treatment parameters to better suit patient safety and application effectiveness. These include the following:

1. *Learning period.* Changing the period of time that the watch observes a patient without the application providing any haptic intervention. Increasing the learning period could be useful if a patient is high-risk, that is, it is highly important that the application understands the nuances of a patient's sleep profile. Resetting the learning period (i.e., starting over) may be deemed necessary for patients who had some issue with their learning period (e.g., ill-fitting watch) or have experienced a large temporal gap in usage, so a sleep profile reset is needed.
2. *Intervention threshold.* After a learning period, the application learns a stress threshold that, when a patient's stress level exceeds the threshold for a given amount of time, an intervention is administered. Doctors can manually change this threshold to make the application more or less responsive to changes in patient stress.

3. *Intervention intensity*. While the application automatically increments and decrements the threshold in response to a patient's responsiveness to the current level, providers often want to enforce a constant level of intervention intensity.
4. *Sleep delay*. Oftentimes providers want their patients to not receive interventions from the application until after sleeping for some amount of time. As such, the delay until the first intervention after falling asleep is also configurable by practitioners.

NightWare is an effective digital therapeutic device, aiming to mitigate traumatic nightmares often encountered in post-traumatic stress disorder (PTSD). Employed via a commercially available smartwatch, NightWare utilizes integrated sensors to monitor users' physiological responses during sleep and creates a sleep profile for each user. Upon detection of potential nightmare-induced stress, the application gently intervenes through subtle vibrations to lessen the nightmare's intensity without rousing the patient completely. The patient's sleep profile continuously updates as their sleep evolves, and ideally improves, over time. The primary objective of NightWare is to contribute to a reduction in both the frequency and severity of traumatic nightmares, with the ultimate aim of enhancing overall sleep quality and, consequently, fostering improved mental health outcomes—both night *and* day.

Important considerations for the usage of sleep-improving wearable devices include the Hawthorne Effect, which describes the alteration of individuals' behavior when they are aware that they are being observed. This effect could manifest in various ways in the context of an application like NightWare. Patients aware that their sleep and nightmares are being monitored and intervened upon by the application might unconsciously change their sleep patterns or their response to nightmares, potentially skewing the application's data and the perceived efficacy of the intervention. For instance, just the knowledge that there is an active effort to reduce nightmare intensity might lead to a placebo effect, where users report a reduction in nightmare severity regardless of the actual impact of the application. Furthermore, this awareness might also result in increased anxiety or stress for some individuals, particularly if they fixate on the need for the application to work, which could paradoxically lead to an increase in nightmares or disrupted sleep. Addressing the Hawthorne Effect in the context of NightWare requires careful consideration to ensure that the data collected is representative of the application's true efficacy, and that users' experiences and reports are not unduly influenced by their awareness of the monitoring and intervention process.

5 Conclusion and Future Research

Nightmare disorder poses a great risk to mental well-being and thus should require clinical attention. Current guidelines have weak or no recommendations for the treatment of nightmares due to limited understanding of nightmare pathophysiology and perhaps, clearly defined research directions. Research on whether treating nightmares could reduce suicide is pre-mature, as nightmares have not been considered by some researchers to be an important risk factor for suicidality. Current studies suggest that if nightmares are treated, there is the possibility to reduce suicidal ideation. It is important to note that nightmare disorders are a potentially modifiable risk factor for suicide, in contrast with other risk factors that cannot be mitigated. Therapies for the prevention of nightmares and improving sleep quality are important to attenuate the development and further exacerbation of comorbid conditions.

The realm of digital therapeutics, particularly in the context of treating traumatic nightmares, remains a vibrant field of active research and innovation, extending beyond the present moment and into the foreseeable future.

One of the future trends important for nightmare prevention is the integration of novel AI methods. The integration of modern AI methodologies, including foundation models capable of emulating physical systems and extensive large language models (LLMs), is creating groundbreaking prospects for the identification and treatment of traumatic nightmares. By incorporating biometric data gleaned from wearables and sensors during sleep, these AI models have the potential to discern patterns and accurately detect occurrences of nightmares. Foundation models are particularly promising as they emulate the body's physiological responses during sleep, capturing intricate variations in heart rate, breathing patterns, body movements, and newly integrated data such as heart rate variability from advanced sensors on devices like the Apple Watch. These nuanced observations are vital for a more precise identification of nightmare episodes.

Parallelly, LLMs play a crucial role in providing immediate post-nightmare support, facilitating guided conversations, and offering personalized coping strategies tailored to the individual's emotional state and historical responses. These models extend their utility to long-term treatment planning, recommending evidence-based interventions and consistently monitoring the individual's recovery trajectory over time. The iterative process of experimenting with alternative machine learning model types and adjusting NightWare's internal models and heuristics based on this expanded dataset ensures continuous improvement and adaptation of the intervention strategies.

Furthermore, the synergy between foundation models and LLMs facilitates the creation of a comprehensive and rich database, significantly enhancing our understanding of nightmares and their triggers. This, in turn, paves the way for the development of more effective, personalized, and adaptive treatment options. In harnessing the capabilities of AI in such a multifaceted manner, we are not only innovating within the realm of mental health care but also demonstrating a deep commitment to providing empathetic and effective solutions for individuals grappling with the challenging repercussions of traumatic experiences, as manifested through nightmares.

References

1. Levier et al: https://www.ncbi.nlm.nih.gov/pmc/articles/PMC5078833/ (2016)
2. Coombs et al: https://www.sciencedirect.com/science/article/pii/S2352827321001221 (2021)
3. Plante, D. T., & Winkelman, J. W. (2006). Parasomnias. *The Psychiatric clinics of North America*, *29*(4), 969. https://doi.org/10.1016/j.psc.2006.08.006
4. Ohayon, M. M., Morselli, P. L., & Guilleminault, C. (1997). Prevalence of nightmares and their relationship to psychopathology and daytime functioning in insomnia subjects. *Sleep*, *20*(5), 340–348. https://doi.org/10.1093/sleep/20.5.340Li
5. Kilpatrick, D. G., Resnick, H. S., Freedy, J. R., Pelcovitz, D., Resick, P., Roth, S., & Kolk, B. (1998). The posttraumatic stress disorder field trial: Evaluation of the PTSD construct: Criteria A through E. *DSM-IV Sourcebook*, *4*, 803–844 7.
6. Li, S. X., Zhang, B., Li, A. M., & Wing, Y. K. (2010). Prevalence and correlates of frequent nightmares: A community-based 2-phase study. *Sleep*, *33*(6), 774–780. https://doi.org/10.1093/sleep/33.6.774
7. Gauchat, A., Séguin, J.R., & Zadra, A. (2014, October). Prevalence and correlates of disturbed dreaming in children. *Pathol Biol (Paris)*, *62*(5), 311–8. https://doi.org/10.1016/j.patbio.2014.05.016. Epub 2014 Aug 6. PMID: 25108315.
8. Levin, R., & Nielsen, T. A. (2007). Disturbed dreaming, posttraumatic stress disorder, and affect distress: A review and neurocognitive model. *Psychol Bull*, *133*, 482–528.
9. Rek, S., Sheaves, B., & Freeman, D. (2017). Nightmares in the general population: Identifying potential causal factors. *Soc Psychiatry Psychiatr Epidemiol*, *52*, 1123–1133.
10. Sandman, N., Valli, K., & Kronholm, E. (2013). Nightmares: Prevalence among the Finnish General Adult Population and War Veterans during 1972–2007. *Sleep*, *36*, 1041–1050.
11. Bjorvatn, B., Grønli, J., & Pallesen, S. (2010). Prevalence of different parasomnias in the general population. *Sleep Med*, *11*, 1031–1034.
12. *Diagnostic and statistical manual of mental disorders: DSM-5* (Fifth). (2013). American Psychiatric Publishing. https://doi.org/10.1176/appi.books.9780890425596
13. Hublin, C., Kaprio, J., & Partinen, M. (1999). Nightmares: Familial aggregation and association with psychiatric disorders in a nationwide twin cohort. *Am J Med Genet*, *88*, 329–336.
14. Janson, C., Gislason, T., & De Backer, W. (1995). Prevalence of sleep disturbances among young adults in three European countries. *Sleep*, *18*, 589–597.
15. Schredl, M. (2010). Nightmare frequency and nightmare topics in a representative German sample. *Eur Arch Psychiatry Clin Neurosci*, *260*, 565–570.
16. Tanskanen, A., Tuomilehto, J., Viinamäki, H., Vartiainen, E., Lehtonen, J., & Puska, P. (2001). Nightmares as predictors of suicide. *Sleep*, *v 1;24(7):844–7. PMID*, 11683487.
17. Horwitz, A. G., Berona, J., & Czyz, E. K. (2017). Positive and Negative Expectations of Hopelessness as Longitudinal Predictors of Depression, Suicidal Ideation, and Suicidal Behavior in High-Risk Adolescents. *Suicide Life Threat Behav*, *47*, 168–176.
18. Li, S. X., Lam, S. P., & Zhang, J. (2016). Sleep Disturbances and Suicide Risk in an 8-Year Longitudinal Study of Schizophrenia-Spectrum Disorders. *Sleep*, *39*, 1275–1282.
19. Sheaves, B., Porcheret, K., & Tsanas, A. (2016). Insomnia, Nightmares, and Chronotype as Markers of Risk for Severe Mental Illness: Results from a Student Population. *Sleep*, *39*, 173–181.
20. Lena Mallon, Jan-Erik Broman, & Jerker Hetta. (2000). Sleeping difficulties in relation to depression and anxiety in elderly adults. *Nordic Journal of Psychiatry*, *54*(5), 355–360. https://doi.org/10.1080/080394800457192
21. Creamer, J. L., Brock, M. S., Matsangas, P., Motamedi, V., & Mysliwiec, V. (2018). Nightmares in United States Military Personnel With Sleep Disturbances. *J Clin Sleep Med JCSM Off Publ Am Acad Sleep Med*, *14(3):419–426*. https://doi.org/10.5664/jcsm.6990.

22. Neylan, T. C., Marmar, C. R., & Metzler, T. J. (1998). Sleep Disturbances in the Vietnam Generation: Findings From a Nationally Representative Sample of Male Vietnam Veterans. *Am J Psychiatry*, *155*, 929–933.
23. Akkaoui, M. A., Lejoyeux, M., & d'Ortho, M.-P. (2020). Nightmares in Patients with Major Depressive Disorder, Bipolar Disorder, and Psychotic Disorders: A Systematic Review. *J Clin Med*, *9*, 3990.
24. Nadorff, M. R., Nadorff, D. K., & Germain, A. (2015). Nightmares: Under-Reported, Undetected, and Therefore Untreated. *J Clin Sleep Med JCSM Off Publ Am Acad Sleep Med*, *11(7)*:747–750. https://doi.org/10.5664/jcsm.4850.
25. Sandman, N., Valli, K., & Kronholm, E. (2015). Nightmares: Risk Factors Among the Finnish General Adult Population. *Sleep*, *38*, 507–514.
26. Pigeon, W. R., Pinquart, M., & Conner, K. (2012). Meta-analysis of sleep disturbance and suicidal thoughts and behaviors. *J Clin Psychiatry*, *73(9):e1160–1167*. https://doi.org/10.4088/JCP.11r07586.
27. Sjöström, N., Waern, M., & Hetta, J. (2007). Nightmares and Sleep Disturbances in Relation to Suicidality in Suicide Attempters. *Sleep*, *30*(1), 91–95. https://doi.org/10.1093/sleep/30.1.91.
28. Agargun, M. Y. (2003). *Nightmares Associated with the Onset of Mania: Three Case Reports 5.*
29. Agargun, M. Y., Besiroglu, L., & Cilli, A. S. (2007). Nightmares, suicide attempts, and melancholic features in patients with unipolar major depression. *J Affect Disord*, *98*, 267–270.
30. Besiroglu, L., & Agargun, M. Y. (2005). Inci R: Nightmares and terminal insomnia in depressed patients with and without melancholic features. *Psychiatry Res*, *133*, 285–287.
31. Lai, Y.-C., Huang, M.-C., & Chen, H.-C. (2014). Familiality and clinical outcomes of sleep disturbances in major depressive and bipolar disorders. *J Psychosom Res*, *76*, 61–67.
32. Marinova, P., Koychev, I., & Laleva, L. (2014). Nightmares and suicide: Predicting risk in depression. *Psychiatr Danub*, *26*, 159–164.
33. Krakow, B., Artar, A., & Warner, T. D. (2000). Sleep Disorder, Depression, and Suicidality in Female Sexual Assault Survivors. *Crisis*, *21*, 163–170.
34. Ağargün, M. Y., Cilli, A. S., & Kara, H. (1998). Repetitive and frightening dreams and suicidal behavior in patients with major depression. *Compr Psychiatry*, *39*, 198–202.
35. Weathers, F. W., Marx, B. P., & Friedman, M. J. (2014). Posttraumatic Stress Disorder in DSM-5: New Criteria, New Measures, and Implications for Assessment. *Psychol Inj Law*, *7*, 93–107.
36. Davis, J., Byrd, P. M., & Rhudy, J. (2007). *Characteristics of Chronic Nightmares in a Trauma-Exposed Treatment-Seeking Sample*.
37. Germain, A., & Nielsen, T. A. (2003). Sleep pathophysiology in posttraumatic stress disorder and idiopathic nightmare sufferers. *Biol Psychiatry*, *54*, 1092–1098.
38. Heim, C., & Nemeroff, C. B. (2009). Neurobiology of posttraumatic stress disorder. *CNS Spectr*, *14*, 13–24.
39. Koffel, E., Khawaja, I. S., & Germain, A. (2016). Sleep Disturbances in Posttraumatic Stress Disorder: Updated Review and Implications for Treatment. *Psychiatr Ann*, *46*, 173–176.
40. Mellman, T. A., & Hipolito, M. M. S. (2006). Sleep disturbances in the aftermath of trauma and posttraumatic stress disorder. *CNS Spectr*, *11*, 611–615.
41. Ross, R. J., Ball, W. A., & Sullivan, K. A. (1989). Sleep disturbance as the hallmark of posttraumatic stress disorder. *Am J Psychiatry*, *146*, 697–707.
42. Nielsen, T. A., Paquette, T., & Solomonova, E. (2010). REM sleep characteristics of nightmare sufferers before and after REM sleep deprivation. *Sleep Med*, *11*, 172–179.
43. Simor, P., Bódizs, R., & Horváth, K. (2013a). Disturbed dreaming and the instability of sleep: Altered nonrapid eye movement sleep microstructure in individuals with frequent nightmares as revealed by the cyclic alternating pattern. *Sleep*, *36*, 413–419.
44. Simor, P., Horváth, K., & Ujma, P. P. (2013b). Fluctuations between sleep and wakefulness: Wake-like features indicated by increased EEG alpha power during different sleep stages in nightmare disorder. *Biol Psychol*, *94*, 592–600.

45. Simor, P., Horváth, K., & Gombos, F. (2012). Disturbed dreaming and sleep quality: Altered sleep architecture in subjects with frequent nightmares. *Eur Arch Psychiatry Clin Neurosci*, *262*, 687–696.
46. Kobayashi, I., Sledjeski, E. M., & Spoonster, E. (2008). Effects of early nightmares on the development of sleep disturbances in motor vehicle accident victims. *J Trauma Stress*, *21*, 548–555.
47. Phelps, A. J., Kanaan, R. A. A., & Worsnop, C. (2018). An Ambulatory Polysomnography Study of the Post-traumatic Nightmares of Post-traumatic Stress Disorder. *Sleep*, *41*.
48. Nielsen, T., & Carr, M. (2017). *Nightmares and nightmare function; Principles and Practice of Sleep Medicine*. Elsevier. https://doi.org/10.1016/B978-0-323-24288-2.00053-2
49. Michels, F., Schilling, C., & Rausch, F. (2014). Nightmare frequency in schizophrenic patients, healthy relatives of schizophrenic patients, patients at high risk states for psychosis, and healthy controls. *Int J Dream Res*, 9–13.
50. Koffel, E., & Watson, D. (2009). Unusual sleep experiences, dissociation, and schizotypy: Evidence for a common domain. *Clin Psychol Rev*, *29*, 548–559.
51. Gehrman, P. R., Harb, G. C., & Cook, J. M. (2015). Sleep diaries of Vietnam War veterans with chronic PTSD: the relationships among insomnia symptoms, psychosocial stress, and nightmares. *Behav Sleep Med*, *13*, 255–264.
52. Sateia, M. J. (2014). International classification of sleep disorders-third edition: Highlights and modifications. *Chest*, *146*, 1387–1394.
53. Derogatis, L. R., Lipman, R. S., & Covi, L. (1973). SCL-90: An outpatient psychiatric rating scale–preliminary report. *Psychopharmacol Bull*, *9*, 13–28.
54. Kellner R: A symptom questionnaire. (1987). *J Clin Psychiatry*, *48*, 268–274.
55. Blake, D. D., Weathers, F. W., & Nagy, L. M. (1995). The development of a Clinician-Administered PTSD Scale. *J Trauma Stress*, *8*, 75–90.
56. Aurora, R. N., Zak, R. S., & Auerbach, S. H. (2010). Best practice guide for the treatment of nightmare disorder in adults. *J Clin Sleep Med JCSM Off Publ Am Acad Sleep Med*, *6*, 389–401.
57. Morgenthaler, T. I., Auerbach, S., & Casey, K. R. (2018). Position Paper for the Treatment of Nightmare Disorder in Adults: An American Academy of Sleep Medicine Position Paper. *J Clin Sleep Med JCSM Off Publ Am Acad Sleep Med*, *14*, 1041–1055.
58. AASM 2010: Standards of Practice Committee, Aurora, R. N., Zak, R. S., Auerbach, S. H., Casey, K. R., Chowdhuri, S., ... & Morgenthaler, T. I. (2010). Best practice guide for the treatment of nightmare disorder in adults. *J Clin Sleep Med*, *6*(4), 389–401.
59. FDA. (2022). https://www.accessdata.fda.gov/drugsatfda_docs/label/2009/017442s033lbl.pdf
60. Boehnlein, J. K., & Kinzie, J. D. (2007). Pharmacologic Reduction of CNS Noradrenergic Activity in PTSD: The Case for Clonidine and Prazosin. *J Psychiatr Pract*, *13*, 72–78.
61. Cranston, C. C., Davis, J. L., & Rhudy, J. L. (2011). Replication and expansion of "Best Practice Guide for the Treatment of Nightmare Disorder in Adults. *J Clin Sleep Med JCSM Off Publ Am Acad Sleep Med*, *7*, 549–553 554–556.
62. Hudson, S. M., Whiteside, T. E., Lorenz, R. A., & Wargo, K. A. (2012). Prazosin for the treatment of nightmares related to posttraumatic stress disorder: a review of the literature. *Prim Care Companion CNS Disord*, *14*(2):PCC.11r01222. https://doi.org/10.4088/PCC.11r01222. Epub 2012 Mar 22. PMID: 22943034; PMCID: PMC3425466.
63. Ferry, D. G., Caplan, N. B., & Cubeddu, L. X. (1986). Interaction Between Antidepressants and Alpha1-Adrenergic Receptor Antagonists on the Binding to Alpha1-Acid Glycoprotein. *J Pharm Sci*, *75*, 146–149.
64. Germain, A., Richardson, R., & Moul, D. E. (2012). Placebo-controlled comparison of prazosin and cognitive-behavioral treatments for sleep disturbances in US Military Veterans. *J Psychosom Res*, *72*, 89–96.
65. Kung, S., Espinel, Z., & Lapid, M. I. (2012). Treatment of Nightmares With Prazosin: A Systematic Review. *Mayo Clin Proc*, *87*, 890–900.

66. Raskind, M. A., Peskind, E. R., Chow, B., Harris, C., Davis-Karim, A., Holmes, H. A., Hart, K. L., McFall, M., Mellman, T. A., Reist, C., Romesser, J., Rosenheck, R., Shih, M. C., Stein, M. B., Swift, R., Gleason, T., Lu, Y., & Huang, G. D. (2018). Trial of Prazosin for Post-Traumatic Stress Disorder in Military Veterans. *N Engl J Med, Feb 8;378(6):507–517.* https://doi.org/10.1056/NEJMoa1507598.
67. Raskind, M. A., Peskind, E. R., & Hoff, D. J. (2007). A parallel group placebo controlled study of prazosin for trauma nightmares and sleep disturbance in combat veterans with post-traumatic stress disorder. *Biol Psychiatry*, *61*, 928–934.
68. Krakow, B., Germain, A., & Warner, T. D. (2001a). The relationship of sleep quality and posttraumatic stress to potential sleep disorders in sexual assault survivors with nightmares, insomnia, and PTSD. *J Trauma Stress*, *14*, 647–665.
69. Krakow, B., Hollifield, M., & Johnston, L. (2001b). Imagery rehearsal therapy for chronic nightmares in sexual assault survivors with posttraumatic stress disorder: A randomized controlled trial. *JAMA*, *286*, 537–545.
70. Krakow, B., Sandoval, D., & Schrader, R. (2001c). Treatment of chronic nightmares in adjudicated adolescent girls in a residential facility. *J Adolesc Health Off Publ Soc Adolesc Med*, *29*, 94–100.
71. Lancee, J., Victor I Spoormaker, Jan van den Bout. (2010). Cognitive-behavioral self-help treatment for nightmares: A randomized controlled trial. *Psychother Psychosom*, *79*, 371–377.
72. Thünker, J., & Pietrowsky, R. (2012). Effectiveness of a manualized imagery rehearsal therapy for patients suffering from nightmare disorders with and without a comorbidity of depression or PTSD. *Behav Res Ther*, *50*, 558–564.
73. Krakow, B., & Zadra, A. (2006). Clinical management of chronic nightmares: Imagery rehearsal therapy. *Behav Sleep Med*, *4*, 45–70.
74. Cook, J. M., Harb, G. C., & Gehrman, P. R. (2010). Imagery rehearsal for posttraumatic nightmares: A randomized controlled trial. *J Trauma Stress*, *23*, 553–563.
75. McCall, W. V., Batson, N., Webster, M., Case, L. D., Joshi, I., Derreberry, T., McDonough, A., & Farris, S. (2013). Nightmares and dysfunctional beliefs about sleep mediate the effect of insomnia symptoms on suicidal ideation. *J Clin Sleep Med*, *Feb 1;9(2):135–40.* https://doi.org/10.5664/jcsm.2408.
76. Shirley X. Li, Siu P. Lam, Joey W. Y. Chan, Mandy W. M. Yu, Yun-Kwok Wing. (2012, 1 August). Residual sleep disturbances in patients remitted from major depressive disorder: a 4-year naturalistic follow-up study. *Sleep*, 35(8),1153–1161. https://doi.org/10.5665/sleep.2008.
77. Sjöström, N., Hetta, J., & Waern, M. (2009). Persistent nightmares are associated with repeat suicide attempt: A prospective study. *Psychiatry Res*, *30;170(2–3):208–11.* https://doi.org/10.1016/j.psychres.2008.09.006.
78. Shi, X., Zhu, Y., Wang, S., Wang, A., Chen, X., Li, Y., & Jiang, L. (2021). The prospective associations between different types of sleep disturbance and suicidal behavior in a large sample of chinese college students. *J Affect Disord*. https://doi.org/10.1016/j.jad.2020.10.019.
79. Liu, X., Yang, Y., Liu, Z. Z., & Jia, C. X. (2021). Longitudinal associations of nightmare frequency and nightmare distress with suicidal behavior in adolescents: Mediating role of depressive symptoms. *Sleep*, *21;44(1):zsaa130.* https://doi.org/10.1093/sleep/zsaa130.
80. Wang, X., Cheng, S., & Xu, H. (2019). Systematic review and meta-analysis of the relationship between sleep disorders and suicidal behaviour in patients with depression. *BMC Psychiatry*, *Oct 17;19(1):303.* https://doi.org/10.1186/s12888-019-2302-5.
81. Harris, L. M., Huang, X., Linthicum, K. P., Bryen, C. P., & Ribeiro, J. D. (2020). Sleep disturbances as risk factors for suicidal thoughts and behaviours: A meta-analysis of longitudinal studies. *Sci Rep*, *Aug 17;10(1):13888.* https://doi.org/10.1038/s41598-020-70866-6.
82. Russell, K., Allan, S., Beattie, L., Bohan, J., MacMahon, K., & Rasmussen, S. (2019). Sleep problem, suicide and self-harm in university students: A systematic review. *Sleep Med Rev*. https://doi.org/10.1016/j.smrv.2018.12.008.

83. Pace-Schott, E. F., Germain, A., & Milad, M. R. (2015a). Effects of sleep on memory for conditioned fear and fear extinction. *Psychol Bull*, *141*, 835–857.
84. Pace-Schott, E. F., Germain, A., & Milad, M. R. (2015b). Sleep and REM sleep disturbance in the pathophysiology of PTSD: the role of extinction memory. *Biol Mood Anxiety Disord*, *5*, 3.
85. Wagner, U., Gais, S., & Born, J. (2001). Emotional memory formation is enhanced across sleep intervals with high amounts of rapid eye movement sleep. *Learn Mem Cold Spring Harb N*, *8*, 112–119.
86. Silvestri, A. J. (2005). REM sleep deprivation affects extinction of cued but not contextual fear conditioning. *Physiol Behav*, *84*, 343–349.
87. Silvestri, A. J., & Root, D. H. (2008). Effects of REM deprivation and an NMDA agonist on the extinction of conditioned fear. *Physiol Behav*, *93*, 274–281.
88. Kobayashi, I., Boarts, J. M., & Delahanty, D. L. (2007). Polysomnographically measured sleep abnormalities in PTSD: A meta-analytic review. *Psychophysiology*, *44*, 660–669.
89. Debiec, J., & LeDoux, J. E. (2006). Noradrenergic signaling in the amygdala contributes to the reconsolidation of fear memory: Treatment implications for PTSD. *Ann N Y Acad Sci*, *1071*, 521–524.
90. Luigi De Gennaro, Cristina Marzano, Fabio Moroni, Giuseppe Curcio, Michele Ferrara, Carlo Cipolli (2010). Recovery sleep after sleep deprivation almost completely abolishes dream recall. *Behav Brain Res*, *206*, 293–298.
91. Lim, J., & Dinges, D. F. (2010). A meta-analysis of the impact of short-term sleep deprivation on cognitive variables. *Psychol Bull*, *136*, 375–389.
92. Suni, Eric. (2022). *How Does Lack of Sleep Effect Cognitive Impairment?* Sleep Foundation. https://www.sleepfoundation.org/sleep-deprivation/lack-of-sleep-and-cognitive-impairment
93. Kana Okano, Jakub R. Kaczmarzyk, Neha Dave, John D E Gabrieli, Jeffrey C. Grossman (2019). Sleep quality, duration, and consistency are associated with better academic performance in college students. *Npj Sci Learn*, *4*, 1–5.
94. Shadmehr, R., & Holcomb, H. H. (1997). Neural correlates of motor memory consolidation. *Science*, *277*, 821–825.
95. Schiller, D., Monfils, M.-H., & Raio, C. M. (2010). Preventing the return of fear in humans using reconsolidation update mechanisms. *Nature*, *463*, 49–53.
96. Gazzaniga, Micheal S. (2000). *The new cognitive neurosciences* (2nd ed.). US, The MIT Press.
97. Bryant, R. A., Creamer, M., & O'Donnell, M. (2009). A study of the protective function of acute morphine administration on subsequent posttraumatic stress disorder. *Biol Psychiatry*, *65*, 438–440.
98. Holbrook, T. L., Galarneau, M. R., & Dye, J. L. (2010). Morphine use after combat injury in Iraq and post-traumatic stress disorder. *N Engl J Med*, *362*, 110–117.
99. Surís, A., North, C., & Adinoff, B. (2010). Effects of exogenous glucocorticoid on combat-related PTSD symptoms. *Ann Clin Psychiatry Off J Am Acad Clin Psychiatr*, *22*, 274–279.
100. Zohar, J., Yahalom, H., & Kozlovsky, N. (2011). High dose hydrocortisone immediately after trauma may alter the trajectory of PTSD: interplay between clinical and animal studies. *Eur Neuropsychopharmacol J Eur Coll Neuropsychopharmacol*, *21*, 796–809
101. Pitman, R. K., Sanders, K. M., & Zusman, R. M. (2002). Pilot study of secondary prevention of posttraumatic stress disorder with propranolol. *Biol Psychiatry*, *51*, 189–192.
102. Stein, M. B., Kerridge, C., & Dimsdale, J. E. (2007). Pharmacotherapy to prevent PTSD: Results from a randomized controlled proof-of-concept trial in physically injured patients. *J Trauma Stress*, *20*, 923–932.
103. Resnick, H., Acierno, R., & Waldrop, A. E. (2007). Randomized controlled evaluation of an early intervention to prevent post-rape psychopathology. *Behav Res Ther*, *45*, 2432–2447.
104. Adler, A. B., Bliese, P. D., & McGurk, D. (2009a). Battlemind debriefing and battlemind training as early interventions with soldiers returning from Iraq: Randomization by platoon. *J Consult Clin Psychol*, *77*, 928–940.

105. Adler, A. B., Castro, C. A., & McGurk, D. (2009b). Time-driven battlemind psychological debriefing: A group-level early intervention in combat. *Mil Med*, *174*, 21–28.
106. Laurence Astill Wright, Marit Sijbrandij, Rob Sinnerton, Catrin Lewis, Neil P Roberts, Jonathan I Bisson. (2019). Pharmacological prevention and early treatment of post-traumatic stress disorder and acute stress disorder: A systematic review and meta-analysis. *Transl Psychiatry*, *9*, 334.
107. Satapathy, Santosh Kumar, Shrey Thakkar, Ayushi Patel, Dharvi Patel, and Divya Patel. 2022. "An Effective EEG Signal-Based Sleep Staging System Using Machine Learning Techniques." In 2022 IEEE 6th Conference on Information and Communication Technology (CICT), 1–6. IEEE.
108. Satapathy, Santosh, D. Loganathan, Hari Kishan Kondaveeti, and Ramakrushna Rath. 2021. "Performance Analysis of Machine Learning Algorithms on Automated Sleep Staging Feature Sets." CAAI Transactions on Intelligence Technology 6 (2): 155–74.
109. Wyawahare, Medha, Rohan Bhole, Vaibhavi Bobade, Akshay Chavan, and Shreya Dehankar. 2023. "EEG-Based Sleep Stage Classification System." In Proceedings of International Conference on Paradigms of Communication, Computing and Data Analytics, 311–21. Springer Nature Singapore.
110. Zhang, Yongqing, Wenpeng Cao, Lixiao Feng, Manqing Wang, Tianyu Geng, Jiliu Zhou, and Dongrui Gao. 2023. "SHNN: A Single-Channel EEG Sleep Staging Model Based on Semi-Supervised Learning." Expert Systems with Applications 213 (March): 119288.
111. Goldberger, A. L., L. A. Amaral, L. Glass, J. M. Hausdorff, P. C. Ivanov, R. G. Mark, J. E. Mietus, G. B. Moody, C. K. Peng, and H. E. Stanley. 2000. "PhysioBank, PhysioToolkit, and PhysioNet: Components of a New Research Resource for Complex Physiologic Signals." Circulation 101 (23): E215–20.
112. Kemp, B., A. H. Zwinderman, B. Tuk, H. A. Kamphuisen, and J. J. Oberyé. 2000. "Analysis of a Sleep-Dependent Neuronal Feedback Loop: The Slow-Wave Microcontinuity of the EEG." IEEE Transactions on Bio-Medical Engineering 47 (9): 1185–94.
113. Kaplan, Katherine A., Prajesh P. Hardas, Susan Redline, Jamie M. Zeitzer, and Sleep Heart Health Study Research Group. 2017. "Correlates of Sleep Quality in Midlife and beyond: A Machine Learning Analysis." Sleep Medicine 34 (June): 162–67.
114. Biedebach, Luka, María Óskarsdóttir, Erna Sif Arnardóttir, Sigridur Sigurdardóttir, Michael Valur Clausen, Sigurveig Þ. Sigurdardóttir, Marta Serwatko, and Anna Sigridur Islind. 2024. "Anomaly Detection in Sleep: Detecting Mouth Breathing in Children." Data Mining and Knowledge Discovery 38 (3): 976–1005.
115. Chinthalachervu, Rohith, Immaneni Teja, M. Ajay Kumar, N. Sai Harshith, and T. Santosh Kumar. 2022. "Driver Drowsiness Detection and Monitoring System Using Machine Learning." Journal of Physics. Conference Series 2325 (1): 012057.
116. canine.org: https://canine.org/news/volunteer-shortage-threatens-service-dog-supply/#:~:text=ADI%20member%20organizations%20%E2%80%93%20which%20last,more%20who%20could%20potentially%20benefit (2023)

www.ingramcontent.com/pod-product-compliance
Lightning Source LLC
Chambersburg PA
CBHW050055161224
19064CB00003B/37

9 783031 682629